AF356831

Hereditary Hemorrhagic Telangiectasia

Hereditary Hemorrhagic Telangiectasia: Recent Advances and Future Challenges

Editors

Hans-Jurgen Mager
Carmelo Bernabeu
Marco Post

MDPI • Basel • Beijing • Wuhan • Barcelona • Belgrade • Manchester • Tokyo • Cluj • Tianjin

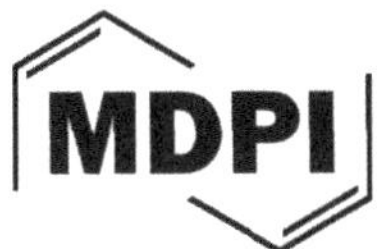

Editors
Hans-Jurgen Mager
St. Antonius Hospital
The Netherlands

Carmelo Bernabeu
Biological Research Centre,
Spanish National Research
Council (CSIC) and Centre for
Biomedical Network Research
on Rare Diseases (CIBERER)
Spain

Marco Post
St. Antonius Hospital and
University Medical Center Utrecht
The Netherlands

Editorial Office
MDPI
St. Alban-Anlage 66
4052 Basel, Switzerland

This is a reprint of articles from the Special Issue published online in the open access journal *Journal of Clinical Medicine* (ISSN 2077-0383) (available at: https://www.mdpi.com/journal/jcm/special_issues/Hereditary_Hemorrhagic_Telangiectasia).

For citation purposes, cite each article independently as indicated on the article page online and as indicated below:

LastName, A.A.; LastName, B.B.; LastName, C.C. Article Title. *Journal Name* **Year**, *Volume Number*, Page Range.

ISBN 978-3-0365-0590-9 (Hbk)
ISBN 978-3-0365-0591-6 (PDF)

Cover image courtesy of Hans-Jurgen Mager.

Contents

About the Editors

Hans-Jurgen Mager MD, Ph.D., is a pulmonologist, working in the St. Antonius Hospital, in Nieuwegein, which is the national HHT center of excellence in the Netherlands. He has more than 20 years experience in HHT care and research. He is chair of the Global Research and Medical Advisory Board of Cure HHT and a member of the HHT working group of VASCERN, the European Reference Network for rare vascular diseases. In addition, he is secretary of the Dutch association of pulmonologists (NVALT).

Carmelo Bernabeu Ph.D., serves as a section editor of the *Journal of Clinical Medicine* (Vascular Medicine). He is a Research Professor at the Biological Research Centre Margarita Salas, Spanish Research Council (CSIC) Madrid, Spain, member of the Centre for Biomedical Network Research on Rare Diseases (CIBERER) of Spain, and Chair Emeritus and current member of the Global Research Medical Advisory Board, Cure HHT Foundation International, US. After receiving his PhD from Autonomous University of Madrid in Spain, he worked, first as a postdoctoral scholar at the Molecular Biology Institute, University of California (UCLA) in Los Angeles, and then as a Research Fellow at the Dana-Farber Cancer Institute, Harvard Medical School, Boston, Massachusetts. Dr. Bernabeu is currently an active researcher with specific interests in the field of vascular biology, namely focused on the rare disease known as hereditary hemorrhagic telangiectasia (HHT) and the two major proteins involved, endoglin and ALK1, their roles as transforming growth factor-beta receptors in endothelial cells, and their involvement in angiogenesis, vascular remodeling, hypertension, cancer and preeclampsia. He has supervised 14 PhD students and is an author of more than 200 peer-reviewed articles (total citations > 15,500; h index = 67) and several international patents.

Marco Post MD, Ph.D., is a Professor in Pulmonary Vascular Disease at the University of Utrecht, the Netherlands. He works as a cardiologist and member of the HHT team in the St. Antonius Hospital, the HHT Center of Excellence in the Netherlands. He is a member of the Global Research Medical Advisory Board of the Cure HHT Foundation International and the HHT working group of the VASCERN, the European Reference Network for Rare Vascular Diseases. He is the author of more than 180 peer-reviewed articles.

Preface to "Hereditary Hemorrhagic Telangiectasia: Recent Advances and Future Challenges"

Hereditary hemorrhagic telangiectasia (HHT) is an autosomal heritable disease, leading to vascular malformations, ranging from mucocutaneous telangiectases to large arteriovenous malformations, which can occur in different organs. HHT is associated with a decreased quality of life and severe complications. If untreated, the disease leads to decreased life expectancy. Recent years have brought advances in diagnosis and treatment, but not a cure for HHT. The exact molecular etiology is still unknown and there is an urgent need for more systematic research. Because understanding the mechanisms of disease is essential for the development of new medicines or therapeutic strategies, this book aims to highlight not only the current knowledge regarding the diagnosis and treatment of HHT, but also the newest insights into the molecular basis of HHT. Among the different contributions, we would like to emphasize: (i) the key role of a systematic screening and treatment of patients at HHT Centers (de Gussem et al. 2020), (ii) the knowledge about genetics, genotype-phenotype correlations, second-hits and circulating biomarkers of HHT (Bernabeu et al. 2020; Cannavicci et al. 2020; Geisthoff et al. 2020; Kilian et al. 2020; Ruiz-Llorente et al. 2020); (iii) advances in imaging and treatment of arteriovenous malformations of the lung, liver and gastrointestinal tract using contrast-enhanced magnetic resonance angiography, computed tomography, endoscopy and embolotherapy (Daniel et al. 2020; Harwin et al. 2020; Mora-Lujan et al. 2020; Majumdar et al. 2020; Van den Heuvel et al. 2020; Schneider et al. 2021), and (iv) pharmacological strategies for HHT-related nose and gastrointestinal bleeding, using well known and repurposed drugs, including bevacizumab, propranolol, tacrolimus, and antithrombotic drugs (Albiñana et al. 2020; Dupuis-Girod et al. 2020; Gaetani et al. 2020; Mei-Zahav et al. 2020; Mora-Lujan et al. 2020).

Hans-Jurgen Mager, Carmelo Bernabeu, Marco Post
Editors

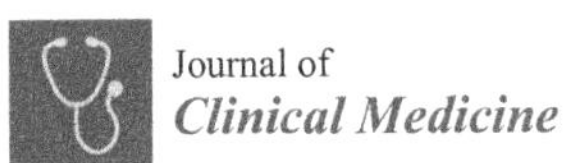

Journal of
Clinical Medicine

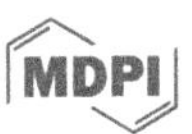

Article

Hereditary Hemorrhagic Telangiectasia (HHT) and Survival: The Importance of Systematic Screening and Treatment in HHT Centers of Excellence

Els M. de Gussem [1,†], Steven Kroon [2,†], Anna E. Hosman [2], Johannes C. Kelder [3], Martijn C. Post [4,5], Repke J. Snijder [2] and Johannes J. Mager [2,*]

1   Department of Internal Medicine, Division of Respirology, University of Manitoba, Grace Hospital, 400 Booth Drive, Winnipeg, MB R3J 3M7, Canada; edegussem@hsc.mb.ca
2   Department of Pulmonology, St Antonius Hospital, Koekoekslaan 1, 3435 CM Nieuwegein, The Netherlands; s.kroon@antoniusziekenhuis.nl (S.K.); a.hosman@antoniusziekenhuis.nl (A.E.H.); r.snijder@antoniusziekenhuis.nl (R.J.S.)
3   Department of Epidemiology and Medical Statistics, St Antonius Hospital, Koekoekslaan 1, 3435 CM Nieuwegein, The Netherlands; keld01@antoniusziekenhuis.nl
4   Department of Cardiology, St Antonius Hospital, Koekoekslaan 1, 3435 CM Nieuwegein, The Netherlands; m.post@antoniusziekenhuis.nl
5   Department of Cardiology, Utrecht University Medical Center, Heidelberglaan 100, 3584 CX Utrecht, The Netherlands
*   Correspondence: j.mager@antoniusziekenhuis.nl; Tel.: +31-(0)-8832-0300; Fax: +31-(0)-883-201-496
†   Both authors contributed equally and both authors share first authorship.

Received: 21 October 2020; Accepted: 3 November 2020; Published: 6 November 2020

Abstract: Hereditary hemorrhagic telangiectasia (HHT), an autosomal dominant disease, is characterized by telangiectases and arteriovenous malformations (AVMs). Untreated AVMs, especially in the lungs—pulmonary AVMs (PAVMs)—can result in morbidity with a decreased life expectancy. We have investigated whether HHT patients, systematically screened for HHT-related organ involvement and treated if needed, have a similar survival as persons without HHT. We included all individuals screened for HHT between 2004 and 2016 with a genetically or clinically confirmed diagnosis (HHT group) or excluded diagnosis (non-HHT control group). The social security number was used to confirm status as dead or alive in December 2019. We included 717 HHT patients and 471 controls. There was no difference in survival between the HHT and the non-HHT control group. The HHT group had a life expectancy of 75.9 years (95% confidence interval (CI) 73.3–78.6), comparable to the control group (79.3 years, 95% CI 74.8–84.0, Mantel–Cox test: $p = 0.29$). In conclusion, the life expectancy of HHT patients systematically screened for HHT-related organ involvement and treated if needed in an HHT center of excellence was similar compared to their controls, justifying systematic screening and treatment in HHT patients.

Keywords: telangiectasia; hereditary hemorrhagic; vascular malformations; survival; life expectancy

---

1. Introduction

Hereditary Hemorrhagic Telangiectasia (HHT) is an autosomal dominant disease, with prevalence rates between 1:5000 and 1:8000 and with approximately 85,000 affected citizens in Europe [1,2]. HHT is characterized by multi-systemic vascular lesions, known as telangiectases, and visceral arteriovenous malformations (AVMs). In approximately 85% of the HHT patients, mutations in the Endoglin (*ENG*) or Activin receptor-like kinase 1 (*ACVRL1*) gene are found, causing HHT type 1 and type 2, respectively [3,4]. Most of the HHT patients suffer from recurrent, spontaneous epistaxis due to rupture of the thin-walled nasal telangiectases. The visceral AVMs are usually asymptomatic but can result in severe morbidity and mortality. The most common visceral localization of the AVMs is the lung (pulmonary AVM (PAVM)). Although much rarer than PAVMs, cerebral vascular malformations (CVMs) can also result in severe morbidity and mortality. The prevalence of PAVMs and CVMs depends on the HHT type: PAVMs occur in up to 60% of patients with HHT type 1 and 5–10% of patients with HHT type 2, and CVMs occur in 8–16% in HHT type 1 and in 0.5–1.5% in HHT type 2 [5]. A PAVM is a direct connection between the pulmonary artery and pulmonary vein with the absence of a normal capillary bed. Due to the absence of the normal capillaries, septic or non-septic emboli can enter the systemic circulation resulting in strokes and brain abscesses [6]. Preventatively, PAVMs can be safely and effectively treated with transcatheter embolotherapy. For patients with CVMs, treatment versus conservative management, should be considered on a case-by-case basis [7].

In the past, HHT patients presented with major complications especially from undiagnosed PAVMs such as hemothorax and paradoxical emboli leading to ischemic stroke or cerebral abscess [6,8]. These complications significantly reduced the quality of life and the life expectancy [9–11]. Several studies have shown a decreased life expectancy in HHT patients that did not receive a systematic HHT screening and treatment [10,12]. According to the current International HHT Guidelines screening and, if indicated, treatment of HHT-related organ involvement is strongly recommended in a center with HHT expertise [7]. The intention of this study is to evaluate if by using this approach the life expectancy of HHT patients is no longer negatively affected.

2. Materials and Methods

2.1. Study Design and Patient Selection

This retrospective cohort study included all consecutive persons who were referred to our HHT outpatient clinic suspected of having HHT between January 2004 and November 2016. This period was chosen because prior to 2004, HHT screening was not standardized in our center. We used the Dutch social security numbers (SSN) of each patient to confirm status alive or deceased, and date of death with the Dutch Ministry of Healthcare. This check was performed on 1 December 2019.

2.2. Patient Selection

We used our HHT database as saved on 14 November 2016 to select the individuals to be included in this study. Patients with a genetic diagnosis (a disease-causing mutation in *ENG*, *ACVRL1* or *SMAD4* gene) and/or clinically confirmed HHT diagnosis according to the Curaçao criteria [3,4], [13,14] were included in the HHT group. Patients without a clinical diagnosis (e.g., none or only 1 criterion) and patients with a possible diagnosis (2 criteria) but without a disease-causing mutation in *ENG*, *ACVLR1* or *SMAD4* (or in the absence of the known HHT family mutation) were included in the non-HHT control group. Patients with two positive clinical criteria but without DNA testing or with a family member with an unknown type of HHT were excluded. The Curaçao criteria include (1) the presence of spontaneous, recurrent epistaxis; (2) multiple mucocutaneous telangiectases at characteristic sites; (3) the presence of visceral AVMs and (4) a first-degree relative with definite HHT [13]. The clinical HHT diagnosis is "unlikely" with less than 2 criteria present, "possible or suspected" with 2 criteria present and "definite" with three or more positive criteria. DNA testing was (usually) only offered to adult patients. We excluded all patients without a known SSN. Patients with a clinical HHT diagnosis (e.g., three or more positive criteria), but negative genetic testing for the known family HHT mutation were excluded because of the uncertainty of their HHT status. To avoid asymptomatic HHT patients being included in the non-HHT control group, any person who had been screened during childhood, but had not been rescreened as an adult or had not undergone DNA testing as a child, was excluded because of age dependent symptom penetrance and the consequently lower sensitivity of the Curaçao criteria in children [15]. Finally, we excluded patients with insufficient data to confirm or reject the HHT diagnosis or patients who did not complete the screening program. We did not exclude patients that were lost to follow-up after completing the initial screening.

2.3. Screening Protocol for HHT

All patients were screened according to our standardized protocol. This protocol for adults entailed a detailed patient interview, a physical examination focused on signs and symptoms of HHT and PAVMs, an inspection of the nasal mucosa by a dedicated HHT Ear, Nose and Throat specialist, laboratory testing for anemia and a transthoracic contrast echocardiography (TTCE) to screen for the presence of a right-to-left shunt secondary to PAVMs. In case of moderate or severe shunt grade on TTCE [16], a non-contrast chest CT-scan was performed. In case of a clinically or genetic confirmed HHT diagnosis, adult patients were advised to undergo further evaluation for CVMs with a non-contrast magnetic resonance imaging of the brain. Screening for other visceral organ involvement was only done on indication. For example, the digestive tract was evaluated in cases with anemia not correlated to epistaxis severity, and screening for hepatic vascular malformations (HVMs) was done in cases with elevated liver enzymes, dyspnea or signs and symptoms associated with liver disease or high-output heart failure. Other aspects of HHT such as epistaxis and anemia were treated accordingly. Children were screened with a different protocol that included a detailed history to detect epistaxis or hypoxemia-related symptoms such as exercise intolerance, poor growth or headaches, a chest radiography and pulse-oximetry. Children were only screened for CVMs on indication. Further investigation with a low-dose chest CT-scan was only performed when abnormalities were found suspect for the presence of a PAVM: a suspect history for PAVMs, saturation with pulse oximetry <96% or a density suspect for a PAVM on the chest radiography [17]. If a treatable PAVM was detected based on a discussion in the multidisciplinary team, embolotherapy of the PAVM with vascular plugs or coils was performed by interventional radiologists specialized in HHT. PAVMs with a feeding artery ≥2–3 mm were regarded as treatable. After embolization of all targeted PAVMs, patients were reviewed in the multidisciplinary team. Follow-up in our institution is standardized and includes a contrast-enhanced chest CT-scan 6 months after embolization, followed by a chest CT-scan every 2 to 5 years in case of sustained occlusion of the embolized PAVM. The follow-up chest CT-scans were discussed in the multidisciplinary team. In case of persistent perfusion or reperfusion of the PAVM on follow-up chest CT-scan, patients were scheduled for repeat embolotherapy. Signs that suggest persistent perfusion or reperfusion include contrast enhancement in the PAVM, no or minimal shrinkage of the PAVM sac or persistence of a large feeding artery or draining vein. Children were followed on a case-by-case basis after embolotherapy, usually with a chest radiography and saturation measurement with pulse oximetry. If a CVM was detected, the patient was subsequently referred to a center with expertise in treating brain vascular malformations in The Netherlands. The need for treatment and follow-up was determined in this center. If no abnormalities were detected with screening in children or adults, rescreening was performed every five years. All children were advised to undergo rescreening with our protocol for adults when they reached the age of 18 years.

2.4. Statistical Methods and Ethics

Statistical analysis was performed using SPSS version 26.0 for Windows (IBM, Armonk, NY, USA) and R version 3.5.3 for Windows (the R Project for Statistical Computing). Data are presented as mean and standard deviation (SD). Continuous variables were compared using the independent samples T-test. The prevalence of anemia, comorbidities and disease complications were compared using Fisher's exact test. Survival was estimated using left-truncated Kaplan–Meier curves. For comparison of survival between groups we used the Mantel–Cox test. Statistical significance was defined at $p < 0.05$. This study was approved by the research ethics board of Medical Research Ethics Committees United (MEC-U) of the St. Antonius Hospital under protocol registration number W16.160.

3. Results

3.1. Patient Selection and Baseline Characteristics

In total, 1541 individuals had been screened for presence of HHT between 2004 and November 2016. From these individuals, 717 patients could be included in the HHT group and 471 in the non-HHT control group. In the HHT group, 319 patients (45%) suffered from HHT type 1, 325 (45%) from HHT type 2, 29 (4%) from juvenile polyposis/HHT overlap syndrome and in 44 patients no disease-causing mutations could be identified. The mean age at presentation in the HHT group was 40.6 years and 54% was female. In the control group the mean age was 40.9 years with 57% female. The mean birthyear for both groups was the year 1969. The control group consisted of family members of HHT patients in whom HHT was ruled out (n = 368), patients with recurrent epistaxis (n = 28) without HHT, patients with mucocutaneous telangiectases without HHT (n = 17) or patients with the suspicion of visceral AVM (n = 58) without HHT. The suspected visceral AVMs (not all were confirmed) were located in the lungs (PAVM: n = 43), digestive tract telangiectases (n = 5), brain (CAVM: n = 4) and four suspected AVMs were located in other organs. In Figure 1 the flowchart of the patient selection is depicted. The demographic characteristics of the included subjects are shown in Table 1.

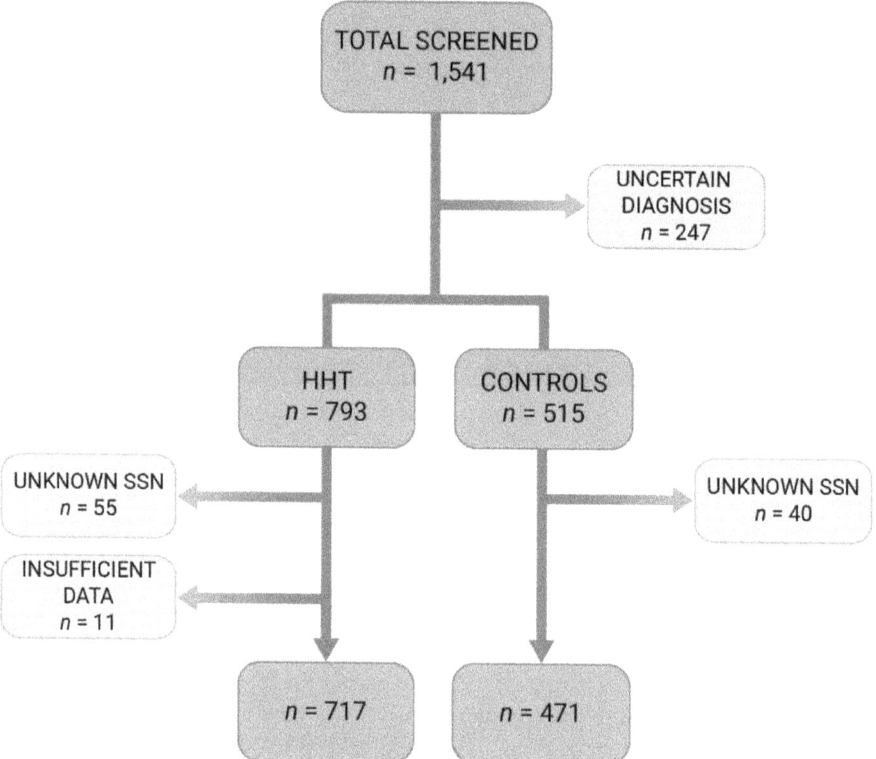

Figure 1. Flowchart of included patients. HHT, Hereditary Hemorrhagic Telangiectasia; SSN, social security number.

Table 1. Demographic characteristics of the included patients. *ACVRL1*, activin receptor-like kinase 1 (HHT type 2); *ENG*, endoglin (HHT type 1); HHT, Hereditary Hemorrhagic Telangiectasia; SD, standard deviation; *SMAD4*, SMAD family member 4 (juvenile polyposis/HHT overlap syndrome).

	HHT Group (n = 717)	Control Group (n = 471)	p-Value
Gender (%)			
Female	384 (54)	268 (57)	0.28
Male	333 (46)	203 (43)	
Genetic mutation (%)			
ENG (HHT type 1)	319 (45)		
ACVRL1 (HHT type 2)	325 (45)	-	-
SMAD4	29 (4)		
Mutation unknown	44 (6)		
Mean age at presentation, years (SD)	40.8 (19.4)	40.6 (17.4)	0.86
ENG (n = 319)	35.7 (19.9)	-	-
ACVRL1 (n = 325)	44.9 (17.8)	-	-
SMAD4 (n = 29)	31.4 (17.2)	-	-
Mutation unknown (n = 44)	54.1 (13.9)	-	-
Mean birth year	1969	1969	-

3.2. Visceral AVMs, Comorbidities and Disease Complications

In Table 2, the number of visceral AVMs, comorbidities and disease complications of the HHT patients and controls are shown. In the HHT group, 255 patients (36%) had PAVMs versus 32 (7%) individuals in the control group. In the HHT group, 60% (432 patients) underwent CVM screening. In 28 out of 432 patients (6%) a CVM was detected. Furthermore, (symptomatic) HVMs and gastrointestinal telangiectases were diagnosed in 75 (11%) and 72 (10%) patients, respectively. The prevalence of anemia was significantly higher in the HHT group compared to the controls ($p < 0.001$). Comorbidities and disease complications were similar between groups with the exception of higher prevalence of pulmonary hypertension (3% vs. <1%, Fisher's exact test: $p = 0.003$) and high-output heart failure (Fisher's exact test: 2% vs. 0%, $p = 0.001$) in the HHT group.

Table 2. Visceral AVMs and comorbidities of the included patients. *ACVRL1*, activin receptor-like kinase 1 (HHT type 2); AVM, arteriovenous malformation; COPD, chronic obstructive pulmonary disease; CVM, cerebrovascular malformations; *ENG*, endoglin (HHT type 1); HHT, Hereditary Hemorrhagic Telangiectasia; HVM, hepatic vascular malformation; SD, standard deviation; *SMAD4*, SMAD family member 4 (juvenile polyposis/HHT overlap syndrome). * For these AVMs, screening is only performed on indication.

	HHT Group (n = 717)	Control Group (n = 471)
PAVM (%)	255 (36)	32 (7)
ENG (n = 319)	176	-
ACVRL1 (n = 325)	47	-
SMAD4 (n = 29)	12	-
Mutation unknown (n = 44)	20	-
PAVM embolotherapy	175	28
CVM (%)		
Yes	28 (4)	4 (2)
No	404 (56)	0
Unknown/not screened	285 (40)	467 (99)

Table 2. *Cont.*

	HHT Group (*n* = 717)	Control Group (*n* = 471)
CVM treatment		
No treatment	14	1
Surgery	5	1
Radiotherapy	3	1
Embolotherapy	2	1
Combination	4	0
HVM (%) *	75 (11)	3 (<1)
Gastrointestinal telangiectases (%) *	72 (10)	6 (1)
Other AVMs (%) *	14 (2)	4 (1)
Spinal	4	0
Pancreatic	3	0
Renal	2	1
Urinary bladder	2	1
Splenic	1	0
Muscular	1	2
Ocular	1	0
Anemia (%)	212 (30)	28 (6)
Comorbidities (%)		
Malignancy	36 (5)	21 (5)
Atrial fibrillation	36 (5)	13 (3)
COPD and bronchiectasis	28 (4)	16 (3)
Acute coronary disease	26 (4)	10 (2)
Venous thromboembolism	25 (4)	8 (2)
Autoimmune disease	21 (3)	23 (5)
Pulmonary hypertension	19 (3)	2 (< 1)
Diabetes mellitus type 2	16 (2)	19 (4)
Peripheral vascular disease	15 (2)	7 (2)
Disease complications (%)		
Cerebrovascular accident	49 (7)	22 (5)
High-output heart failure	14 (2)	0 (0)
Brain abscess	11 (2)	3 (1)

3.3. Survival of HHT Patients and Controls

In Table 3, the number of patients, and the age and cause of death are shown. In the HHT group 57 patients (8%) had died versus 24 (5%) in the control group. The most frequent cause of death in the HHT was infectious disease, followed by malignancy. The cause of death in the control group was not recorded. There was no difference in survival between the HHT and the non-HHT control group (Mantel–Cox test: $p = 0.29$; Figure 2). The survival of patients with HHT type 1 did not differ from patients with HHT type 2 (Mantel–Cox test: $p = 0.28$; Figure 3A). Compared to the non-HHT control group, the survival of both patients with HHT type 1 (Mantel-Cox test: $p = 0.28$) and patients with HHT type 2 (Mantel–Cox test: $p = 0.85$) did not differ (Figure 3B,C). The mean life expectancy of the HHT population was 75.9 years (95% CI 73.3–78.6 years), comparable to the non-HHT control group (79.3 years, 95% CI 74.8–84.0 years). The mean life expectancy for patients with HHT type 1 was 76.4 years (95% CI 71.6–82.3 years) and 77.9 years (95% CI 74.5–81.3 years) for patients with HHT type 2. The survival of patients with a genetically confirmed HHT diagnosis (HHT type 1, type 2 or juvenile polyposis/HHT overlap syndrome) was comparable to the survival of their relatives in whom HHT was ruled out (e.g., a known family mutation, the individual did not inhere the specific mutation) (Mantel–Cox test: $p = 0.43$; Figure 3D). There was no significant difference in survival of men and women with HHT (Mantel–Cox test: $p = 0.10$; Figure 4A). HHT patients with visceral AVMs had a worse survival compared to HHT patients without visceral AVMs (Mantel–Cox test: $p = 0.017$). The survival in HHT patients with and without PAVM, CVM or gastrointestinal telangiectases did not differ, only patients with HVM had significantly worse survival compared to HHT patients without HVM (see Figure 4B–F). HHT patients without anemia showed a tendency to a better survival (see Figure 4G).

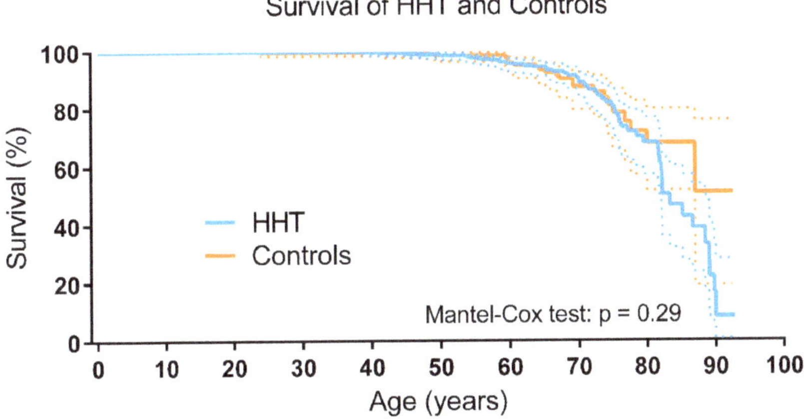

Figure 2. Left-truncated Kaplan–Meier curve of HHT and controls. The dotted lines represent the 95% confidence intervals. HHT, Hereditary Hemorrhagic Telangiectasia.

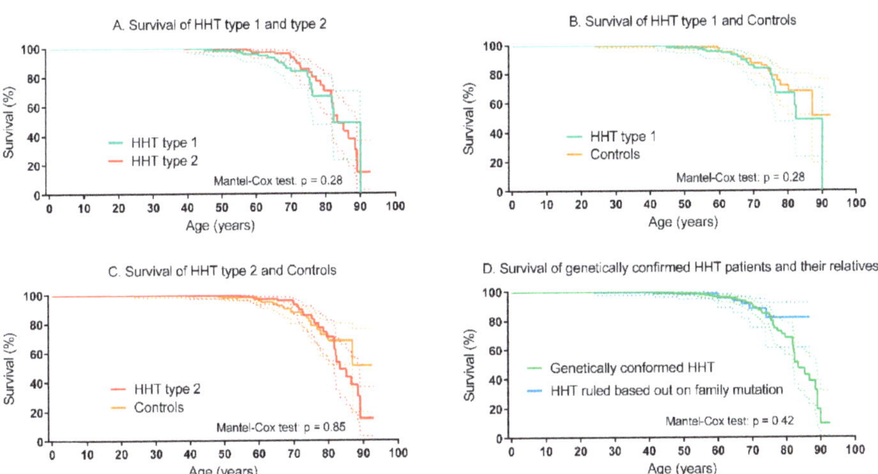

Figure 3. Left-truncated Kaplan–Meier curves of HHT subtypes and controls (**A**) HHT type 1 and HHT type 2. (**B**) HHT type 1 and controls. (**C**) HHT type 2 and controls. (**D**) Patients with genetically confirmed HHT (HHT type 1, type 2 and juvenile polyposis/HHT overlap syndrome) and their relatives without HHT. The dotted lines represent the 95% confidence intervals. HHT, Hereditary Hemorrhagic Telangiectasia.

Table 3. Number of deceased patients, age and cause of death. HHT, Hereditary Hemorrhagic Telangiectasia; SD, standard deviation.

	HHT Group (*n* = 717)	Control Group (*n* = 471)	*p*-Value
Deceased (%)	57 (8)	24 (5)	0.06
Mean age death, years (SD)	69.7 (13.3)	64.3 (13.7)	0.1
Cause of death			
Infection	15		
Heart failure	9		
Malignancy	8		
Severe anemia	4		
Thromboembolism	2	-	-
Postoperative complications	2		
Hemorrhagic stroke	1		
Unknown	1		
	17		

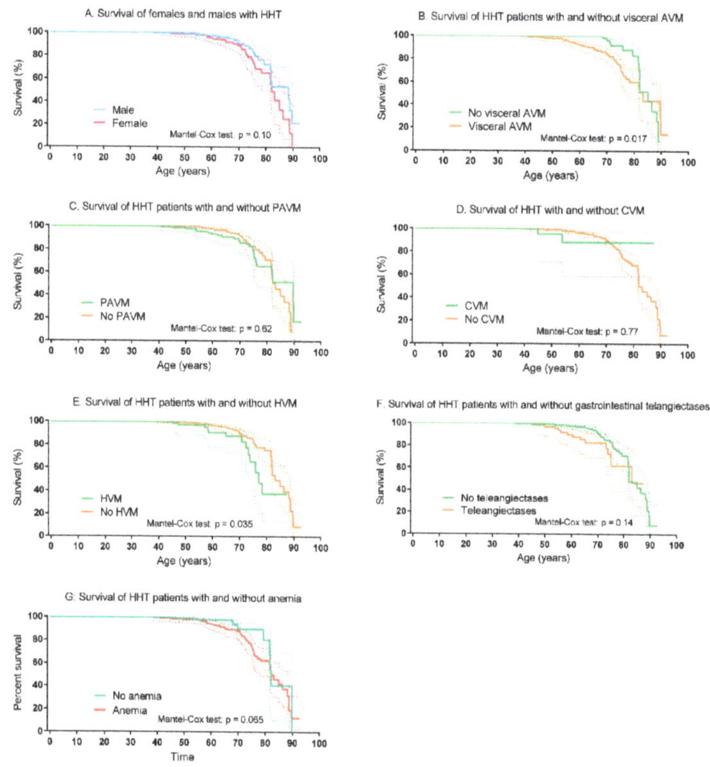

Figure 4. Left-truncated Kaplan–Meier curves of HHT patients. (**A**) Survival of females and males with HHT. (**B**) Survival of HHT patients with and without visceral AVM. (**C**) Survival of HHT patients with and without PAVM. (**D**) Survival of HHT patients with and without CVM. (**E**) Survival of HHT patients with and without HVM. (**F**) Survival of HHT patients with and without gastrointestinal telangiectases. (**G**) Survival of HHT patients with and without anemia. The dotted lines represent the 95% confidence intervals. AVM, arteriovenous malformation; CVM, cerebrovascular malformation; HHT, Hereditary Hemorrhagic Telangiectasia; HVM, hepatic vascular malformation.

4. Discussion

We found that the life expectancy of patients with HHT who have been systematically screened for HHT-related organ involvement, treated if needed and followed in a center with HHT expertise did not differ from the life expectancy of the non-HHT control group. These results emphasize the importance of systematic screening of HHT patients, treatment and follow-up in an HHT expertise center.

Previous studies have shown conflicting results on life expectancy in patients with HHT. A study with 73 patients with HHT and 218 controls with a 20-year follow-up did not reveal any significant differences in survival between both groups [18]. However, two studies assessing survival in parents of a current HHT population showed worse survival in these parents with HHT compared to their non-HHT partners [10,12]. Since the population of the latter studies was comprised of parents with HHT, these studies concerned a largely unscreened and untreated population. In the study by De Gussem et al., patients with HHT type 1 had especially worse survival compared to non-HHT partners. The authors stated that this was probably caused by the higher prevalence of (untreated) PAVMs and CVMs and subsequent complications [10]. Donaldson et al. observed higher risks of stroke, cerebral abscess and bleeding complications and showed poorer survival in a study on a primary care database including almost 700 HHT patients in comparison to age and sex matched controls [9]. However, as emphasized by the authors, many of the HHT-related complications were amenable to intervention, early diagnosis and treatment. Their study also showed a higher mortality rate in the time period closest to the diagnosis of HHT. This might be related to the fact that some patients presented with HHT-related complications at the time of diagnosis. Once patients have been diagnosed with HHT, they are followed and treated for organ involvement to reduce morbidity and mortality.

Our study shows that the life expectancy of patients, who are screened for HHT-related organ involvement and if needed, treated in a center with HHT expertise, is similar to the life expectancy of their relatives without HHT. We did not observe difference in survival between HHT type 1 and type 2. This is an important finding because a previous study by our group showed worse survival in (largely untreated) HHT type 1 population [10]. In addition, survival of men and women with HHT and HHT patients with and without PAVMs, CVMs or gastrointestinal telangiectases did not differ. We observed a significant difference in HHT patients with and without visceral AVMs and patients with and without HVMs. This is probably caused by the fact that screening for HVMs is only done on indication in our center and thus the majority of these patients probably suffered from symptomatic HVMs.

This improvement in survival of HHT patients in comparison to previous publications is most likely due to the benefit of screening for the presence of PAVMs and PAVM treatment if indicated. Additionally, screening methods and treatment options for PAVMs, CVMs, epistaxis, gastro-intestinal bleeding and subsequent anemia have improved over the years, which most likely benefits survival as well. In addition to this, several studies have suggested that patients with HHT possibly have a natural protection against certain cancers and myocardial infarction, possibly benefiting survival rates [19,20]. While we did not observe a negative effect of HHT on the survival in this study, it is important to realize that the quality of life in these patients will probably still be lower compared to their controls even if optimal screening and treatment was performed. Two studies investigated the quality of life in an HHT population screened and treated in two different HHT centers. The authors observed that the HHT-related symptoms and organ involvement had a major negative effect on the quality of life [21,22].

We have not compared the survival of the HHT patients and controls to the Dutch population. However, we think that they are in line with each other. The life expectancy of Dutch people born in 1969 was 73.54 years [23]. We observed a slightly higher life expectancy of our HHT patients and controls, most likely because the patients included in this study already lived to an average age of approximately 40 years. The comorbidities were comparable between the HHT group and the controls with the exception of anemia, higher rates of pulmonary hypertension and high-output heart failure in the HHT group. It would be very informative to compare our HHT group, to HHT patients that did not receive screening; however, this is not ethically possible.

We acknowledge that there is selection bias of the patients who passed away prior to the HHT diagnosis and were thus not included in this study. Additionally, there is a small chance of presence of undiagnosed HHT patients in the non-HHT control group. However, in view of the number of patients and non-HHT controls in this study and in view of the convincing results, it seems unlikely that this would influence the outcomes significantly. Strengths of this study are the use of consecutive data in a large patient population. Although the control group also consists of patients that were referred to our hospital with visceral AVMs, the largest part of the controls included first-degree family members of HHT patients. Therefore, the lifestyle and socio-economic conditions are to some degree comparable which makes the non-HHT controls a better control group than the Dutch population for evaluation the influence of HHT on life expectancy.

In conclusion, the survival of patients with HHT is not negatively affected by HHT if the HHT patients have been systematically screened and treated for HHT-related organ involvement in a center with HHT expertise. These findings demonstrate the importance of systematic screening of HHT patients and treatment of PAVMs and other HHT-related organ involvement.

Author Contributions: Study concept and design: E.M.d.G., A.E.H., J.C.K., R.J.S., J.J.M. Acquisition of the data: E.M.d.G., S.K., A.E.H., J.C.K., R.J.S., J.J.M. Analysis and Interpretation of data: E.M.d.G., S.K., A.E.H., J.C.K., M.C.P., R.J.S., J.J.M. Critical writing of the manuscript: E.M.d.G., S.K., A.E.H. Revising the intellectual content: A.E.H., J.C.K., M.C.P., R.J.S., J.J.M. Final approval of the version to be published: E.M.d.G., S.K., A.E.H., J.C.K., M.C.P., R.J.S., J.J.M. All authors have read and agreed to the published version of the manuscript.

Funding: This research received no external funding.

Conflicts of Interest: The authors declare no conflict of interest.

Abbreviations

ACVRL1: activin receptor-like kinase 1; AVM, arteriovenous malformation; CI, confidence interval; CT, computed tomography; CVM, cerebral vascular malformation; *ENG*, endoglin; HHT, Hereditary Hemorrhagic Telangiectasia; HVM, hepatic vascular malformation; PAVM, pulmonary arteriovenous malformation; SD, standard deviation; SSN, social security number; TTCE, transthoracic contrast echocardiography; VM, vascular malformation.

References

1. Govani, F.S.; Shovlin, C.L. Hereditary haemorrhagic telangiectasia: A clinical and scientific review. *Eur. J. Hum. Genet.* **2009**, *17*, 860–871. [CrossRef] [PubMed]
2. Shovlin, C.L.; Buscarini, E.; Kjeldsen, A.D.; Mager, H.J.; Sabba, C.; Droege, F.; Geisthoff, U.; Ugolini, S.; Dupuis-Girod, S. European Reference Network for Rare Vascular Diseases (VASCERN) Outcome Measures for Hereditary Haemorrhagic Telangiectasia (HHT). *Orphanet J. Rare Dis.* **2018**, *13*, 1–5. [CrossRef] [PubMed]
3. McAllister, K.A.; Grogg, K.M.; Johnson, D.W.; Gallione, C.J.; Baldwin, M.A.; Jackson, C.E.; Helmbold, E.A.; Markel, D.S.; McKinnon, W.C.; Murrell, J. Endoglin, a TGF-beta binding protein of endothelial cells, is the gene for hereditary haemorrhagic telangiectasia type 1. *Nat. Genet.* **1994**, *8*, 345–351. [CrossRef] [PubMed]
4. Johnson, D.W.; Berg, J.N.; Baldwin, M.A.; Gallione, C.J.; Marondel, I.; Yoon, S.-J.; Stenzel, T.T.; Speer, M.; Pericak-Vance, M.A.; Diamond, A.; et al. Mutations in the activin receptor-like kinase 1 gene in hereditary haemorrhagic telangiectasia type 2. *Nat. Genet.* **1996**, *13*, 189–195. [CrossRef] [PubMed]
5. Kroon, S.; Snijder, R.J.; Faughnan, M.E.; Mager, H.J. Systematic screening in hereditary hemorrhagic telangiectasia: A review. *Curr. Opin. Pulm. Med.* **2018**, *24*, 260–268. [CrossRef] [PubMed]
6. Khurshid, I.; Downie, G.H. Pulmonary arteriovenous malformation. *Postgrad. Med. J.* **2002**, *78*, 191–197. [CrossRef] [PubMed]
7. Faughnan, M.E.; Palda, V.A.; Garcia-Tsao, G.; Geisthoff, U.W.; McDonald, J.; Proctor, D.D.; Spears, J.; Brown, D.H.; Chesnutt, M.S.; Cottin, V.; et al. International guidelines for the diagnosis and management of hereditary haemorrhagic telangiectasia. *J. Med. Genet.* **2011**, *48*, 73–87. [CrossRef]

8. Boother, E.J.; Brownlow, S.; Tighe, H.C.; Bamford, K.B.; Jackson, J.E.; Shovlin, C.L. Cerebral Abscess Associated with Odontogenic Bacteremias, Hypoxemia, and Iron Loading in Immunocompetent Patients with Right-to-Left Shunting Through Pulmonary Arteriovenous Malformations. *Clin. Infect. Dis.* **2017**, *65*, 595–603. [CrossRef]

9. Donaldson, J.W.; McKeever, T.M.; Hall, I.P.; Hubbard, R.B.; Fogarty, A.W. Complications and mortality in hereditary hemorrhagic telangiectasia. *Neurology* **2015**, *84*, 1886–1893. [CrossRef]

10. de Gussem, E.M.; Edwards, C.P.; Hosman, A.E.; Westermann, C.J.J.; Snijder, R.J.; Faughnan, M.E.; Mager, J.J. Life expectancy of parents with Hereditary Haemorrhagic Telangiectasia. *Orphanet J. Rare Dis.* **2016**, *11*, 46. [CrossRef]

11. Droege, F.; Thangavelu, K.; Stuck, B.A.; Stang, A.; Lang, S.; Geisthoff, U. Life expectancy and comorbidities in patients with hereditary hemorrhagic telangiectasia. *Vasc. Med.* **2018**, *23*, 377–383. [CrossRef]

12. Sabbà, C.; Pasculli, G.; Suppressa, P.; D'Ovidio, F.; Lenato, G.M.; Resta, F.; Assennato, G.; Guanti, G. Life expectancy in patients with hereditary haemorrhagic telangiectasia. *QJM Mon. J. Assoc. Physicians* **2006**, *99*, 327–334. [CrossRef] [PubMed]

13. Shovlin, C.L.; Guttmacher, A.E.; Buscarini, E.; Faughnan, M.E.; Hyland, R.H.; Westermann, C.J.; Kjeldsen, A.D.; Plauchu, H. Diagnostic criteria for hereditary hemorrhagic telangiectasia (Rendu-Osler-Weber syndrome). *Am. J. Med. Genet.* **2000**, *91*, 66–67. [CrossRef]

14. Gallione, C.J.; Richards, J.A.; Letteboer, T.G.W.; Rushlow, D.; Prigoda, N.L.; Leedom, T.P.; Ganguly, A.; Castells, A.; van Amstel, J.K.P.; Westermann, C.J.J.; et al. SMAD4 mutations found in unselected HHT patients. *J. Med. Genet.* **2006**, *43*, 793–797. [CrossRef]

15. Pahl, K.S.; Choudhury, A.; Wusik, K.; Hammill, A.; White, A.; Henderson, K.; Pollak, J.; Kasthuri, T.S. Applicability of the Curaçao Criteria for the Diagnosis of Hereditary Hemorrhagic Telangiectasia in the Pediatric Population. *J. Pediatr.* **2018**, *197*, 207–213. [CrossRef] [PubMed]

16. van Gent, M.W.F.; Post, M.C.; Luermans, J.G.L.M.; Snijder, R.J.; Westermann, C.J.J.; Plokker, H.W.M.; Overtoom, T.T.; Mager, J.J. Screening for pulmonary arteriovenous malformations using transthoracic contrast echocardiography: A prospective study. *Eur. Respir. J.* **2009**, *33*, 85–91. [CrossRef] [PubMed]

17. Hosman, A.E.; de Gussem, E.M.; Balemans, W.A.F.; Gauthier, A.; Westermann, C.J.J.; Snijder, R.J.; Post, M.C.; Mager, J.J. Screening children for pulmonary arteriovenous malformations: Evaluation of 18 years of experience. *Pediatr. Pulmonol.* **2017**, *52*, 1206–1211. [CrossRef]

18. Kjeldsen, A.; Aagaard, K.S.; Tørring, P.M.; Möller, S.; Green, A. 20-year follow-up study of Danish HHT patients—Survival and causes of death. *Orphanet J. Rare Dis.* **2016**, *11*, 1–8. [CrossRef]

19. Hosman, A.E.; Devlin, H.L.; Silva, B.M.; Shovlin, C.L. Specific cancer rates may differ in patients with hereditary haemorrhagic telangiectasia compared to controls. *Orphanet J. Rare Dis.* **2013**, *8*, 1–15. [CrossRef]

20. Shovlin, C.L.; Awan, I.; Cahilog, Z.; Abdulla, F.N.; Guttmacher, A.E. Reported cardiac phenotypes in hereditary hemorrhagic telangiectasia emphasize burdens from arrhythmias, anemia and its treatments, but suggest reduced rates of myocardial infarction. *Int. J. Cardiol.* **2016**, *215*, 179–185. [CrossRef] [PubMed]

21. Geirdal, A.Ø.; Dheyauldeen, S.; Bachmann-Harildstad, G.; Heimdal, K. Quality of life in patients with hereditary hemorrhagic telangiectasia in Norway: A population based study. *Am. J. Med. Genet. A* **2012**, *158A*, 1269–1278. [CrossRef]

22. Zarrabeitia, R.; Farinas-Alvarez, C.; Santibanez, M.; Senaris, B.; Fontalba, A.; Botella, L.M.; Parra, J.A. Quality of life in patients with hereditary haemorrhagic telangiectasia (HHT). *Health Qual. Life Outcomes* **2017**, *15*, 19. [CrossRef] [PubMed]

23. The World Bank—Life Expectancy at Birth, Total (Years)—Netherlands. 2020. Available online: https://data.worldbank.org/indicator/SP.DYN.LE00.IN?locations=NL (accessed on 18 October 2020).

Publisher's Note: MDPI stays neutral with regard to jurisdictional claims in published maps and institutional affiliations.

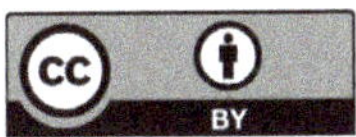

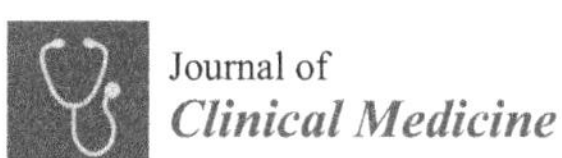 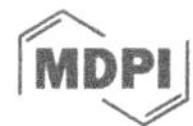

Journal of
Clinical Medicine

Review

Potential Second-Hits in Hereditary Hemorrhagic Telangiectasia

Carmelo Bernabeu [1,*], Pinar Bayrak-Toydemir [2,3], Jamie McDonald [3,4] and Michelle Letarte [5]

[1] Centro de Investigaciones Biológicas Margarita Salas, Consejo Superior de Investigaciones Científicas (CSIC) and Centro de Investigación Biomédica en Red de Enfermedades Raras (CIBERER), 28040 Madrid, Spain

[2] ARUP Institute for Clinical and Experimental Pathology, Salt Lake City, UT 84108, USA; pinar.bayrak-toydemir@aruplab.com

[3] Department of Pathology, University of Utah, Salt Lake City, UT 84132, USA; Jamie.mcdonald@hsc.utah.edu

[4] Department of Radiology, University of Utah, Salt Lake City, UT 84132, USA

[5] Molecular Medicine, Hospital for Sick Children, and Department of Immunology, University of Toronto, Toronto, ON M5G 0A4, Canada; michelle.letarte@sickkids.ca

* Correspondence: bernabeu.c@cib.csic.es

Received: 4 October 2020; Accepted: 2 November 2020; Published: 5 November 2020

Abstract: Hereditary hemorrhagic telangiectasia (HHT) is an autosomal dominant genetic disorder that presents with telangiectases in skin and mucosae, and arteriovenous malformations (AVMs) in internal organs such as lungs, liver, and brain. Mutations in *ENG* (endoglin), *ACVRL1* (ALK1), and *MADH4* (Smad4) genes account for over 95% of HHT. Localized telangiectases and AVMs are present in different organs, with frequencies which differ among affected individuals. By itself, HHT gene heterozygosity does not account for the focal nature and varying presentation of the vascular lesions leading to the hypothesis of a "second-hit" that triggers the lesions. Accumulating research has identified a variety of triggers that may synergize with HHT gene heterozygosity to generate the vascular lesions. Among the postulated second-hits are: mechanical trauma, light, inflammation, vascular injury, angiogenic stimuli, shear stress, modifier genes, and somatic mutations in the wildtype HHT gene allele. The aim of this review is to summarize these triggers, as well as the functional mechanisms involved.

Keywords: hereditary hemorrhagic telangiectasia (HHT), second-hit; arteriovenous malformation (AVM); endoglin; ALK1; Smad4; inflammation; shear stress; vascular injury; somatic mutation; cell adhesion; angiogenesis; vascular endothelial growth factor (VEGF); transforming growth factor beta (TGF-β)

---

1. Clinical Characteristics of HHT

Hereditary hemorrhagic telangiectasia (HHT) is an autosomal dominant vascular disorder that exhibits age-related penetrance and extensive clinical variability, including intra-familial variability [1]. The characteristic vascular lesions range from 1 to 2 mm punctate mucocutaneous telangiectases to arteriovenous malformations (AVMs) several centimeters in diameter within visceral organs, particularly the lungs, liver, and brain. Telangiectases close to the surface of the skin and mucous membranes are fragile and frequently rupture and bleed upon slight trauma. Spontaneous and recurrent nose-bleeding (epistaxis) typically begins in mid-childhood and is the most common clinical manifestation; although occurring in over 90% of patients, the severity varies from an infrequent few drops to brisk bleeds multiple times daily. Gastrointestinal (GI) bleeding due to mucosal telangiectases affects approximately 25% of patients, almost always presenting after the age of 50. Many HHT patients have iron-deficiency anemia secondary to chronic bleeding of telangiectases, more often from nasal than GI lesions [2,3].

Solid organ AVMs are direct connections between artery and vein which bypass capillary beds and result in life-threatening complications more often related to the shunting of blood per se through these low resistance pathways, than to hemorrhage. For example, pulmonary AVMs (PAVMs), which occur in about 50% of HHT patients overall, result in high-flow continuous intrapulmonary right-to-left shunts with significant related risk for stroke or brain abscess [4,5]. The majority of PAVMs (70% or more) occur in HHT patients, but approximately 20% are acquired and associated with trauma, cardiothoracic surgery, hepatic cirrhosis, metastatic cancer, mitral stenosis, infection, amyloidosis, and chronic thromboembolic disease [6]. The frequency of hepatic vascular malformations was approximately 75% in two studies that systematically imaged the liver of affected individuals using computed tomography (CT) [7,8] and 41% in another study using ultrasound examination [9], although only a minority (8% in the CT study) were symptomatic. When symptomatic, hepatic vascular malformations associated with HHT typically present in later adulthood as high output heart failure, due to significantly increased blood flow through shunting pathways in the liver [10]. Intracranial hemorrhage is the risk posed by brain AVMs, which are typically congenital and occur in about 10% of those with HHT [11,12].

The clinical diagnosis of HHT is based on the Curaçao Criteria: (i) recurrent and spontaneous nosebleeds (epistaxis), (ii) cutaneous or mucosal telangiectases on the skin of the hands, lips, or face, or inside of the nose or oral cavity, (iii) visceral AVMs or telangiectases in one or more of the internal organs, including lungs, brain, liver, gastrointestinal tract, and spinal cord, and (iv) family history of HHT (i.e., first-degree relative with a definite HHT clinical or genetic diagnosis). The HHT diagnosis is considered definite if three criteria are present, possible or suspected with two criteria, and unlikely if only one is present [3,13]. It is of note that the disease experts who initially created and twenty years later confirmed these consensus clinical criteria for HHT, believe that the locations of telangiectases and AVMs are specific in HHT. In fact, multiple telangiectases or an AVM in a location other than those considered characteristic actually argue against the diagnosis of HHT.

Overall, the phenotype and age of onset of manifestations is highly variable in HHT and this variability seems to depend on HHT subtype, as well as genetic background and/or environmental triggers (second-hits) to which each individual is exposed.

2. Genetics of HHT: The Germline Mutation

Heterozygous mutations in several genes are known to cause HHT. Endoglin (*ENG*) mutations cause what is referred to as HHT1 (OMIM #187300) [14], activin receptor-like kinase 1 (*ACVRL1*) mutations cause HHT2 (OMIM #600376) [15], while mothers against decapentaplegic homolog 4 (*MADH4* or *SMAD4*) mutations cause a syndrome which combines familial juvenile polyposis and HHT (JP/HT; OMIM #175050) [16]. Also, mutations in the *GDF2* gene, encoding bone morphogenetic protein 9 (BMP9), were described as the cause of an HHT-like syndrome [17], also named as HHT5 (OMIM #615506). Two further loci have been found by linkage analyses on chromosomes 5 (HHT3) and 7 (HHT4), but their corresponding coding genes have not been identified [18,19].

ENG and *ACVRL1* are the predominant genes mutated in HHT, each responsible for almost half of cases. A mutation in one of these two genes is detected in over 95% of individuals who meet Curaçao diagnostic criteria, and a mutation in *SMAD4* is detected in an additional 1–2% [20,21]. Although the phenotypes generated by mutations in *ENG* or *ACVRL1* are similar enough that they cannot be reliably distinguished in the clinical setting, pulmonary and cerebral AVMs are more frequent in HHT1 patients while GI bleeding and liver AVMs are more common in HHT2 [22,23]. Studies suggest that solid organ AVMs in JP/HHT are at least as common as in HHT1 and HHT2, and that pulmonary AVMs may be more frequent [16,21,24,25]. Overall, Curaçao diagnostic criteria for HHT are highly predictive of a pathogenic variant in *ENG* (HHT1) or *ACVRL1* (HHT2) but cannot distinguish between these two genotypes [21]. Furthermore, the genetic heterogeneity does not explain the striking variable expression observed within families.

There are no common disease-causing mutations or mutation hot spots in any of the HHT genes. Both *ENG* and *ACVRL1* mutations that cause HHT are dispersed almost equally throughout the genes except in a couple of exons. Mutations of all types have been reported [20,26]. The frequency of single or several exon deletions/duplications is up to 10%. Mutations causing sequence changes are slightly more common in the *ENG* than *ACVRL1*. Missense mutations account for more than half of mutations detected, however, nonsense, deletions, insertions, and splice site mutations have also been reported. Mutant *ENG* and *ACVRL1* proteins, including the products of multiple missense mutations, were shown to be expressed at the 50% level, in accordance to the haploinsufficiency model [20].

All the genes mutated in HHT encode proteins involved in the signaling pathway of the transforming growth factor beta (TGF-β) superfamily, including bone morphogenetic proteins (BMPs) (Figure 1). The most likely affected pathway in HHT involves the auxiliary receptor endoglin associated with the signaling serine/threonine kinase receptor ALK1. Both proteins are able to bind the ligands BMP9 and BMP10 [27–29], which form a heterodimeric complex that provides most of their BMP biological activity in plasma [30,31]. Upon ligand binding, ALK1 phosphorylates Smad1/5/8 followed by their nuclear translocation in complex with Smad4 [32–35]. Because endoglin and ALK1 are predominantly expressed in endothelial cells, which respond to circulating BMP9, they are widely accepted as the target cells most affected in HHT.

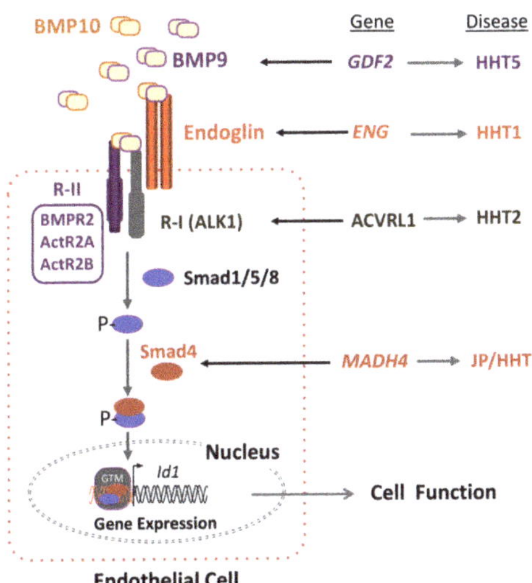

Figure 1. Hereditary hemorrhagic telangiectasia (HHT) and the transforming growth factor beta (TGF-β) signaling pathway in endothelial cells. Heterodimers of bone morphogenetic protein 9 (BMP9) and BMP10, among other members of the TGF-β family, bind to an endothelial cell surface receptor complex composed by the type I (R-I) receptor named ALK1 and the type II (R-II; BMPR2, ActR2A, ActR2B) receptor, both serine/threonine kinases, as well as the auxiliary receptor endoglin. The heterodimeric association between different R-I and R-II determines the specificity of the ligand signaling. Upon ligand binding, the R-II transphosphorylates ALK1, which subsequently propagates the signal by phosphorylating the receptor-regulated Smad (R-Smad) family of proteins, Smad1/5/8. Once phosphorylated (P-), R-Smads form heteromeric complexes with a cooperating homologue named Smad4 and translocate into the nucleus, where they regulate the transcriptional activity of different target genes, in turn modulating endothelial cell function. The involvement of other components of the TGF-β pathway has been omitted for simplification [32]. BMP9, Endoglin, ALK1, and Smad4 proteins are encoded by *GDF2*, *ENG*, *ACVRL1*, and *MADH4* genes, whose pathogenic mutations give rise to HHT5, HHT1, HHT2, and JPHT, respectively. BMP, bone morphogenetic protein; GTM, general transcription machinery. Adapted from Ruiz-Llorente et al. [34].

It is worth noting that within the TGF-β system, endoglin is known to participate in several receptor complexes, not necessarily including ALK1, and is capable of binding different ligands [36–39]. In addition, endoglin has been reported to be involved in several pathways relevant to vascular homeostasis. Endoglin was shown to regulate the organization of the actin cytoskeleton in endothelial cells via the interaction of its cytoplasmic domain with zyxin and zyxin-related protein 1 (ZRP1) [40,41]. Upon interacting with these members of the zyxin family, endoglin coordinates matrix-dependent cues with actin dynamics like stress fibers and focal adhesions. In primary cultures of endothelial cells from HHT1 patients, endoglin deficiency appears to lead to a disorganized F-actin cytoskeleton and abnormal tube formation [42]. This is in agreement with the fragile mucocutaneous telangiectases that easily break, leading to the frequent nose and gastrointestinal bleedings present in HHT patients. An active search for novel endoglin-specific interactors has allowed the identification of multiple proteins, suggesting the involvement of endoglin in ALK1-independent pathways; nonetheless, the functional characterization and relevance of the novel interactors to the HHT1 field remains to be established [39,43]. Overall, it can be postulated that the phenotypic differences between HHT1 and HHT2 could arise, at least in part, from a subthreshold endoglin participation in these ALK1-independent signaling pathways.

3. Pathogenic Mechanisms in HHT: The Second-Hit Hypothesis

A deficient expression of the HHT genes underlies the molecular basis of disease pathogenesis. Mono-allelic loss of expression leading to haploinsufficiency of the respective HHT1 and HHT2 proteins has been shown to dysregulate TGF-β/BMP signaling in endothelial cells negatively impacting cell proliferation, migration, and recruitment during vascular remodeling and angiogenesis [20,34,44,45].

Different *Eng* or *Acvrl1* genetic mouse models of HHT have been described by several groups during the last three decades [45]. Mice lacking functional endoglin [46–48] or ALK1 [49,50] were generated by germline gene-targeting. In all cases, global embryonic loss of endoglin or ALK1 expression leads to cardiovascular defects, enlarged fragile vessels, and embryonic lethality by mid-gestation. These early models suggested that both endoglin and ALK1 were essential for cardiovascular development and homeostasis and that a further decrease in the level of these essential proteins could lead to vascular abnormalities.

The second-hit hypothesis, also known as Knudson hypothesis, was first described to explain the progression of cancer [51]. It was suggested that the first event of tumorigenesis in familiar cancers would be due to germline inactivation of one allele, followed by somatic inactivation of the second allele. Recently, using next-generation sequencing, Snellings et al. [52] have been able to demonstrate the presence of low-frequency somatic mutations in telangiectases of HHT1 and HHT2 patients, suggesting that the bi-allelic loss of *ENG* or *ACVRL1* was required for the development of vascular lesions. Overall, haploinsufficiency is widely accepted as the underlying cause of HHT1 and HHT2 pathogenicity [20,34,53], although a dominant negative effect has been described in a few *ENG* and *ACVRL1* pathogenic mutations [54–57]. Nonetheless, neither haploinsufficiency nor a dominant negative effect by itself can account for the localized generation of vascular lesions in HHT patients. It is intriguing that the vascular HHT lesions appear only at distinct sites within certain organs, rather than being present throughout the body and in all organs/tissues. This paradox has been explained, as in many other genetic diseases, by postulating the need for a second-hit.

The second-hit hypothesis has evolved over the years in order to explain how multiple factors, either environmental or genetic (modifier genes or somatic mutations), can contribute to complex diseases with phenotypic heterogeneity. In the case of HHT, external or physiological triggers such as vascular injury, inflammation, and angiogenic stimuli could account for the generation of AVMs. We will first describe the environmental factors proposed for HHT and their effects on endothelial cell functions. We will then describe how modifier genes or a somatic mutation in the normal HHT allele may synergize with a background of deficient endoglin or ALK1 expression/activity to generate vascular lesions [58] (Figure 2).

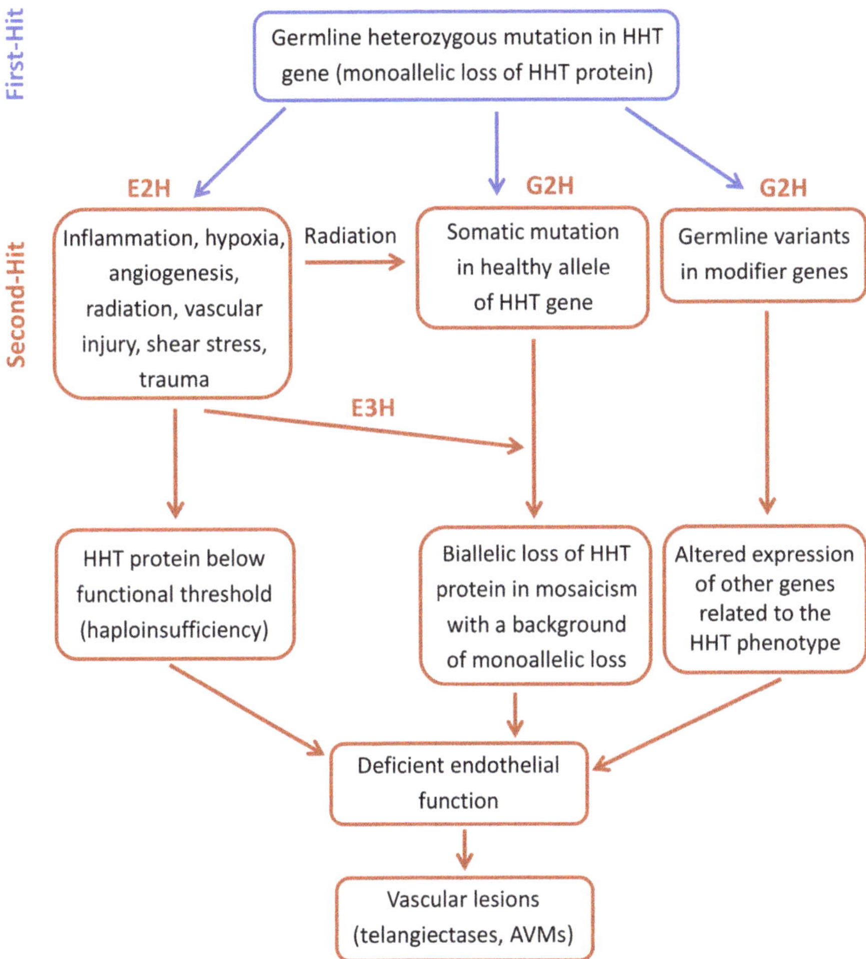

Figure 2. Hypothetical second-hit model in hereditary hemorrhagic telangiectasia (HHT). The germline heterozygous mutation in the HHT gene leads to a monoallelic loss of the encoded HHT protein in endothelial cells (First-hit). A subsequent environmental stimulus like inflammation, hypoxia, neoangiogenesis, vascular injury, radiation, shear stress, or trauma (environmental second-hit; E2H), can induce the expression/activation of mediators, which generate a microenvironment where HHT protein levels are below the needed functional threshold. This drop in the HHT functional protein can also be generated by a somatic mutation in the normal allele (genetic second-hit; G2H), leading to a focal protein loss in lesions. One possible cause of somatic mutation is sunlight radiation, especially in skin telangiectases. A somatic mutation could also synergize with an environmental third-hit (E3H). Modifier genes (G2H) could also contribute to focal vascular lesions by affecting HHT protein level and activity. In all cases, the result is an impaired endothelial cell function, leading to the generation of telangiectases or arteriovenous malformations (AVMs).

3.1. Environmental Second-Hits

The underlying pathogenic mechanisms leading to new telangiectases and AVMs in HHT are not completely understood. The variability in severity of symptoms and age of onset amongst patients, even within members of the same family, suggests that the HHT phenotype involves the contribution of environmental factors, which can be external or physiological.

3.1.1. Mechanical and Light-Induced Triggers

It is widely recognized that disease progression worsens with a patient's age [1,59]. An increased number of telangiectases in hands and lips from older patients have been observed, a finding compatible with the assumption that aged patients have been subjected to more cutaneous insults over time than younger patients. To further confirm this hypothesis, a recent study has assessed the influence of environmental triggers (mechanical or light-induced) on the number of cutaneous telangiectases in HHT patients, taking into account their dominant hand and exposure to sunlight [60]. Overall, HHT patients developed more telangiectases on their dominant hand, suggesting that mechanical stress induced by manual work may account for this increase. They also developed more telangiectases on their lower lip than on the upper lip. This preferential location could be explained by the fact that the lower lip is subjected to more physical damage than the upper lip; for example, it is in contact with the upper incisor teeth, and gravity naturally increases the chances of food touching the lower lip. In addition, HHT patients, who claimed to have had excessive sun exposure in the past, exhibited a higher number of telangiectases on both lips. While sunlight comprises a spectrum of light with varying wavelengths (ultraviolet (UV), visible, and infrared), the induction of telangiectases is likely caused predominantly by the damaging UV light with shorter wavelength (100–400 nm) [60]. Taken together, these results show that mechanical and sunlight-induced trauma strongly influence the formation of telangiectases in HHT patients, suggesting potential implications in preventive measures for HHT [60].

The effect of tissue wounding, mechanical stimulation, or radiation has been analyzed in several HHT animal models. Upon skin wounding, conditional knockout mouse models, in which both copies of *Eng* [61], *Acvrl1* [62], or *Smad4* [63] were postnatally deleted, developed vascular malformations. Also, it has been reported that defective fluid shear stress mechano-transduction mediates the formation of AVMs in HHT2 animal models [64,65]. The underlying mechanism appears to involve the BMP9/endoglin/ALK1/Smad4 pathway [66]. Thus, ALK1 expression requires blood flow [64], and fluid shear stress potentiates BMP9 activation of ALK1 signaling, which correlates with enhanced association of ALK1 and endoglin. It is noteworthy that vascular injury stimulates gene expression of endoglin and ALK1 via activation of the stress-inducible transcription factor KLF6 (Kruppel-like factor 6) [67,68], suggesting the protective functional involvement of endoglin and ALK1 under stress in healthy conditions. In fact, endoglin modulates shear-induced collateral artery growth and prevents vascular malformation by regulating flow-induced cell migration and specification [69,70]. Moreover, ALK1 is needed for BMP9 and flow responses and mediates both inhibition of endothelial proliferation and recruitment of mural cells, favoring vascular stabilization [65]. Thus, it is expected that a decreased endoglin or ALK1 expression in HHT would be detrimental for the vasculature under shear stress conditions.

Furthermore, SMAD4 is an essential effector of BMP9/ALK1 signaling that affects AVM pathogenesis via regulation of casein kinase 2 and its expression prevents flow-induced AVMs [71]. The role of endoglin in response to flow was also analyzed using zebrafish embryonic development as a model to study blood vessel expansion and contraction [72]. Interestingly, in loss of function endoglin mutants, blood vessels abnormally enlarge in response to flow and exacerbate pre-existing embryonic arterial-venous shunts, suggesting that endoglin controls blood vessel diameter in response to hemodynamic cues [73]. In addition, a subset of HHT patients present with polymicrogyria, a condition characterized by abnormal development of the brain with vascular regions experiencing low fluid shear stress during corticogenesis in utero, leading to a brain surface with many ridges or folds, called gyri. In HHT, polymicrogyria appears exclusively associated with a subset of pathogenic variants in endoglin that is involved in blood flow-related mechano-transduction [74]. Taken together, these findings suggest that the interplay between the BMP9/endoglin/ALK1 pathway and blood flow-induced mechano-transduction signals plays a critical role during development of HHT lesions [64–66,72,73].

The effect of ionizing radiation in the formation of telangiectases has also been analyzed in an HHT1 mouse model [75]. Kidneys of *Endoglin* heterozygous (*Eng*$^{+/-}$) or wild-type mice were irradiated with 16 Gy and mice were sacrificed after 20 weeks. Intriguingly, *Eng*$^{+/-}$ mice displayed reduced telangiectasia formation in the irradiated kidney compared to controls [75]. While the nature of the ionizing radiation used and the tissue irradiated were different in these studies, their results are at variance with the expected increased number of telangiectases induced by sunlight in HHT patients [60].

3.1.2. Modulators of Endothelial Function

The major HHT gene products (endoglin and ALK1) are predominantly expressed on endothelial cells which are recognized as the target cells in this disorder. Therefore, HHT-induced changes in endothelial cell function, including the monoallelic loss of expression of either HHT gene, are likely to impact vascular homeostasis and the response to external environmental hits as well as to physiological stimuli, leading to lesions such as telangiectases and AVMs.

VEGF-Dependent Angiogenic Stimuli

The Vascular Endothelial Growth Factor (VEGF) family of growth factors targets endothelial cells by preferentially binding to VEGF receptor 1 (VEGFR1), stimulating cell proliferation and migration and thereby promoting angiogenesis and vascular remodeling. The wound-induced de novo AVM formation in HHT animal models involves angiogenic processes with active extension of arterial blood vessels, meeting growing venous branches [61]. Furthermore, VEGF levels were shown to be elevated in skin telangiectases and plasma of HHT patients [76–78], leading several research teams to investigate the role of VEGF in the generation of HHT vascular lesions. The delivery of recombinant human VEGF165 (AdhVEGF) into basal ganglia led to increased micro-vessel density in both *Eng* heterozygous (*Eng*$^{+/-}$) and *Eng*$^{+/+}$ mice, as expected from the pro-angiogenic activity of VEGF. However, confocal microscopic examination revealed grossly abnormal micro-vessels in *Eng*$^{+/-}$ mouse brains that were not observed in *Eng*$^{+/+}$ mice. Abnormal micro-vessels featured enlargement, clustering, twist, or spirals [79]. Similar results were obtained using a Cre transgenic mouse line where *Eng* was deleted in smooth muscle and endothelial cells. Ectopic expression of VEGF into the brain to induce focal angiogenesis promoted the formation of AVMs [80]. These two HHT1 brain AVM models show that VEGF induces AVMs in the *Eng* heterozygous adult mouse brain, suggesting that VEGF stimulation may play a pivotal role in the initiation and development of vascular malformations in states of endoglin insufficiency present in HHT1 patients [79,80].

The triggering role of VEGF in AVM formation was also observed in *Acvrl1*-deficient mice; although, comparative studies showed that upon angiogenic stimulation with VEGF, deletion of *Eng* induces a more severe cerebrovascular dysplasia per copy than that of *Acvrl1* [62,81]. Also, a distinct pulmonary and hepatic angiogenic profile and response to anti-VEGF treatment was found between *Eng* and *Acvrl1* heterozygous mice [82]. It is noteworthy that in wound-induced skin AVMs of *Acvrl1*-deficient adult mice, VEGF neutralizing antibody can prevent AVM formation and ameliorate internal bleeding. In addition, with topical applications at different stages of AVM development, the VEGF blockade can prevent both the formation of AVMs and cease their progression [62]. These observations not only show that VEGF-dependent angiogenesis is a key event during AVM formation, but also suggest that VEGF inhibition could be an effective therapy for prevention of AVM development. In fact, Bevacizumab (Avastin), a humanized monoclonal antibody to VEGF and potent anti-angiogenic drug, has been used to treat HHT patients with severe epistaxis, GI-bleeding, or high-output cardiac failure/hepatic AVMs [83].

ALK1 Signaling and the Notch Pathway

In recent years, an increased interest has been devoted to the crosstalk between endothelial ALK1 and Notch in the development of AVMs and their possible involvement in HHT [84,85]. The Notch pathway is an intercellular signaling pathway, where both receptor and ligand are membrane-bound on adjacent cells. Signaling initiates when cell surface Notch receptors engage ligands like Delta-like 4 (Dll4) or Jagged1 (JAG1) on opposing cells, leading to the cleavage of Notch and the release of Notch Intercellular Domain (NICD) into the cytoplasm. Then, NICD translocates into the nucleus to initiate the transcription of the downstream targets HEY1 and HEY2, transcriptional repressors involved in VEGF-dependent signaling and arterial cell fate, among others [85,86]. Previous studies had shown that arteriovenous shunts occur in mouse and zebrafish mutants for components of the Notch signaling pathway [87,88], a finding that prompted the investigation of a role for the Notch pathway in AVM pathogenesis of HHT [84]. In *Acvrl1* knockout mouse models of HHT2, AVMs show decreased Notch signaling with loss of ALK1 causing expansion of the shunt through endothelial cell proliferation. Also, by cooperating with the Notch pathway, expression of ALK1 inhibits angiogenesis, and blocking ALK1 signaling during postnatal development in mice leads to retinal hypervascularization and the appearance of AVMs. Furthermore, combined blockade of ALK1 and Notch signaling exacerbates hypervascularization, whereas activation of ALK1 by its high-affinity ligand BMP9 rescues hyper-sprouting induced by Notch inhibition. The molecular basis of this regulation appears to involve ALK1-dependent Smad signaling in synergy with activated Notch in stalk endothelial cells to induce expression of the Notch targets HEY1 and HEY2, which, in turn, repress VEGF signaling, tip endothelial cell formation, and endothelial sprouting [84]. These results demonstrate a direct link between ALK1 and Notch signaling routes during vascular morphogenesis that may be relevant to the pathogenesis of HHT [85]. It can be postulated that dysregulation of ALK1 signaling, achieved upon ALK1 or endoglin haploinsufficiency, may act as a second-hit, impairing the ALK1/Notch collaboration and leading to the formation of the vascular lesions in HHT.

Proliferation and Apoptosis Stimuli

Endoglin is markedly upregulated in the proliferating endothelium of tissues undergoing angiogenesis. This is in agreement with the fact that the endoglin/ALK1 pathway promotes endothelial cell proliferation and opposes TGF-β1/ALK5-dependent responses, including inhibition of cellular proliferation [58,89]. Furthermore, neutralizing anti-endoglin antibodies or silencing endoglin enhances the inhibitory effect of TGF-β on proliferation and migration, whereas ectopic endoglin expression counteracts the anti-proliferative effect of TGF-β1 in endothelial cells [90,91]. Moreover, inhibition of endoglin expression on endothelial cells increases the anti-proliferative effect of TGF-β1 and enhances endothelial cell apoptosis induced by hypoxia and TGF-β1 [90,92]. It is worth noting that apoptosis can be induced by chemotherapeutic drugs or UV irradiation [93], with UV light being one of the potential second-hits described in HHT patients [60]. These results demonstrate that the endoglin/ALK1 pathway not only promotes proliferation, but also counteracts the hypoxia/TGF-β-induced apoptosis of endothelial cells. This role in endothelial cell survival suggests that in the presence of anti-proliferative and/or pro-apoptotic stimuli, decreased activity of the endoglin/ALK1/Smad4 route, as occurs in HHT patients, may lead to reduced cell proliferation and/or apoptosis in capillaries, leading to the vascular lesion. Conversely, the endothelial proliferation associated with triggers of angiogenesis, such as vascular injury, ischemia, or trauma, may synergize with the loss of expression of HHT genes as their products may not reach the necessary threshold to cope with the vascular remodeling required [58]. It should be noted that BMP9 and ALK1 have been described both as pro- and anti-angiogenic factors depending on the cellular context [84,89,94,95]. In this regard, BMP signaling strongly induces expression of the helix-loop-helix transcription factor Id1, which promotes endothelial proliferation and migration [96]; but, paradoxically, BMP9 has been reported to inhibit VEGF- and fibroblast growth factor (FGF)-induced proliferation [27,97] and has been described as a vascular quiescence factor.

Inflammation and Endothelial Cell Adhesion and Nitric Oxide Regulation

Inflammation is a complex biological response to harmful stimuli, such as pathogens, tissue damage, or irritants, involving blood vessels, immune cells, and molecular mediators. The inflammatory context is associated with an upregulated expression of endothelial endoglin, and with an inflammatory cell infiltrate [58,98]. It is noteworthy that HHT skin telangiectases and internal AVMs show a perivascular mononuclear cell infiltrate, including lymphocytes and monocytes/macrophages [99,100], suggesting that both endoglin function and leukocyte infiltration are involved in the vascular repair/remodeling process whose dysregulation may lead to AVM formation in HHT. Indeed, it has been reported that endoglin plays a crucial role in leukocyte-mediated vascular repair in HHT [101], in agreement with the pro-active role of leukocyte infiltration during angiogenesis and vascular remodeling [102]. Several in vivo and in vitro models of inflammation and vascular repair have shown that *Endoglin* heterozygosity leads to an abnormal leukocyte infiltration and function [82,101,103–107]. In a mouse model of dextran sodium sulfate (DSS)-induced chronic colitis, increased leukocyte infiltration of the gut and more severe colitis was observed in $Eng^{+/-}$ relative to control mice [82,103,105]. Also, upon myocardial infarction, a greater deterioration in cardiac function was observed in $Eng^{+/-}$ compared to control mice, although host inflammatory leukocyte numbers in the infarct area were similar; however, defects in vessel formation and heart function in $Eng^{+/-}$ mice were rescued by injection of leukocytes from healthy human donors, but not by leukocytes from HHT1 patients [101]. Using a distal middle cerebral artery occlusion model, $Eng^{+/-}$ mice showed larger infarct/atrophic volumes associated with fewer infiltrating macrophages, suggesting that endoglin deficiency impairs brain injury recovery by inhibiting macrophage homing, delaying inflammation resolution, and reducing angiogenesis [106]. In addition, decreased inflammation-induced leukocyte trafficking to the peritoneum and lungs was found in $Eng^{+/-}$ mice treated with the inflammatory stimuli carrageenan or lipopolysaccharide (LPS), respectively [104].

The underlying molecular mechanism by which endothelial endoglin is involved can be explained at least in part by its capacity to act as a counter-receptor of leukocyte integrins [104,108,109], thus regulating not only endothelium-leukocyte adhesion, but also leukocyte extravasation [104,110]. These processes appear to be mediated by pro-inflammatory molecules such as the chemokine CXCL12, an integrin activator, which strongly promotes leukocyte adhesion to endothelial endoglin or to purified endoglin. Moreover, both endoglin-dependent cellular adhesion and transmigration processes involve the leukocyte integrin $\alpha_5\beta_1$ via the endoglin arginine-glycine-aspartic acid (RGD) motif [104]. Based on these results, it can be postulated that the function of endothelial endoglin as an adhesion counter-receptor for leukocyte integrins is involved in HHT1 pathogenesis. According to this hypothetical model, in healthy subjects, the capillary network subjected to an inflammatory stimulus is infiltrated with leukocytes that contribute to the vascular repair/remodeling. By contrast, in HHT1 patients, deficient endoglin expression impairs leukocyte infiltration, leading to defective vascular repair/remodeling. As a consequence, the capillary network would disappear and only a preferential channel would remain to eventually become the arterio-venous shunt [110]. While these results may explain the role of endothelial endoglin in leukocyte adhesion within the HHT1 context, the putative cell adhesion-related function of the other HHT gene products, especially ALK1, remains to be explored. Because the kinase ALK1 can interact and target the endoglin cytoplasmic domain for serine and threonine phosphorylation, it can be speculated that this phosphorylation may activate or enhance the binding of endoglin to integrins by inside-out signaling [111,112]. Interestingly, the expression of integrin β_8 subunit, whose complex with the integrin alpha V binds ligands via the RGD motif, is reduced in sporadic human brain AVMs. In addition, focal deletion of integrin β_8, combined with an angiogenic VEGF stimulus, enhances vascular dysplasia and hemorrhage in the brain of adult *Acvrl1* heterozygous mice [113]. Further studies are needed to assess the involvement of ALK1 in integrin-dependent cell adhesion.

Inflammation and oxidative stress induced by reactive oxygen species (ROS) are closely related pathophysiological processes in cardiovascular disease [114]. Tissue injuries and infections activate the immune response by infiltrating circulating mononuclear cells into tissues where they can release ROS, in turn stimulating inflammation. ROS are reactive derivatives of O_2 metabolism that reduce levels of the vasodilator nitric oxide (NO). In endothelial cells, the major enzymatic sources of ROS are respiratory enzymes of the mitochondria, nicotinamide adenine dinucleotide phosphate (NADPH) oxidases, and uncoupled endothelial nitric oxide synthase (eNOS). Several lines of evidence support the involvement of endoglin and AlK1 in the regulation of eNOS-derived ROS. Endoglin positively regulates the expression and function of eNOS [39,115,116] and forms a complex with eNOS in caveolae, providing a stabilizing function for eNOS. Upon Ca^{2+}-induced activation, $Eng^{+/-}$ endothelial cells show reduced eNOS/Hsp90 association, produce less NO, and generate more eNOS-derived superoxide ($O_2{}^{2-}$), indicating that endoglin is an important regulator in the coupling of eNOS activity. Resistance arteries from $Eng^{+/-}$ mice display an eNOS-dependent enhancement in endothelium-dependent dilatation and impairment in the myogenic response, and treatment with an $O_2{}^-$ scavenger reverses these vasomotor abnormalities [116]. Both endoglin and ALK1 haploinsufficiency lead to eNOS-derived ROS, oxidative stress, and endothelial dysfunction, with potential pathogenic consequences in HHT [117,118]. Relatedly, to reduce telangiectasia-derived bleeding in HHT patients, therapeutic interventions with the antioxidant, N-acetyl cysteine, aiming to decrease ROS bioavailability, have yielded promising results [119,120].

3.2. Genetic Second-Hits

3.2.1. Germline Modifier Variants/Genes

Modifier genes are those in which a genetic variation modifies the effects of mutation at a major gene locus and in so doing, affect disease severity. That modifier genes affected the phenotype in HHT was initially suggested by the study of heterozygous *Eng* and *Acvrl1* mice. The first animal model of HHT was generated in *Eng* heterozygous ($Eng^{+/-}$) mice of the 129/Ola inbred strain that were subsequently backcrossed onto the C57BL/6 strain [46]. Early observations of these *Eng* heterozygous mice revealed that disease manifestations were associated with the 129/Ola background, suggesting that other gene(s) contributed to the generation of vascular lesions. Analysis of a large number of mice over a period of one-year established disease prevalence at 72% in 129/Ola, intermediate in backcrosses (36%), and low in C57BL/6 (7%) [121]. Multiple signs of HHT were detected, such as ear telangiectasia, hemorrhage, dilated vessels, liver and lung congestion, brain and heart ischemia, and even cerebral AVMs [121,122]. Disease sequelae included stroke, fatal hemorrhage, and congestive heart failure. Interestingly, 129/Ola inbred mice had previously been shown to carry significant alterations in liver and lung vasculature, such as portal shunting and reduction/truncation of peripheral vessels, when compared to C57BL/6 mice [123,124]. These vascular features might have contributed to the more severe HHT manifestations observed in the $Eng^{+/-}$ 129/Ola mice. These results strongly suggested that the genetic background via alterations of pathways critical to vascular function in the context of reduced endoglin (and/or ALK1) expression can modify the outcome of disease [44].

Similar to the HHT1 animal model, *Acvrl1* heterozygous mice have dilated vessels and HHT-like vascular lesions in liver, nailbed, intestine, or skin that develop between 7 and 20 months [125]. However, these lesions occur with partial penetrance (approximately 40%). Both $Eng^{+/-}$ and $Acvrl1^{+/-}$ adult mice present normal blood vessels, suggesting there are no major vascular defects during developmental angiogenesis [45]. This finding agrees with the observation that the majority of the vasculature in HHT patients functions normally while vascular lesions are localized and sporadic. In addition, animal models with systemic or endothelial-specific deletion of *Eng*, *Acvrl1*, or *Smad4* in adulthood lead to vascular malformations compatible with an HHT phenotype [45,61,63,80,126–128].

The search for human modifier genes of HHT was initiated by looking for genetic regions syntenic to the mouse modifier loci, *Tgfbm's*, that modify the lethal vascular phenotype of $Tgfb1^{-/-}$ mice [129]. The rationale was that endoglin is a co-receptor for TGF-β1 and that *Eng* null mice have an embryonic lethal phenotype similar to that of the *Tgfb1* null mice. This study led to the identification of human polymorphic variants of the protein, non-receptor tyrosine phosphatase 14 (PTPN14), in the *Tgfbm2* region, showing genetic association with the presence of PAVMs in HHT1 and HHT2 patients in two independent populations. PTPN14 was shown to modulate angiogenesis in endothelial cell culture and to alter the expression of EphrinB2, important in arteriovenous specification [129].

It was subsequently shown that genetic variation within the functional *ENG* allele inherited from the non-affected parent was associated with the presence of pulmonary AVMs in HHT1 patients [130]. Expression of the pulmonary AVM at-risk *ENG* variant, *rs10987746*-C, correlated with *ENG* mRNA levels in a panel of lymphoblastoid cell lines. Furthermore, expression quantitative trait loci (eQTL) analysis showed association between the *rs10987746*-C variant and higher expression of *PTPN14* in a panel of angiogenically active lung adenocarcinoma samples, but not in normal lungs. Quantitative TaqMan® expression analysis in a panel of normal lung tissues from genetically heterogeneous interspecific backcross mice, demonstrated a strong correlation between expression levels of *Eng*, *Acvrl1*, and *Ptpn14*, further suggesting a related role for these genes in lung biology [130]. *PTPN14* has also been shown to be a negative regulator of Yap/Taz signaling, implicated in mechano-transduction, suggesting a potential link between endoglin/ALK1 signaling and shear stress [130].

Variants of ADAM17, which maps within the *Tgfbm3* region, have also been shown to associate with the presence of PAVMs in HHT1 but not HHT2 [131]. ADAM17 is known to downregulate Smad2 signaling by shedding the extracellular domain of TGF-β receptor I (ALK5), and therefore would not affect an ALK1-dependent pathway.

Common polymorphisms in HHT genes other than the disease-causing mutation can be associated with differences in HHT phenotype severity, and specifically, the presence of AVMs. For example, the *ACVRL1 c.314-35A>G* common variant was shown to be associated with sporadic brain AVMs [132,133], and also subsequently with PAVMs as well as vascular malformations overall in patients with *ENG* mutations, but not in patients with *ACVRL1* mutations [134].

Furthermore, a recent analysis found the number of deleterious variants in angiogenesis-related genes to be significantly higher in HHT patients versus healthy individuals. A comparison of the frequencies of variants in these angiogenesis-related genes in a 100-exome dataset from HHT samples with those from publicly available population frequency datasets suggests that the combination of several modifying variants contribute to the phenotypic heterogeneity of HHT (Bayrak-Toydemir et al., unpublished data). Another study analyzed 11 candidate variants of *Tgfbm* loci in 752 HHT patients and could not find any association with the presence of PAVMs. They also did not find significant associations between variants reported in sporadic AVMs and vascular malformations in HHT [135]. Further investigations are needed to elucidate the role of modifier genes in the phenotypic heterogeneity of HHT. It is likely that such a complex disorder is influenced by genetic modifiers, as has been observed in other diseases such as cystic fibrosis [136,137].

3.2.2. Somatic Mutations in the Second Allele of the HHT Genes

The original second-hit hypothesis refers to a familial form of cancer caused by the germline inactivation of one allele, followed by the somatic inactivation of the second allele [51]. In the context of a germline mutation, random somatic mutations are much more likely to lead to biallelic loss, explaining the multiple tumors that characterize familial cancers. The second-hit mechanism is accepted for tumors and has also been reported for vascular malformations. The first vascular malformation syndrome in which a somatic second-hit was described is the cerebral cavernous malformation (CCM) [138]. Familial CCM samples carry a somatic second mutation in one of the *CCM* genes [139]. Mouse models also support this mechanism, as the loss of both alleles of a *CCM* gene is required for CCM lesions [140]. In the last several years, there have been multiple publications demonstrating the somatic second-hit as part of the disease mechanism to explain the development of multifocal vascular lesions. These include somatic mutations in *RASA1* in lesions from patients with capillary malformation-arteriovenous malformation (CM-AVM) and *TIE2 (TEK)* somatic mutations in lesions from patients with venous malformations as predominant examples [141–143].

The ability to detect somatic mutations in very low frequency has been aided by the advent of next-generation sequencing (NGS). Using NGS, Snellings et al. [52] have been able to demonstrate the presence of low-frequency somatic mutations in telangiectases of HHT1 and HHT2 patients, suggesting that the bi-allelic loss of *ENG* or *ACVRL1* was required for the development of vascular lesions. Somatic mutations in either *ENG* or *ACVRL1* could be identified in skin telangiectasia tissue from a small number of patients with HHT [52]. They studied 3 mm skin biopsies from telangiectases obtained from one patient with an *ENG* germline mutation and 4 patients with different *ACVRL1* mutations. Somatic mutations were only identified in 47% of samples (9 of 19 samplings from 5 patients) from 4 of 5 patients studied. These second mutations were different from the patient's germline mutation and were located on the other allele. Dermal telangiectasia tissues showed loss of function mutations with complete loss of the protein function. These second mutations were also different on distinct telangiectasia biopsies of the same individual. Somatic second-hit mutation frequency in the tissue was up to 2.3% on all of these samples. Possible explanations for this low frequency include telangiectases being highly mosaic for the somatic mutation, a high percentage of normal tissue present in the biopsy, or variable cellular composition in distinct biopsies where the genetic second-hit is restricted to a cell type of low abundance within the lesions. The observation that somatic mutations were not seen in every biopsy sample tested may suggest that not all telangiectases carry a somatic mutation and that an environmental tertiary-hit might still be required for a vascular lesion to occur. Of note, the telangiectases used for this study were of the skin, a tissue which undergoes a lifetime of exposure to sunlight radiation, a known mutagen that could generate some of the HHT somatic mutations (Figure 2). Overall, these preliminary observations need to be extended and confirmed in additional genes such as *SMAD4*, and in additional tissues, including visceral AVMs.

The pathogenic mechanism by which the biallelic loss, triggered by a somatic mutation, leads to the HHT phenotype has been experimentally addressed in some knockout animal models. By itself, the loss of function of both alleles does not appear to be sufficient to develop the vascular lesions. Interestingly, in adult knockout mouse models for the three major HHT genes (*Eng*, *Acvrl1*, and *Smad4*), the HHT phenotype appears to develop upon local injury or an angiogenic stimulus, such as VEGF [61–63,144]. In addition, the appearance of vascular lesions in embryos and adult *Eng* and *Acvrl1* knockout mice in the absence of external stimuli suggests that internal physiological cues such as angiogenesis or shear stress may also contribute to their HHT phenotype [126,127]. Accordingly, it can be postulated that compared to a monoallelic loss (heterozygous background), the localized biallelic loss generated by a somatic mutation may give rise to a faster and more severe HHT phenotype in the presence of an environmental or physiological additional hit.

4. Conclusions

The two-hit hypothesis has been widely accepted for many years as a plausible explanation for the phenotypic variability found in HHT. Here, we have reviewed some of the reported environmental and genetic second-hits (Figure 2). Thus, germline heterozygous mutations in HHT genes (first-hit) result in a monoallelic protein loss in endothelial cells. A subsequent environmental stimulus (second-hit) like inflammation, hypoxia, neoangiogenesis, vascular injury, shear stress, radiation, or trauma, can induce the expression/activation of mediators, which generate a microenvironment where HHT protein levels are below the needed functional threshold. Furthermore, the existence of a genetic second-hit (somatic mutation in the normal HHT allele), combined with an environmental trigger (tertiary-hit), and/or the presence of modifier variants, can set a much lower threshold for disease development. In all cases, the consequence is an impaired endothelial cell function that leads to the generation of telangiectases and AVMs. Overall, the current clinical data, as well as in vivo and in vitro experimental results, support the second-hit hypothesis to explain why certain individuals with HHT genotypes develop earlier and/or more severe clinical phenotypes than other family members. Also, the organ-specific location of telangiectases and AVMs in HHT, and the differing age of presentation for lesions at each site, suggest that the required second-hits may be tissue-specific. However, major gaps in our knowledge remain, particularly in delineating the exact role of the different second-hits that lead to the development of clinically relevant symptoms in HHT, and how this information can be applied in the clinical practice. Further studies to better understand the pathological mechanisms of HHT, including identification of novel potential second-hits, are needed, as well as the translation of this knowledge into preventive clinical measures and treatments.

Author Contributions: Conceptualization, C.B. and M.L.; formal analysis, C.B., P.B.-T., J.M. and M.L.; resources, C.B.; writing—original draft preparation, C.B.; writing—review and editing, C.B., P.B.-T., J.M., and M.L.; visualization, C.B., P.B.-T., J.M. and M.L.; supervision, C.B., P.B.-T., J.M. and M.L.; project administration, C.B.; funding acquisition, C.B. All authors have read and agreed to the published version of the manuscript.

Funding: This research was funded by Consejo Superior de Investigaciones Científicas of Spain (CSIC; grant 201920E022 to C.B.).

Acknowledgments: CIBERER is an initiative of the Instituto de Salud Carlos III (ISCIII) of Spain supported by European Regional Development (FEDER) funds. We acknowledge support of the publication fee by the CSIC Open Access Publication Support Initiative through its Unit of Information Resources for Research (URICI).

Conflicts of Interest: The authors declare no conflict of interest.

References

1. Plauchu, H.; de Chadarevian, J.P.; Bideau, A.; Robert, J.M. Age-related clinical profile of hereditary hemorrhagic telangiectasia in an epidemiologically recruited population. *Am. J. Med. Genet.* **1989**, *32*, 291–297. [CrossRef] [PubMed]
2. Faughnan, M.E.; Palda, V.A.; Garcia-Tsao, G.; Geisthoff, U.W.; McDonald, J.; Proctor, D.D.; Spears, J.; Brown, D.H.; Buscarini, E.; Chesnutt, M.S.; et al. International guidelines for the diagnosis and management of hereditary haemorrhagic telangiectasia. *J. Med. Genet.* **2011**, *48*, 73–87. [CrossRef] [PubMed]
3. Faughnan, M.E.; Mager, J.J.; Hetts, S.W.; Palda, V.A.; Lang-Robertson, K.; Buscarini, E.; Deslandres, E.; Kasthuri, R.S.; Lausman, A.; Poetker, D.; et al. Second International Guidelines for the Diagnosis and Management of Hereditary Hemorrhagic Telangiectasia. *Ann. Intern. Med.* **2020**. Online ahead of print. [CrossRef] [PubMed]
4. Cottin, V.; Chinet, T.; Lavolé, A.; Corre, R.; Marchand, E.; Reynaud-Gaubert, M.; Plauchu, H.; Cordier, J.F.; Groupe d'Etudes et de Recherche sur les Maladies "Orphelines" Pulmonaires (GERM"O"P). Pulmonary arteriovenous malformations in hereditary hemorrhagic telangiectasia: A series of 126 patients. *Medicine* **2007**, *86*, 1–17. [CrossRef]
5. Dupuis-Girod, S.; Cottin, V.; Shovlin, C.L. The Lung in Hereditary Hemorrhagic Telangiectasia. *Respiration* **2017**, *94*, 315–330. [CrossRef]
6. Majumdar, S.; McWilliams, J.P. Approach to Pulmonary Arteriovenous Malformations: A Comprehensive Update. *J. Clin. Med.* **2020**, *9*, 1927. [CrossRef]
7. Ianora, A.A.; Memeo, M.; Sabba, C.; Cirulli, A.; Rotondo, A.; Angelelli, G. Hereditary hemorrhagic telangiectasia: Multi-detector row helical CT assessment of hepatic involvement. *Radiology* **2004**, *230*, 250–259. [CrossRef]
8. Memeo, M.; Stabile Ianora, A.A.; Scardapane, A.; Suppressa, P.; Cirulli, A.; Sabbà, C.; Rotondo, A.; Angelelli, G. Hereditary haemorrhagic telangiectasia: Study of hepatic vascular alterations with multi-detector row helical CT and reconstruction programs. *Radiol. Med.* **2005**, *109*, 125–138. [PubMed]
9. Buscarini, E.; Danesino, C.; Olivieri, C.; Lupinacci, G.; De Grazia, F.; Reduzzi, L.; Blotta, P.; Gazzaniga, P.; Pagella, F.; Grosso, M.; et al. Doppler ultrasonographic grading of hepatic vascular malformations in hereditary hemorrhagic telangiectasia—Results of extensive screening. *Ultraschall Med.* **2004**, *25*, 348–355. [CrossRef] [PubMed]
10. Garcia-Tsao, G.; Korzenik, J.R.; Young, L.; Henderson, K.J.; Jain, D.; Byrd, B.; Pollak, J.S.; White, R.I., Jr. Liver disease in patients with hereditary hemorrhagic telangiectasia. *N. Engl. J. Med.* **2000**, *343*, 931–936. [CrossRef]
11. Kim, H.; Nelson, J.; Krings, T.; terBrugge, K.G.; McCulloch, C.E.; Lawton, M.T.; Young, W.L.; Faughnan, M.E.; Brain Vascular Malformation Consortium HHT Investigator Group. Hemorrhage rates from brain arteriovenous malformation in patients with hereditary hemorrhagic telangiectasia. *Stroke* **2015**, *46*, 1362–1364. [CrossRef] [PubMed]

12. Brinjikji, W.; Iyer, V.N.; Yamaki, V.; Lanzino, G.; Cloft, H.J.; Thielen, K.R.; Swanson, K.L.; Wood, C.P. Neurovascular Manifestations of Hereditary Hemorrhagic Telangiectasia: A Consecutive Series of 376 Patients during 15 Years. *AJNR Am. J. Neuroradiol.* **2016**, *37*, 1479–1486. [CrossRef]

13. Shovlin, C.L.; Guttmacher, A.E.; Buscarini, E.; Faughnan, M.E.; Hyland, R.H.; Westermann, C.J.; Kjeldsen, A.D.; Plauchu, H. Diagnostic criteria for hereditary hemorrhagic telangiectasia (Rendu-Osler-Weber syndrome). *Am. J. Med. Genet.* **2000**, *91*, 66–67. [CrossRef]

14. McAllister, K.A.; Grogg, K.M.; Johnson, D.W.; Gallione, C.J.; Baldwin, M.A.; Jackson, C.E.; Helmbold, E.A.; Markel, D.S.; McKinnon, W.C.; Murrel, J.; et al. Endoglin, a TGF-β binding protein of endothelial cells, is the gene for hereditary haemorrhagic telangiectasia type 1. *Nat. Genet.* **1994**, *8*, 345–351. [CrossRef] [PubMed]

15. Johnson, D.W.; Berg, J.N.; Baldwin, M.A.; Gallione, C.J.; Marondel, I.; Yoon, S.J.; Stenzel, T.T.; Speer, M.; Pericak-Vance, M.A.; Diamond, A.; et al. Mutations in the activin receptor-like kinase 1 gene in hereditary haemorrhagic telangiectasia type. *Nat. Genet.* **1996**, *13*, 189–195. [CrossRef] [PubMed]

16. Gallione, C.J.; Repetto, G.M.; Legius, E.; Rustgi, A.K.; Schelley, S.L.; Tejpar, S.; Mitchell, G.; Drouin, E.; Westermann, C.J.; Marchuk, D.A. A combined syndrome of juvenile polyposis and hereditary haemorrhagic telangiectasia associated with mutations in MADH4 (SMAD4). *Lancet* **2004**, *363*, 852–859. [CrossRef]

17. Wooderchak-Donahue, W.L.; McDonald, J.; O'Fallon, B.; Upton, P.D.; Li, W.; Roman, B.L.; Young, S.; Plant, P.; Fülöp, G.T.; Langa, C.; et al. BMP9 mutations cause a vascular-anomaly syndrome with phenotypic overlap with hereditary hemorrhagic telangiectasia. *Am. J. Hum. Genet.* **2013**, *93*, 530–537. [CrossRef]

18. Cole, S.G.; Begbie, M.E.; Wallace, G.M.; Shovlin, C.L. A new locus for hereditary haemorrhagic telangiectasia (HHT3) maps to chromosome 5. *J. Med. Genet.* **2005**, *42*, 577–582. [CrossRef]

19. Bayrak-Toydemir, P.; McDonald, J.; Akarsu, N.; Toydemir, R.M.; Calderon, F.; Tuncali, T.; Tang, W.; Miller, F.; Mao, R. A fourth locus for hereditary hemorrhagic telangiectasia maps to chromosome 7. *Am. J. Med. Genet. A* **2006**, *140*, 2155–2162. [CrossRef]

20. Abdalla, S.A.; Letarte, M. Hereditary haemorrhagic telangiectasia: Current views on genetics and mechanisms of disease. *J. Med. Genet.* **2006**, *43*, 97–110. [CrossRef]

21. McDonald, J.; Bayrak-Toydemir, P.; DeMille, D.; Wooderchak-Donahue, W.; Whitehead, K. Curaçao diagnostic criteria for hereditary hemorrhagic telangiectasia is highly predictive of a pathogenic variant in ENG or ACVRL1 (HHT1 and HHT2). *Genet. Med.* **2020**, *22*, 1201–1205. [CrossRef]

22. Bossler, A.D.; Richards, J.; George, C.; Godmilow, L.; Ganguly, A. Novel mutations in ENG and ACVRL1 identified in a series of 200 individuals undergoing clinical genetic testing for hereditary hemorrhagic telangiectasia (HHT): Correlation of genotype with phenotype. *Hum. Mutat.* **2006**, *27*, 667–675. [CrossRef]

23. Bayrak-Toydemir, P.; McDonald, J.; Markewitz, B.; Lewin, S.; Miller, F.; Chou, L.S.; Gedge, F.; Tang, W.; Coon, H.; Mao, R. Genotype-phenotype correlation in hereditary hemorrhagic telangiectasia: Mutations and manifestations. *Am. J. Med. Genet. A* **2006**, *140*, 463–470. [CrossRef]

24. Jelsig, A.M.; Tørring, P.M.; Kjeldsen, A.D.; Qvist, N.; Bojesen, A.; Jensen, U.B.; Andersen, M.K.; Gerdes, A.M.; Brusgaard, K.; Ousager, L.B. JP-HHT phenotype in Danish patients with SMAD4 mutations. *Clin. Genet.* **2016**, *90*, 55–62. [CrossRef]

25. McDonald, N.M.; Ramos, G.P.; Sweetser, S. SMAD4 mutation and the combined juvenile polyposis and hereditary hemorrhage telangiectasia syndrome: A single center experience. *Int. J. Colorectal Dis.* **2020**, *35*, 1963–1965. [CrossRef]

26. Gedge, F.; McDonald, J.; Phansalkar, A.; Chou, L.S.; Calderon, F.; Mao, R.; Lyon, E.; Bayrak-Toydemir, P. Clinical and analytical sensitivities in hereditary hemorrhagic telangiectasia testing and a report of de novo mutations. *J. Mol. Diagn.* **2007**, *9*, 258–265. [CrossRef]

27. Scharpfenecker, M.; van Dinther, M.; Liu, Z.; van Bezooijen, R.L.; Zhao, Q.; Pukac, L.; Löwik, C.W.; ten Dijke, P. BMP-9 signals via ALK1 and inhibits bFGF-induced endothelial cell proliferation and VEGF-stimulated angiogenesis. *J. Cell Sci.* **2007**, *120*, 964–972. [CrossRef]

28. Castonguay, R.; Werner, E.D.; Matthews, R.G.; Presman, E.; Mulivor, A.W.; Solban, N.; Sako, D.; Pearsall, R.S.; Underwood, K.W.; Seehra, J.; et al. Soluble endoglin specifically binds bone morphogenetic proteins 9 and 10 via its orphan domain, inhibits blood vessel formation, and suppresses tumor growth. *J. Biol. Chem.* **2011**, *286*, 30034–30046. [CrossRef]

29. Alt, A.; Miguel-Romero, L.; Donderis, J.; Aristorena, M.; Blanco, F.J.; Round, A.; Rubio, V.; Bernabeu, C.; Marina, A. Structural and functional insights into endoglin ligand recognition and binding. *PLoS ONE* **2012**, *7*, e29948. [CrossRef] [PubMed]

30. Tillet, E.; Bailly, S. Emerging roles of BMP9 and BMP10 in hereditary hemorrhagic telangiectasia. *Front. Genet.* **2015**, *5*, 456. [CrossRef] [PubMed]

31. Tillet, E.; Ouarné, M.; Desroches-Castan, A.; Mallet, C.; Subileau, M.; Didier, R.; Lioutsko, A.; Belthier, G.; Feige, J.J.; Bailly, S. A heterodimer formed by bone morphogenetic protein 9 (BMP9) and BMP10 provides most BMP biological activity in plasma. *J. Biol. Chem.* **2018**, *293*, 10963–10974. [CrossRef]

32. Santibañez, J.F.; Quintanilla, M.; Bernabeu, C. TGF-β/TGF-β receptor system and its role in physiological and pathological conditions. *Clin. Sci.* **2011**, *121*, 233–251. [CrossRef] [PubMed]

33. Roman, B.L.; Hinck, A.P. ALK1 signaling in development and disease: New paradigms. *Cell. Mol. Life Sci.* **2017**, *74*, 4539–4560. [CrossRef] [PubMed]

34. Ruiz-Llorente, L.; Gallardo-Vara, E.; Rossi, E.; Smadja, D.M.; Botella, L.M.; Bernabeu, C. Endoglin and alk1 as therapeutic targets for hereditary hemorrhagic telangiectasia. *Expert. Opin. Ther. Targets* **2017**, *21*, 933–947. [CrossRef]

35. Wood, J.H.; Guo, J.; Morrell, N.W.; Li, W. Advances in the molecular regulation of endothelial BMP9 signalling complexes and implications for cardiovascular disease. *Biochem. Soc. Trans.* **2019**, *47*, 779–791. [CrossRef]

36. Barbara, N.P.; Wrana, J.L.; Letarte, M. Endoglin is an accessory protein that interacts with the signaling receptor complex of multiple members of the transforming growth factor-beta superfamily. *J. Biol. Chem.* **1999**, *274*, 584–594. [CrossRef] [PubMed]

37. Guerrero-Esteo, M.; Sanchez-Elsner, T.; Letamendia, A.; Bernabeu, C. Extracellular and cytoplasmic domains of endoglin interact with the transforming growth factor-beta receptors I and II. *J. Biol. Chem.* **2002**, *277*, 29197–29209. [CrossRef]

38. Bernabeu, C.; Conley, B.A.; Vary, C.P. Novel biochemical pathways of endoglin in vascular cell physiology. *J. Cell Biochem.* **2007**, *102*, 1375–1388. [CrossRef]

39. Xu, G.; Barrios-Rodiles, M.; Jerkic, M.; Turinsky, A.L.; Nadon, R.; Vera, S.; Voulgaraki, D.; Wrana, J.L.; Toporsian, M.; Letarte, M. Novel protein interactions with endoglin and activin receptor-like kinase 1: Potential role in vascular networks. *Mol. Cell. Proteom.* **2014**, *13*, 489–502. [CrossRef]

40. Conley, B.A.; Koleva, R.; Smith, J.D.; Kacer, D.; Zhang, D.; Bernabéu, C.; Vary, C.P. Endoglin controls cell migration and composition of focal adhesions: Function of the cytosolic domain. *J. Biol. Chem.* **2004**, *279*, 27440–27449. [CrossRef]

41. Sanz-Rodriguez, F.; Guerrero-Esteo, M.; Botella, L.M.; Banville, D.; Vary, C.P.; Bernabéu, C. Endoglin regulates cytoskeletal organization through binding to ZRP-1, a member of the Lim family of proteins. *J. Biol. Chem.* **2004**, *279*, 32858–32868. [CrossRef]

42. Fernandez-L, A.; Sanz-Rodriguez, F.; Zarrabeitia, R.; Pérez-Molino, A.; Hebbel, R.P.; Nguyen, J.; Bernabéu, C.; Botella, L.M. Blood outgrowth endothelial cells from Hereditary Haemorrhagic Telangiectasia patients reveal abnormalities compatible with vascular lesions. *Cardiovasc. Res.* **2005**, *68*, 235–248. [CrossRef]

43. Gallardo-Vara, E.; Ruiz-Llorente, L.; Casado-Vela, J.; Ruiz-Rodríguez, M.J.; López-Andrés, N.; Pattnaik, A.K.; Quintanilla, M.; Bernabeu, C. Endoglin Protein Interactome Profiling Identifies TRIM21 and Galectin-3 as New Binding Partners. *Cells* **2019**, *8*, 1082. [CrossRef]

44. Bourdeau, A.; Faughnan, M.E.; Letarte, M. Endoglin-deficient mice, a unique model to study hereditary hemorrhagic telangiectasia. *Trends Cardiovasc. Med.* **2000**, *10*, 279–285. [CrossRef]

45. Tual-Chalot, S.; Oh, S.P.; Arthur, H.M. Mouse models of hereditary hemorrhagic telangiectasia: Recent advances and future challenges. *Front. Genet.* **2015**, *6*, 25. [CrossRef] [PubMed]

46. Bourdeau, A.; Dumont, D.J.; Letarte, M. A murine model of hereditary hemorrhagic telangiectasia. *J. Clin. Investig.* **1999**, *104*, 1343–1351. [CrossRef]

47. Li, D.Y.; Sorensen, L.K.; Brooke, B.S.; Urness, L.D.; Davis, E.C.; Taylor, D.G.; Boak, B.B.; Wendel, D.P. Defective angiogenesis in mice lacking endoglin. *Science* **1999**, *284*, 1534–1537. [CrossRef] [PubMed]

48. Arthur, H.M.; Ure, J.; Smith, A.J.; Renforth, G.; Wilson, D.I.; Torsney, E.; Charlton, R.; Parums, D.V.; Jowett, T.; Marchuk, D.A.; et al. Endoglin, an ancillary TGFbeta receptor, is required for extraembryonic angiogenesis and plays a key role in heart development. *Dev. Biol.* **2000**, *217*, 42–53. [CrossRef]

49. Oh, S.P.; Seki, T.; Goss, K.A.; Imamura, T.; Yi, Y.; Donahoe, P.K.; Li, L.; Miyazono, K.; ten Dijke, P.; Kim, S.; et al. Activin receptor-like kinase 1 modulates transforming growth factor-b1 signaling in the regulation of angiogenesis. *Proc. Natl. Acad. Sci. USA* **2000**, *97*, 2626–2631. [CrossRef] [PubMed]

50. Urness, L.D.; Sorensen, L.K.; Li, D.Y. Arteriovenous malformations in mice lacking activin receptor-like kinase-1. *Nat. Genet.* **2000**, *26*, 328–331. [CrossRef]

51.   Maris, J.M.; Knudson, A.G. Revisiting tissue specificity of germline cancer predisposing mutations. *Nat. Rev. Cancer* **2015**, *15*, 65–66. [CrossRef]

52.   Snellings, D.A.; Gallione, C.J.; Clark, D.S.; Vozoris, N.T.; Faughnan, M.E.; Marchuk, D.A. Somatic Mutations in Vascular Malformations of Hereditary Hemorrhagic Telangiectasia Result in Bi-allelic Loss of ENG or ACVRL1. *Am. J. Hum. Genet.* **2019**, *105*, 894–906. [CrossRef]

53.   Shovlin, C.L.; Hughes, J.M.; Scott, J.; Seidman, C.E.; Seidman, J.G. Characterization of endoglin and identification of novel mutations in hereditary hemorrhagic telangiectasia. *Am. J. Hum. Genet.* **1997**, *61*, 68–79. [CrossRef] [PubMed]

54.   Lux, A.; Attisano, L.; Marchuk, D.A. Assignment of transforming growth factor beta1 and beta3 and a third new ligand to the type I receptor ALK-1. *J. Biol. Chem.* **1999**, *274*, 9984–9992. [CrossRef]

55.   Gu, Y.; Jin, P.; Zhang, L.; Zhao, X.; Gao, X.; Ning, Y.; Meng, A.; Chen, Y.G. Functional analysis of mutations in the kinase domain of the TGF-beta receptor ALK1 reveals different mechanisms for induction of hereditary hemorrhagic telangiectasia. *Blood* **2006**, *107*, 1951–1954. [CrossRef] [PubMed]

56.   Förg, T.; Hafner, M.; Lux, A. Investigation of endoglin wild-type and missense mutant protein heterodimerisation using fluorescence microscopy based IF, BiFC and FRET analyses. *PLoS ONE* **2014**, *9*, e102998. [CrossRef]

57.   Mallet, C.; Lamribet, K.; Giraud, S.; Dupuis-Girod, S.; Feige, J.J.; Bailly, S.; Tillet, E. Functional analysis of endoglin mutations from hereditary hemorrhagic telangiectasia type 1 patients reveals different mechanisms for endoglin loss of function. *Hum. Mol. Genet.* **2015**, *24*, 1142–1154. [CrossRef]

58.   López-Novoa, J.M.; Bernabeu, C. The physiological role of endoglin in the cardiovascular system. *Am. J. Physiol. Heart Circ. Physiol.* **2010**, *299*, H959–H974. [CrossRef]

59.   Gonzalez, C.D.; Cipriano, S.D.; Topham, C.A.; Stevenson, D.A.; Whitehead, K.J.; Vanderhooft, S.; Presson, A.P.; McDonald, J. Localization and age distribution of telangiectases in children and adolescents with hereditary hemorrhagic telangiectasia: A retrospective cohort study. *J. Am. Acad. Dermatol.* **2019**, *81*, 950–955. [CrossRef] [PubMed]

60.   Geisthoff, U.; Nguyen, H.L.; Lefering, R.; Maune, S.; Thangavelu, K.; Droege, F. Trauma Can Induce Telangiectases in Hereditary Hemorrhagic Telangiectasia. *J. Clin. Med.* **2020**, *9*, 1507. [CrossRef]

61.   Park, S.O.; Wankhede, M.; Lee, Y.J.; Choi, E.J.; Fliess, N.; Choe, S.W.; Oh, S.H.; Walter, G.; Raizada, M.K.; Sorg, B.S.; et al. Real-time imaging of de novo arteriovenous malformation in a mouse model of hereditary hemorrhagic telangiectasia. *J. Clin. Investig.* **2009**, *119*, 3487–3496. [CrossRef]

62.   Han, C.; Choe, S.W.; Kim, Y.H.; Acharya, A.P.; Keselowsky, B.G.; Sorg, B.S.; Lee, Y.J.; Oh, S.P. VEGF neutralization can prevent and normalize arteriovenous malformations in an animal model for hereditary hemorrhagic telangiectasia 2. *Angiogenesis* **2014**, *17*, 823–830. [CrossRef]

63.   Kim, Y.H.; Choe, S.W.; Chae, M.Y.; Hong, S.; Oh, S.P. SMAD4 Deficiency Leads to Development of Arteriovenous Malformations in Neonatal and Adult Mice. *J. Am. Heart Assoc.* **2018**, *7*, e009514. [CrossRef]

64.   Corti, P.; Young, S.; Chen, C.Y.; Patrick, M.J.; Rochon, E.R.; Pekkan, K.; Roman, B.L. Interaction between alk1 and blood flow in the development of arteriovenous malformations. *Development* **2011**, *138*, 1573–1582. [CrossRef]

65.   Baeyens, N.; Larrivée, B.; Ola, R.; Hayward-Piatkowskyi, B.; Dubrac, A.; Huang, B.; Ross, T.D.; Coon, B.G.; Min, E.; Tsarfati, M.; et al. Defective fluid shear stress mechanotransduction mediates hereditary hemorrhagic telangiectasia. *J. Cell Biol.* **2016**, *214*, 807–816. [CrossRef] [PubMed]

66.   Hiepen, C.; Mendez, P.L.; Knaus, P. It Takes Two to Tango: Endothelial TGFβ/BMP Signaling Crosstalk with Mechanobiology. *Cells* **2020**, *9*, 1965. [CrossRef]

67.   Botella, L.M.; Sánchez-Elsner, T.; Sanz-Rodriguez, F.; Kojima, S.; Shimada, J.; Guerrero-Esteo, M.; Cooreman, M.P.; Ratziu, V.; Langa, C.; Vary, C.P.; et al. Transcriptional activation of endoglin and transforming growth factor-beta signaling components by cooperative interaction between Sp1 and KLF6: Their potential role in the response to vascular injury. *Blood* **2002**, *100*, 4001–4010. [CrossRef]

68.   Garrido-Martín, E.M.; Blanco, F.J.; Roque, M.; Novensa, L.; Tarocchi, M.; Lang, U.E.; Suzuki, T.; Friedman, S.L.; Botella, L.M.; Bernabeu, C. Vascular injury triggers Krüppel-like factor 6 mobilization and cooperation with specificity protein 1 to promote endothelial activation through upregulation of the activin receptor-like kinase 1 gene. *Circ. Res.* **2013**, *112*, 113–127. [CrossRef]

69. Seghers, L.; de Vries, M.R.; Pardali, E.; Hoefer, I.E.; Hierck, B.P.; ten Dijke, P.; Goumans, M.J.; Quax, P.H. Shear induced collateral artery growth modulated by endoglin but not by ALK1. *J. Cell. Mol. Med.* **2012**, *16*, 2440–2450. [CrossRef]

70. Jin, Y.; Muhl, L.; Burmakin, M.; Wang, Y.; Duchez, A.C.; Betsholtz, C.; Arthur, H.M.; Jakobsson, L. Endoglin prevents vascular malformation by regulating flow-induced cell migration and specification through VEGFR2 signalling. *Nat. Cell Biol.* **2017**, *19*, 639–652. [CrossRef]

71. Ola, R.; Künzel, S.H.; Zhang, F.; Genet, G.; Chakraborty, R.; Pibouin-Fragner, L.; Martin, K.; Sessa, W.; Dubrac, A.; Eichmann, A. SMAD4 Prevents Flow Induced Arteriovenous Malformations by Inhibiting Casein Kinase 2. *Circulation* **2018**, *138*, 2379–2394. [CrossRef]

72. Sugden, W.W.; Meissner, R.; Aegerter-Wilmsen, T.; Tsaryk, R.; Leonard, E.V.; Bussmann, J.; Hamm, M.J.; Herzog, W.; Jin, Y.; Jakobsson, L.; et al. Endoglin controls blood vessel diameter through endothelial cell shape changes in response to haemodynamic cues. *Nat. Cell Biol.* **2017**, *19*, 653–665. [CrossRef] [PubMed]

73. Sugden, W.W.; Siekmann, A.F. Endothelial cell biology of Endoglin in hereditary hemorrhagic telangiectasia. *Curr. Opin. Hematol.* **2018**, *25*, 237–244. [CrossRef]

74. Klostranec, J.M.; Chen, L.; Mathur, S.; McDonald, J.; Faughnan, M.E.; Ratjen, F.; Krings, T. A theory for polymicrogyria and brain arteriovenous malformations in HHT. *Neurology* **2019**, *92*, 34–42. [CrossRef]

75. Scharpfenecker, M.; Floot, B.; Russell, N.S.; Ten Dijke, P.; Stewart, F.A. Endoglin haploinsufficiency reduces radiation-induced fibrosis and telangiectasia formation in mouse kidneys. *Radiother. Oncol.* **2009**, *92*, 484–491. [CrossRef]

76. Sadick, H.; Naim, R.; Sadick, M.; Hörmann, K.; Riedel, F. Plasma level and tissue expression of angiogenic factors in patients with hereditary hemorrhagic telangiectasia. *Int. J. Mol. Med.* **2005**, *15*, 591–596. [CrossRef]

77. Sadick, H.; Naim, R.; Gossler, U.; Hormann, K.; Riedel, F. Angiogenesis in hereditary hemorrhagic telangiectasia: VEGF165 plasma concentration in correlation to the VEGF expression and microvessel density. *Int. J. Mol. Med.* **2005**, *15*, 15–19. [CrossRef]

78. Botella, L.M.; Albiñana, V.; Ojeda-Fernandez, L.; Recio-Poveda, L.; Bernabéu, C. Research on potential biomarkers in hereditary hemorrhagic telangiectasia. *Front. Genet.* **2015**, *6*, 115. [CrossRef]

79. Xu, B.; Wu, Y.Q.; Huey, M.; Arthur, H.M.; Marchuk, D.A.; Hashimoto, T.; Young, W.L.; Yang, G.Y. Vascular endothelial growth factor induces abnormal microvasculature in the endoglin heterozygous mouse brain. *J. Cereb. Blood Flow Metab.* **2004**, *24*, 237–244. [CrossRef]

80. Choi, E.J.; Chen, W.; Jun, K.; Arthur, H.M.; Young, W.L.; Su, H. Novel brain arteriovenous malformation mouse models for type 1 hereditary hemorrhagic telangiectasia. *PLoS ONE* **2014**, *9*, e88511. [CrossRef] [PubMed]

81. Hao, Q.; Zhu, Y.; Su, H.; Shen, F.; Yang, G.Y.; Kim, H.; Young, W.L. VEGF Induces More Severe Cerebrovascular Dysplasia in Endoglin than in Alk1 Mice. Version 2. *Transl. Stroke Res.* **2010**, *1*, 197–201. [CrossRef]

82. Ardelean, D.S.; Jerkic, M.; Yin, M.; Peter, M.; Ngan, B.; Kerbel, R.S.; Foster, F.S.; Letarte, M. Endoglin and activin receptor-like kinase 1 heterozygous mice have a distinct pulmonary and hepatic angiogenic profile and response to anti-VEGF treatment. *Angiogenesis* **2014**, *17*, 129–146. [CrossRef]

83. Buscarini, E.; Botella, L.M.; Geisthoff, U.; Kjeldsen, A.D.; Mager, H.J.; Pagella, F.; Suppressa, P.; Zarrabeitia, R.; Dupuis-Girod, S.; Shovlin, C.L.; et al. Safety of thalidomide and bevacizumab in patients with hereditary hemorrhagic telangiectasia. *Orphanet J. Rare Dis.* **2019**, *14*, 28. [CrossRef] [PubMed]

84. Larrivée, B.; Prahst, C.; Gordon, E.; del Toro, R.; Mathivet, T.; Duarte, A.; Simons, M.; Eichmann, A. ALK1 signaling inhibits angiogenesis by cooperating with the Notch pathway. *Dev. Cell* **2012**, *22*, 489–500. [CrossRef]

85. Peacock, H.M.; Caolo, V.; Jones, E.A. Arteriovenous malformations in hereditary haemorrhagic telangiectasia: Looking beyond ALK1-NOTCH interactions. *Cardiovasc Res.* **2016**, *109*, 196–203. [CrossRef] [PubMed]

86. Fischer, A.; Schumacher, N.; Maier, M.; Sendtner, M.; Gessler, M. The Notch target genes Hey1 and Hey2 are required for embryonic vascular development. *Genes Dev.* **2004**, *18*, 901–911. [CrossRef] [PubMed]

87. Lawson, N.D.; Scheer, N.; Pham, V.N.; Kim, C.H.; Chitnis, A.B.; Campos-Ortega, J.A.; Weinstein, B.M. Notch signaling is required for arterial-venous differentiation during embryonic vascular development. *Development* **2001**, *128*, 3675–3683.

88. Krebs, L.T.; Shutter, J.R.; Tanigaki, K.; Honjo, T.; Stark, K.L.; Gridley, T. Haploinsufficient lethality and formation of arteriovenous malformations in Notch pathway mutants. *Genes Dev.* **2004**, *18*, 2469–2473. [CrossRef] [PubMed]

89. Lebrin, F.; Goumans, M.J.; Jonker, L.; Carvalho, R.L.; Valdimarsdottir, G.; Thorikay, M.; Mummery, C.; Arthur, H.M.; ten Dijke, P. Endoglin promotes endothelial cell proliferation and TGF-beta/ALK1 signal transduction. *EMBO J.* **2004**, *23*, 4018–4028. [CrossRef]

90. Li, C.; Hampson, I.N.; Hampson, L.; Kumar, P.; Bernabeu, C.; Kumar, S. CD105 antagonizes the inhibitory signaling of transforming growth factor beta1 on human vascular endothelial cells. *FASEB J.* **2000**, *14*, 55–64. [CrossRef]

91. She, X.; Matsuno, F.; Harada, N.; Tsai, H.; Seon, B.K. Synergy between anti-endoglin (CD105) monoclonal antibodies and TGF-beta in suppression of growth of human endothelial cells. *Int. J. Cancer* **2004**, *108*, 251–257. [CrossRef]

92. Li, C.; Issa, R.; Kumar, P.; Hampson, I.N.; Lopez-Novoa, J.M.; Bernabeu, C.; Kumar, S. CD105 prevents apoptosis in hypoxic endothelial cells. *J. Cell Sci.* **2003**, *116*, 2677–2685. [CrossRef]

93. Nivet, A.; Schlienger, M.; Clavère, P.; Huguet, F. Effects of high-dose irradiation on vascularization: Physiopathology and clinical consequences. *Cancer Radiother.* **2019**, *23*, 161–167. [CrossRef]

94. David, L.; Mallet, C.; Keramidas, M.; Lamandé, N.; Gasc, J.M.; Dupuis-Girod, S.; Plauchu, H.; Feige, J.J.; Bailly, S. Bone morphogenetic protein-9 is a circulating vascular quiescence factor. *Circ. Res.* **2008**, *102*, 914–922. [CrossRef]

95. Suzuki, Y.; Ohga, N.; Morishita, Y.; Hida, K.; Miyazono, K.; Watabe, T. BMP-9 induces proliferation of multiple types of endothelial cells in vitro and in vivo. *J. Cell Sci.* **2010**, *123*, 1684–1692. [CrossRef]

96. Valdimarsdottir, G.; Goumans, M.J.; Rosendahl, A.; Brugman, M.; Itoh, S.; Lebrin, F.; Sideras, P.; ten Dijke, P. Stimulation of Id1 expression by bone morphogenetic protein is sufficient and necessary for bone morphogenetic protein-induced activation of endothelial cells. *Circulation* **2002**, *106*, 2263–2270. [CrossRef]

97. David, L.; Mallet, C.; Mazerbourg, S.; Feige, J.J.; Bailly, S. Identification of BMP9 and BMP10 as functional activators of the orphan activin receptor-like kinase 1 (ALK1) in endothelial cells. *Blood* **2007**, *109*, 1953–1961. [CrossRef]

98. Torsney, E.; Charlton, R.; Parums, D.; Collis, M.; Arthur, H.M. Inducible expression of human endoglin during inflammation and wound healing in vivo. *Inflamm. Res.* **2002**, *51*, 464–470. [CrossRef]

99. Braverman, I.M.; Keh, A.; Jacobson, B.S. Ultrastructure and three-dimensional organization of the telangiectases of hereditary hemorrhagic telangiectasia. *J. Investig. Dermatol.* **1990**, *95*, 422–427. [CrossRef]

100. Zhang, R.; Hanc, Z.; Degos, V.; Shen, F.; Choi, E.J.; Sun, Z.; Kang, S.; Wong, M.; Zhu, W.; Zhan, L.; et al. Persistent infiltration and pro-inflammatory differentiation of monocytes cause unresolved inflammation in brain arteriovenous malformation. *Angiogenesis* **2016**, *19*, 451–461. [CrossRef]

101. Van Laake, L.W.; van den Driesche, S.; Post, S.; Feijen, A.; Jansen, M.A.; Driessens, M.H.; Mager, J.J.; Snijder, R.J.; Westermann, C.J.; Doevendans, P.A.; et al. Endoglin has a crucial role in blood cell-mediated vascular repair. *Circulation* **2006**, *114*, 2288–2297. [CrossRef] [PubMed]

102. Jaipersad, A.S.; Lip, G.Y.; Silverman, S.; Shantsila, E. The role of monocytes in angiogenesis and atherosclerosis. *J. Am. Coll. Cardiol.* **2014**, *63*, 1–11. [CrossRef]

103. Jerkic, M.; Peter, M.; Ardelean, D.; Fine, M.; Konerding, M.A.; Letarte, M. Dextran sulfate sodium leads to chronic colitis and pathological angiogenesis in Endoglin heterozygous mice. *Inflamm. Bowel Dis.* **2010**, *16*, 1859–1870. [CrossRef]

104. Rossi, E.; Sanz-Rodriguez, F.; Eleno, N.; Düwell, A.; Blanco, F.J.; Langa, C.; Botella, L.M.; Cabañas, C.; Lopez-Novoa, J.M.; Bernabeu, C. Endothelial endoglin is involved in inflammation: Role in leukocyte adhesion and transmigration. *Blood* **2013**, *121*, 403–415. [CrossRef]

105. Peter, M.R.; Jerkic, M.; Sotov, V.; Douda, D.N.; Ardelean, D.S.; Ghamami, N.; Lakschevitz, F.; Khan, M.A.; Robertson, S.J.; Glogauer, M.; et al. Impaired resolution of inflammation in the Endoglin heterozygous mouse model of chronic colitis. *Mediat. Inflamm.* **2014**, *2014*, 767185. [CrossRef] [PubMed]

106. Shen, F.; Degos, V.; Chu, P.L.; Han, Z.; Westbroek, E.M.; Choi, E.J.; Marchuk, D.; Kim, H.; Lawton, M.T.; Maze, M.; et al. Endoglin deficiency impairs stroke recovery. *Stroke* **2014**, *45*, 2101–2106. [CrossRef]

107. Han, Z.; Shaligram, S.; Faughnan, M.E.; Clark, D.; Sun, Z.; Su, H. Reduction of endoglin receptor impairs mononuclear cell-migration. *Explor. Med.* **2020**, *1*, 136–148. [CrossRef]

108. Rossi, E.; Smadja, D.M.; Boscolo, E.; Langa, C.; Arevalo, M.A.; Pericacho, M.; Gamella-Pozuelo, L.; Kauskot, A.; Botella, L.M.; Gaussem, P.; et al. Endoglin regulates mural cell adhesion in the circulatory system. *Cell. Mol. Life Sci.* **2016**, *73*, 1715–1739. [CrossRef]

109. Rossi, E.; Pericacho, M.; Bachelot-Loza, C.; Pidard, D.; Gaussem, P.; Poirault-Chassac, S.; Blanco, F.J.; Langa, C.; González-Manchón, C.; Lopez-Novoa, J.M.; et al. Human endoglin as a potential new partner involved in platelet-endothelium interactions. *Cell. Mol. Life Sci.* **2018**, *75*, 1269–1284. [CrossRef]

110. Rossi, E.; Lopez-Novoa, J.M.; Bernabeu, C. Endoglin involvement in integrin-mediated cell adhesion as a putative pathogenic mechanism in hereditary hemorrhagic telangiectasia type 1 (HHT1). *Front. Genet.* **2015**, *5*, 457. [CrossRef]

111. Koleva, R.I.; Conley, B.A.; Romero, D.; Riley, K.S.; Marto, J.A.; Lux, A.; Vary, C.P. Endoglin structure and function: Determinants of endoglin phosphorylation by transforming growth factor-beta receptors. *J. Biol. Chem.* **2006**, *281*, 25110–25123. [CrossRef]

112. Blanco, F.J.; Santibanez, J.F.; Guerrero-Esteo, M.; Langa, C.; Vary, C.P.; Bernabeu, C. Interaction and functional interplay between endoglin and ALK-1, two components of the endothelial transforming growth factor-beta receptor complex. *J. Cell. Physiol.* **2005**, *204*, 574–584. [CrossRef]

113. Ma, L.; Shen, F.; Jun, K.; Bao, C.; Kuo, R.; Young, W.L.; Nishimura, S.L.; Su, H. Integrin β8 Deletion Enhances Vascular Dysplasia and Hemorrhage in the Brain of Adult Alk1 Heterozygous Mice. *Transl. Stroke Res.* **2016**, *7*, 488–496. [CrossRef] [PubMed]

114. Incalza, M.A.; D'Oria, R.; Natalicchio, A.; Perrini, S.; Laviola, L.; Giorgino, F. Oxidative stress and reactive oxygen species in endothelial dysfunction associated with cardiovascular and metabolic diseases. *Vascul. Pharmacol.* **2018**, *100*, 1–19. [CrossRef]

115. Jerkic, M.; Rivas-Elena, J.V.; Prieto, M.; Carrón, R.; Sanz-Rodríguez, F.; Pérez-Barriocanal, F.; Rodríguez-Barbero, A.; Bernabéu, C.; López-Novoa, J.M. Endoglin regulates nitric oxide-dependent vasodilatation. *FASEB J.* **2004**, *18*, 609–611. [CrossRef]

116. Toporsian, M.; Gros, R.; Kabir, M.G.; Vera, S.; Govindaraju, K.; Eidelman, D.H.; Husain, M.; Letarte, M. A role for endoglin in coupling eNOS activity and regulating vascular tone revealed in hereditary hemorrhagic telangiectasia. *Circ. Res.* **2005**, *96*, 684–692. [CrossRef] [PubMed]

117. Jerkic, M.; Letarte, M. Contribution of oxidative stress to endothelial dysfunction in hereditary hemorrhagic telangiectasia. *Front. Genet.* **2015**, *6*, 34. [CrossRef]

118. Jerkic, M.; Sotov, V.; Letarte, M. Oxidative stress contributes to endothelial dysfunction in mouse models of hereditary hemorrhagic telangiectasia. *Oxid. Med. Cell Longev.* **2012**, *2012*, 686972. [CrossRef]

119. De Gussem, E.M.; Snijder, R.J.; Disch, F.J.; Zanen, P.; Westermann, C.J.; Mager, J.J. The effect of N-acetylcysteine on epistaxis and quality of life in patients with HHT: A pilot study. *Rhinology* **2009**, *47*, 85–88.

120. Albiñana, V.; Cuesta, A.M.; Rojas-P., I.; Gallardo-Vara, E.; Recio-Poveda, L.; Bernabéu, C.; Botella, L.M. Review of Pharmacological Strategies with Repurposed Drugs for Hereditary Hemorrhagic Telangiectasia Related Bleeding. *J. Clin. Med.* **2020**, *9*, 1766. [CrossRef]

121. Bourdeau, A.; Faughnan, M.E.; McDonald, M.L.; Paterson, A.D.; Wanless, I.R.; Letarte, M. Potential role of modifier genes influencing transforming growth factor-beta1 levels in the development of vascular defects in endoglin heterozygous mice with hereditary hemorrhagic telangiectasia. *Am. J. Pathol.* **2001**, *158*, 2011–2020. [CrossRef]

122. Satomi, J.; Mount, R.J.; Toporsian, M.; Paterson, A.D.; Wallace, M.C.; Harrison, R.V.; Letarte, M. Cerebral vascular abnormalities in a murine model of hereditary hemorrhagic telangiectasia. *Stroke* **2003**, *34*, 783–789. [CrossRef]

123. Coulson, P.S.; Wilson, R.A. Portal shunting and resistance to Schistosoma mansoni in 129 strain mice. *Parasitology* **1989**, *99*, 383–389. [CrossRef]

124. Elsaghier, A.A.; McLaren, D.J. Schistosoma mansoni: Evidence that vascular abnormalities correlate with the 'non-permissive' trait in 129/Ola mice. *Parasitology* **1989**, *99*, 377–381. [CrossRef]

125. Srinivasan, S.; Hanes, M.A.; Dickens, T.; Porteous, M.E.; Oh, S.P.; Hale, L.P.; Marchuk, D.A. A mouse model for hereditary hemorrhagic telangiectasia (HHT) type 2. *Hum. Mol. Genet.* **2003**, *12*, 473–482. [CrossRef] [PubMed]

126. Sorensen, L.K.; Brooke, B.S.; Li, D.Y.; Urness, L.D. Loss of distinct arterial and venous boundaries in mice lacking endoglin, a vascular-specific TGFbeta coreceptor. *Dev. Biol.* **2003**, *261*, 235–250. [CrossRef]

127. Mahmoud, M.; Allinson, K.R.; Zhai, Z.; Oakenfull, R.; Ghandi, P.; Adams, R.H.; Fruttiger, M.; Arthur, H.M. Pathogenesis of arteriovenous malformations in the absence of endoglin. *Circ. Res.* **2010**, *106*, 1425–1433. [CrossRef]

128. Garrido-Martin, E.M.; Nguyen, H.L.; Cunningham, T.A.; Choe, S.W.; Jiang, Z.; Arthur, H.M.; Lee, Y.J.; Oh, S.P. Common and distinctive pathogenetic features of arteriovenous malformations in hereditary hemorrhagic telangiectasia 1 and hereditary hemorrhagic telangiectasia 2 animal models–brief report. *Arterioscler. Thromb. Vasc. Biol.* **2014**, *34*, 2232–2236. [CrossRef] [PubMed]

129. Benzinou, M.; Clermont, F.F.; Letteboer, T.G.; Kim, J.H.; Espejel, S.; Harradine, K.A.; Arbelaez, J.; Luu, M.T.; Roy, R.; Quigley, D.; et al. Mouse and human strategies identify PTPN14 as a modifier of angiogenesis and hereditary haemorrhagic telangiectasia. *Nat. Commun.* **2012**, *3*, 616. [CrossRef]

130. Letteboer, T.G.; Benzinou, M.; Merrick, C.B.; Quigley, D.A.; Zhau, K.; Kim, I.J.; To, M.D.; Jablons, D.M.; van Amstel, J.K.; Westermann, C.J.; et al. Genetic variation in the functional ENG allele inherited from the non-affected parent associates with presence of pulmonary arteriovenous malformation in hereditary hemorrhagic telangiectasia 1 (HHT1) and may influence expression of PTPN14. *Front. Genet.* **2015**, *6*, 67. [CrossRef]

131. Kawasaki, K.; Freimuth, J.; Meyer, D.S.; Lee, M.M.; Tochimoto-Okamoto, A.; Benzinou, M.; Clermont, F.F.; Wu, G.; Roy, R.; Letteboer, T.G.; et al. Genetic variants of Adam17 differentially regulate TGFβ signaling to modify vascular pathology in mice and humans. *Proc. Natl. Acad. Sci. USA* **2014**, *111*, 7723–7728. [CrossRef]

132. Pawlikowska, L.; Tran, M.N.; Achrol, A.S.; Ha, C.; Burchard, E.; Choudhry, S.; Zaroff, J.; Lawton, M.T.; Castro, R.; McCulloch, C.E.; et al. Polymorphisms in transforming growth factor-beta-related genes ALK1 and ENG are associated with sporadic brain arteriovenous malformations. *Stroke* **2005**, *36*, 2278–2280. [CrossRef]

133. Simon, M.; Franke, D.; Ludwig, M.; Aliashkevich, A.F.; Köster, G.; Oldenburg, J.; Boström, A.; Ziegler, A.; Schramm, J. Association of a polymorphism of the ACVRL1 gene with sporadic arteriovenous malformations of the central nervous system. *J. Neurosurg.* **2006**, *104*, 945–949. [CrossRef]

134. Pawlikowska, L.; Nelson, J.; Guo, D.E.; McCulloch, C.E.; Lawton, M.T.; Young, W.L.; Kim, H.; Faughnan, M.E.; Brain Vascular Malformation Consortium HHT Investigator Group. The ACVRL1 c.314-35A>G polymorphism is associated with organ vascular malformations in hereditary hemorrhagic telangiectasia patients with ENG mutations, but not in patients with ACVRL1 mutations. *Am. J. Med. Genet. A* **2015**, *167*, 1262–1267. [CrossRef]

135. Pawlikowska, L.; Nelson, J.; Guo, D.E.; McCulloch, C.E.; Lawton, M.T.; Kim, H.; Faughnan, M.E.; Brain Vascular Malformation Consortium HHT Investigator Group. Association of common candidate variants with vascular malformations and intracranial hemorrhage in hereditary hemorrhagic telangiectasia. *Mol. Genet. Genom. Med.* **2018**, *6*, 350–356. [CrossRef]

136. Davies, J.C.; Griesenbach, U.; Alton, E. Modifier genes in cystic fibrosis. *Pediatr. Pulmonol.* **2005**, *39*, 383–391. [CrossRef]

137. Kormann, M.S.D.; Dewerth, A.; Eichner, F.; Baskaran, P.; Hector, A.; Regamey, N.; Hartl, D.; Handgretinger, R.; Antony, J.S. Transcriptomic profile of cystic fibrosis patients identifies type I interferon response and ribosomal stalk proteins as potential modifiers of disease severity. *PLoS ONE* **2017**, *12*, e0183526. [CrossRef]

138. Rigamonti, D.; Hadley, M.N.; Drayer, B.P.; Johnson, P.C.; Hoenig-Rigamonti, K.; Knight, J.T.; Spetzler, R.F. Cerebral cavernous malformations. Incidence and familial occurrence. *N. Engl. J. Med.* **1988**, *319*, 343–347. [CrossRef]

139. Akers, A.L.; Johnson, E.; Steinberg, G.K.; Zabramski, J.M.; Marchuk, D.A. Biallelic somatic and germline mutations in cerebral cavernous malformations (CCMs): Evidence for a two-hit mechanism of CCM pathogenesis. *Hum. Mol. Genet.* **2009**, *18*, 919–930. [CrossRef] [PubMed]

140. Chan, A.C.; Drakos, S.G.; Ruiz, O.E.; Smith, A.C.; Gibson, C.C.; Ling, J.; Passi, S.F.; Stratman, A.N.; Sacharidou, A.; Revelo, M.P.; et al. Mutations in 2 distinct genetic pathways result in cerebral cavernous malformations in mice. *J. Clin. Investig.* **2011**, *121*, 1871–1881. [CrossRef] [PubMed]

141. Limaye, N.; Wouters, V.; Uebelhoer, M.; Tuominen, M.; Wirkkala, R.; Mulliken, J.B.; Eklund, L.; Boon, L.M.; Vikkula, M. Somatic mutations in angiopoietin receptor gene TEK cause solitary and multiple sporadic venous malformations. *Nat. Genet.* **2009**, *41*, 118–124. [CrossRef] [PubMed]

142. Macmurdo, C.F.; Wooderchak-Donahue, W.; Bayrak-Toydemir, P.; Le, J.; Wallenstein, M.B.; Milla, C.; Teng, J.M.; Bernstein, J.A.; Stevenson, D.A. RASA1 somatic mutation and variable expressivity in capillary malformation/arteriovenous malformation (CM/AVM) syndrome. *Am. J. Med. Genet. A* **2016**, *170*, 1450–1454. [CrossRef]

143. Cai, R.; Liu, F.; Liu, Y.; Chen, H.; Lin, X. RASA-1 somatic "second hit" mutation in capillary malformation-arteriovenous malformation. *J. Dermatol.* **2018**, *45*, 1478–1480. [CrossRef]
144. Choi, E.J.; Walker, E.J.; Shen, F.; Oh, S.P.; Arthur, H.M.; Young, W.L.; Su, H. Minimal homozygous endothelial deletion of Eng with VEGF stimulation is sufficient to cause cerebrovascular dysplasia in the adult mouse. *Cerebrovasc. Dis.* **2012**, *33*, 540–547. [CrossRef] [PubMed]

Publisher's Note: MDPI stays neutral with regard to jurisdictional claims in published maps and institutional affiliations.

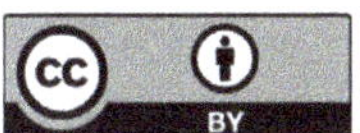

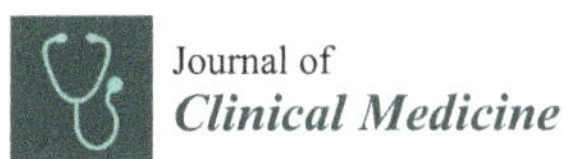

Journal of
Clinical Medicine

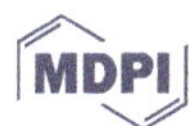

Article

Trauma Can Induce Telangiectases in Hereditary Hemorrhagic Telangiectasia

Urban Geisthoff [1,2], Ha-Long Nguyen [3], Rolf Lefering [4], Steffen Maune [5], Kruthika Thangavelu [1] and Freya Droege [6,*]

1   Department of Otorhinolaryngology, Head and Neck Surgery, University Hospital Marburg, Philipps-Universität Marburg, Baldingerstrasse, 35043 Marburg, Germany; geisthof@med.uni-marburg.de (U.G.); kruthika.thangavelu@gmail.com (K.T.)
2   Morbus Osler-Selbsthilfe e.V. (German HHT Self-Help Group), 89264 Weissenhorn, Germany
3   Laboratory of Human Molecular Genetics, de Duve Institute, Université catholique de Louvain, 1200 Brussels, Belgium; ha-long.nguyen@uclouvain.be
4   Institute for Research in Surgical Medicine (IFOM), University of Witten/Herdecke, Campus Merheim, 51109 Cologne, Germany; rolf.lefering@uni-wh.de
5   Department of Otorhinolaryngology, Hospitals of the City of Cologne, University of Witten/Herdecke, 51067 Cologne, Germany; maunes@kliniken-koeln.de
6   Department of Otorhinolaryngology, Head and Neck Surgery, Essen University Hospital, University Duisburg-Essen, Hufelandstrasse 55, 45122 Essen, Germany
*   Correspondence: freya.droege@uk-essen.de; Tel.: +49-201-723-85832; Fax: +49-201-723-5903

Received: 15 April 2020; Accepted: 14 May 2020; Published: 17 May 2020

Abstract: Hereditary hemorrhagic telangiectasia (HHT) is an autosomal dominant disease of the fibrovascular tissue resulting in visceral vascular malformations and (muco-) cutaneous telangiectases with recurrent bleedings. The mechanism behind the disease is not fully understood; however, observations from HHT mouse models suggest that mechanical trauma may induce the formation of abnormal vessels. To assess the influence of environmental trauma (mechanical or light induced) on the number of telangiectases in patients with HHT, the number of telangiectases on the hands, face, and lips were counted on 103 HHT patients possessing at least three out of four Curaçao criteria. They were then surveyed for information concerning their dominant hand, exposure to sunlight, and types of regular manual work. Patients developed more telangiectases on their dominant hand and lower lip (Wilcoxon rank sum test: $p < 0.001$). Mechanical stress induced by manual work led to an increased number of telangiectases on patients' hands (Mann–Whitney U test: $p < 0.001$). There was also a positive correlation between sun exposure and the number of telangiectases on the lips (Mann–Whitney U test: 0.027). This study shows that mechanical and UV-induced trauma strongly influence the formation of telangiectases in HHT patients. This result has potential implications in preventive measures and on therapeutic approaches for HHT.

Keywords: hereditary hemorrhagic telangiectasia (HHT); telangiectases; mechanical damage; sun-induced trauma; vascular malformations; Endoglin; activin-receptor-like kinase 1

---

1. Introduction

Hereditary hemorrhagic telangiectasia (HHT) is a rare autosomal dominantly inherited disorder that affects the vasculature. The predominant vascular defects range from small telangiectases within nearly all cutaneous and mucocutaneous membranes to larger AV malformations (AVM) within the lungs, liver and brain. Diagnosis of HHT is established either by genetic testing or the fulfillment of at least three of the four Curaçao criteria (recurrent epistaxis, multiple telangiectases at characteristic sites, AVM in visceral lesions, and a family history) [1,2].

About 50–80% of HHT patients form (muco-)cutaneous telangiectases, predominantly on the mucosa of the nose and mouth, tongue, lips, face and fingers [1–3]. Since the dilated vessels are compromised, they are prone to rupture. Recurrent bleedings, especially epistaxis, can lead to severe anemia that can impair patients' daily routine and quality of life [4–6]. An age-dependent penetrance of the disease [7] and highly variable clinical phenotypes are described. The age of onset, the severity and the location of the vascular lesions differ among each patient [8,9].

The mechanisms leading to new AVMs are not completely understood. In animal models for HHT mechanical stress like wounding or fluid shear stress induced new arteriovenous malformations [10,11]. However, to our knowledge, this has never been confirmed in adults with HHT. The aim of this study was to evaluate the influence of mechanical or sun-induced trauma on the number of telangiectases in patients with HHT.

2. Experimental Section

In 103 consecutive patients who fulfilled at least three out of four Curaçao criteria [1], telangiectases on both hands as well as the upper and lower lip were quantitated. Afterwards, they were surveyed about their dominant hand, level/type of regular manual labor involving strain on the hands (low, medium, high) and exposure to sunlight (low, medium, high). Examples were given to facilitate a graded assessment: medium strain by manual work would be a person from time to time but not daily having a wound on the hand due to mechanical stress from manual work. Medium sun exposure would be a person who frequently would get tanned but rarely had sunburns. Patients who have had laser therapy of their hands (one patient) or lips (17 patients) in the past were excluded from the analysis.

Description of the study population included number of patients (n), mean ± standard deviation (SD), t test, and 95% confidence intervals (95% CI). A Pearson correlation coefficient was performed to analyze patients' age and number of telangiectases. The Mann–Whitney U test and Kruskal–Wallis test were used for comparisons between patients, while paired tests (Wilcoxon rank sum; sign test) were used for intra-individual comparisons. A 5% significance level was determined. Statistical analyses were performed with IBM Corp. IBM SPSS Statistics for Windows, version 23.0. Armonk, NY, United States.

Study Approval

The authors assert that all procedures contributing to this work comply with the ethical standards of the Helsinki Declaration. The submission of the manuscript has been approved by the institutional review board ("Studienkommission") of the hospitals of the city of Cologne (180920171130). Data was provided voluntarily by HHT patients.

3. Results

The study cohort consisted of 61 females (59%) and 42 males (41%), ranging from age 9 to 83 years. No observable difference in the number of telangiectases was found between female and male patients (telangiectases on hands: men (m ± SD): 85 ± 126, women (m ± SD): 78 ± 94; Mann–Whitney U test: $p = 0.536$; telangiectases on lips: men (m ± SD): 15 ± 14, women (m ± SD): 19 ± 20; Mann–Whitney U test: $p = 0.423$).

There was a positive correlation between advanced age and the number of telangiectases on hands ($r = 0.429$, $p < 0.001$). Patients developed more telangiectases on their dominant hand (dominant hand, mean: 47 telangiectases, 95% CI: 35–60; non-dominant hand, mean: 37 telangiectases, 95% CI: 27–47; Wilcoxon rank sum test: $p < 0.001$; see also Table 1 and Figure 1). Those patients were significantly older than those with telangiectases distributed equally on both hands and those with more telangiectases on the non-dominant hand (average age: more telangiectases on dominant hand (m ± SD): 55 ± 15 years, equally distributed: (m ± SD): 39 ± 16 years, more telangiectases on non-dominant hand: (m ± SD): 50 ± 17 years; Kruskal–Wallis test: $p = 0.010$).

Table 1. Patients classified by handedness and number of telangiectases.

	Right Handed (*n*)	Ambidextrous (*n*)	Left Handed (*n*)	Total
more TAE on dominant hand (*n*)	67	0	2	69
equal number of TAE (*n*)	13	2	1	16
more TAE on non-dominant hand (*n*)	14	2	1	17
Total	94	4	4	

n: number of patients (total: 102), TAE: telangiectases, two patients were ambidextrous and had an unequal number of TAE on the hands.

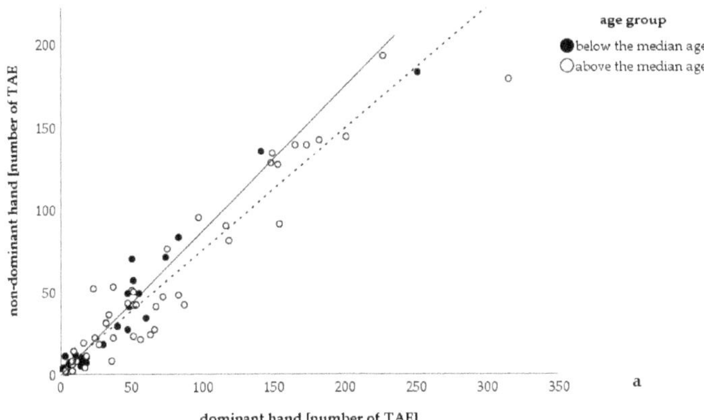

Figure 1. Correlation between number of telangiectases on the dominant and non-dominant hand. Number of telangiectases counted on the dominant hand correlated with the number of telangiectases on the non-dominant hand. The number of telangiectases on the dominant hand was significantly higher than on the non-dominant hand (Wilcoxon rank sum test: $p < 0.001$). The median age was 53 years (minimum: 9 years, maximum 83 years, $n = 102$). The continuous line is the bisectrix, dots lying on this line represent patients' equal numbers of telangiectases on both hands; the dashed line is the tendency line. TAE: telangiectases.

A typical example is shown in Figure 2. Additionally, patients reporting medium or high level of manual work in the past ($n = 21$, mean ± SD: 24 ± 34) showed significantly more telangiectases on their hands than patients with low levels of manual work ($n = 77$, mean ± SD: 7 ± 14; numbers add up to 98 as the four ambidextrous patients were excluded from the analysis) (Mann–Whitney U test: $p < 0.01$).

In evaluating the telangiectases on patients' lips, 86 of the 103 patients were examined; 17 were excluded due to having had laser therapy on the lips in the past. Opposed to the findings in the hands, there was no statistically significant correlation between advanced age and the number of lip telangiectases, but only a tendency ($r = 0.191$, $p = 0.078$). More telangiectases were found on the lower lip in 75 patients and on the upper lip in two; three had an equal number on both lips, and six patients did not have any telangiectases (sign test: $p < 0.001$, lower lip: mean: 14 telangiectases 95% CI: 10–17; upper lip: mean: 4 telangiectases 95% CI: 3-5; Wilcoxon rank sum test < 0.001; numbers add up to 86 as 17 patients from 103 had laser therapy (Figure 3)). Of those 86 only 76 were able to describe their sun exposure sufficiently. It was also found that those reporting medium or high sun exposure ($n = 9$, mean ± SD: 14 ± 10) had more telangiectases on their lips than patients with low exposure to the sun ($n = 67$, mean ± SD: 9 ± 11) (Mann–Whitney U test: 0.027).

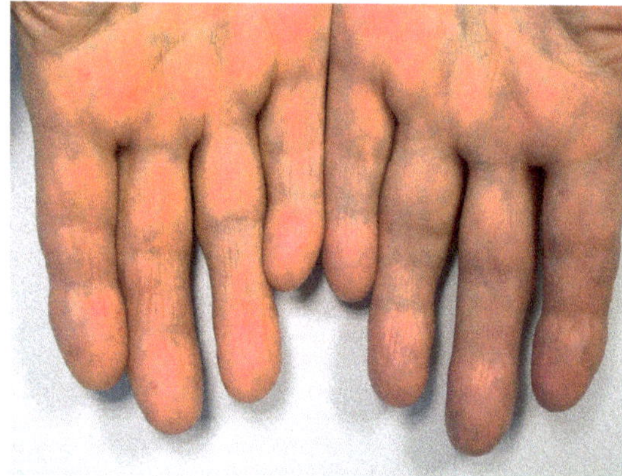

Figure 2. Photo of patient's hands with more telangiectases on the right dominant hand. The hands of a right-handed female patient of 68 years are shown. Her hands were exposed to relatively low mechanical strain in the past. A total of 36 telangiectases were counted on her right and eight telangiectases on her left hand (only some of them are visible in the photo). She experienced two episodes of bleeding of telangiectases on her right hand, however, never on the left hand.

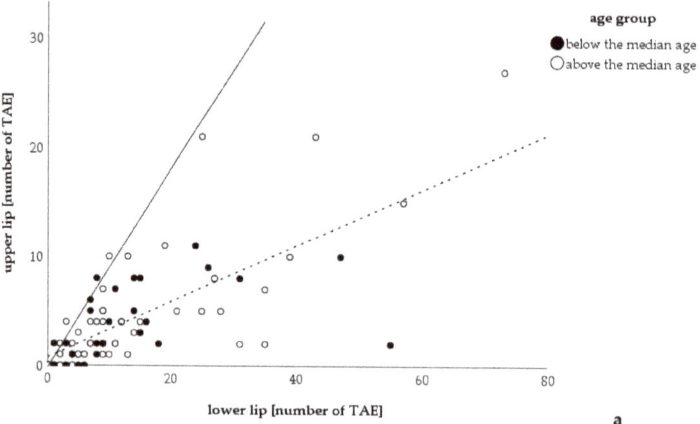

Figure 3. Correlation between number of telangiectases on the upper and lower lip. Number of telangiectases counted on the upper lip correlated with the number of telangiectases on the lower lip ($n = 86$). The number of telangiectases of the lower lip was significantly higher than the number on the upper lip (Wilcoxon rank sum test: $p < 0.001$; mean number of TAE: upper lip = 4 TAE, lower lip = 13 TAE). The median age was 54 years (minimum: 9 years, maximum 83 years, $n = 86$). The continuous line is the bisectrix, dots lying on this line represent patients with equal numbers of telangiectases on both lips; the dashed line is the tendency line. TAE: telangiectases.

To emphasize the influence that the sun's UV insult can have on formation of malformations in HHT, we note an anecdotal finding of a 65-year-old male patient who exhibited asymmetric distribution of telangiectases on his forehead. He informed us of his daily after-work ritual whereby he would sit on a bench on his balcony and read the newspaper. The sun would always shine on his left forehead, the side with more telangiectases (Figure 4).

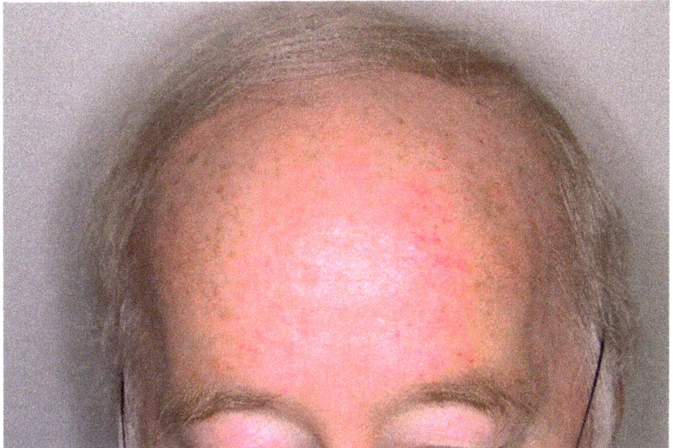

Figure 4. Photo of a patient's head with more telangiectases on the left forehead after sun exposure. This patient (65 years old) reported that he usually sat on the same bench in the afternoon. The sun used to shine from the left side. He did not report on any mechanical stress in that region.

4. Discussion

The underlying pathogenic HHT mechanism remains unclear. The wide variability in age of onset and severity of symptoms amongst patients, even within the same family, suggests several factors contribute to the complexity of this disease. There does not appear to be gender propensity amongst HHT patients. Underscoring this point, no correlation between a patient's sex and the number of telangiectases counted was found in this study. It has been observed that disorder progression worsens along with a patient's age [12–14]. In accordance, we observed more telangiectases within older patients' hands, and to some degree, lips. This could be due to the presumption that advanced aged patients have experienced more daily (muco-)cutaneous insults over time than younger patients.

Patients are heterozygous for germline, loss-of-function mutations in certain members of the transforming growth factor-ß (TGF-ß) signaling pathway; most notably, endoglin (HHT1) or activin-like kinase receptor-1 (HHT2) [7,15,16]. It has been postulated that a homozygous state is not viable [17], which is supported by animal models [18,19]. It was initially presumed that haploinsufficiency of relevant HHT genes is responsible for development of vascular lesions. However, the unpredictable, focal nature of defects does not completely support this theory. Several other types of vascular malformations, such as inherited subsets of venous malformations and cerebral cavernous malformations, with a similar pattern of clinical manifestations were found to follow Knudson's two-hit mechanism in which complete bi-allelic, localized loss of function of a gene of interest is required for formation of vascular lesions [20–22]. Recently, it was shown that HHT may also follow this trend rather than haploinsufficiency, as low-frequency somatic (mosaic) mutations were found in about half of the telangiectases isolated from HHT patients [23]. However, conditional mouse models in which both copies of ENG were deleted postnatally within endothelial cells also required a pro-angiogenic stimulus in order to develop vascular malformations. Conditional knockout models of ALK1 and SMAD4 formed vascular defects more consistently but inducing angiogenesis made lesions more robust. Hence, the mouse models suggest that loss of any of the HHT genes alone is not sufficient to form vascular lesions and that an external factor, such as in the form of wounding and shear/biomechanical stress, that triggers angiogenesis is needed [10,11,24–31]. A potential explanation is that since ALK-1 and ENG are increased in response to environmental and other physiological insults, such as fluid shear stress, vascular injury, inflammation, infection, ischemia, and angiogenic stimuli, the levels of wild type ALK-1 or ENG left is not sufficient for a vascular bed's need to maintain homeostasis [11,32,33].

To our knowledge, this study is the first to confirm the influence that environmental factors play on lesion development in human patients. We assume that each patient in our cohort has a predisposing mutation in one of the HHT-associated genes; however, we cannot appropriately speculate the consequences of the loss of function as we did not have their genotypes. Our data in which more telangiectases were found on a patient's dominant hand, and within patients whom performed more manual labor, indicates that triggers acting as an angiogenic stimulus play a vital role in the development of abnormal vessels in HHT. Patients in our cohort had more telangiectases on the lower, rather than the upper lip. One contributing factor could be that the lower lip is subjected to more physical insults than the upper lip; for example, it is in contact with the upper incisor teeth, or gravity naturally increases the chances of food touching the lower lip [34,35]. However, other environmental stimuli are likely be involved as well. The most probable cause is related to the fact that squamous cell carcinoma in the lower lip is more frequent than the upper lip. In oral oncology it is an accepted concept that the lower lip is more exposed to the sun. Additionally, surface area of the lower lip is larger in most individuals [36–39]. Similarly, HHT patients who claimed to have had excessive sun exposure in the past exhibited a higher number of telangiectases on the lips. In addition, one patient in the study displayed asymmetric distribution of telangiectases on his forehead, which corresponded to the side of his head that was predominantly exposed to the sun as he sat on his balcony. Thus, our data indicates that sunlight is able to stimulate development of new telangiectases; therefore, HHT patients should be advised to take extra precautions regarding sun protection when outdoors.

Beyond the cosmetic concerns, recurrent bleedings may lead to functional impairment in patients' professional and daily life [40]. Prevention of mechanical trauma and destruction of existing telangiectases are the main strategies in treating recurrent epistaxis. Nasal humidification is recommended to limit crust formation and mechanical trauma to the mucosa [41,42]. Alternatively, destruction of telangiectases can be performed, usually by laser therapy [43,44]. Cutaneous telangiectases, the vascular stigmata of HHT [45], are easily identifiable and accessible to treatment. A retrospective survey of patients treated with endonasal Nd:YAG laser treatment revealed that the duration of the interval between treatment sessions increased with the number of interventions [46]. Nevertheless, some of our patients stated that epistaxis worsened after commencing endonasal treatment (unpublished results from the outpatient clinics of the authors), indicating that this approach is not reliably effective for all patients.

Sunlight is comprised of a spectrum of light (UV, visible, and infrared) with varying wavelengths. The induction of telangiectases is presumably caused by widely reported damaging UV light (within the shorter wavelengths from 100 to 400 nm) [47]. It remains unclear whether light-induced trauma of longer wavelengths, such as within the infrared region, has as much of an influence in stimulating telangiectasia development. Light from the Nd:YAG laser (wavelength = 1064 nm) is used to destroy a vascular lesion and may lead to more scar formation, antagonizing induction of new telangiectases [48]. There is still evidence lacking if laser treatment could prevent the development of new telangiectases. Hence, before elective laser treatment patients should be informed about a possible long-term deterioration by induction of new telangiectases. Additionally, the concomitant therapy with drugs which might compensate for the genetic loss, e.g., tranexamic acid [49], during the period of wound healing could be discussed with the patients.

In conclusion, we could demonstrate that in patients with HHT mechanical and light-induced trauma promote the formation of telangiectases. Preventing these traumata might also prevent the formation of new telangiectases.

Study Limitations

It should be noted that a limitation of the study was the difficulty in grading both sunlight exposure and strain by manual work. The method chosen (giving general examples for each grade level) was quite vague, and several patients did not fully understand how to self-assess themselves. However, a more quantitative categorization (e.g., estimated intensity combined with mean daily hours of sun light exposure or manual work) proved to be impractical or more complicated based on discussions with patients during the study preparation stage. Additionally, exposition to the discussed factors did not occur under controlled conditions. Other unknown factors might have played a role, too, so that uncertainties in the hypothesized chain of causation remain.

Author Contributions: Conceptualization, U.G.; methodology, U.G.; software, U.G.; F.D.; validation, F.D., R.L.; U.G.; formal analysis, U.G.; H.-L.N.; R.L.; F.D.; investigation, U.G.; F.D.; data curation, U.G.; F.D.; writing—original draft preparation, U.G.; H.-L.N.; F.D.; writing—review and editing, U.G.; H.-L.N.; R.L.; S.M.; K.T.; F.D.; visualization, U.G.; F.D.; supervision, U.G., F.D.; project administration, U.G.; F.D.; All authors have read and agreed to the published version of the manuscript.

Funding: This research did not receive any specific grant from funding agencies in the public, commercial, or not-for-profit sectors.

Acknowledgments: We are indebted to the HHT patients for their participation in the study, and the physician assistant Ms. Monika Hentschel for her help in data acquisition. Part of this study was presented at the IX. International Scientific HHT meeting in Kemer, Turkey, 20.-24.5.2011, the annual meeting of the German society for otorhinolaryngology 1.-5.6.2011 and has been published as abstract in Hematology Reports 2011; 3(s2): 33. We acknowledge support by the Open Access Publication Fund of the University of Duisburg-Essen.

References

1. Shovlin, C.L.; Guttmacher, A.E.; Buscarini, E.; Faughnan, M.E.; Hyland, R.H.; Westermann, C.J.; Kjeldsen, A.D.; Plauchu, H. Diagnostic criteria for hereditary hemorrhagic telangiectasia (Rendu-Osler-Weber syndrome). *Am. J. Med. Genet.* **2000**, *91*, 66–67. [CrossRef]
2. Osler, W. On a family form of recurring epistaxis associated with multiple telangiectases of the skin and mucous membranes. *Johns Hopkins Hosp. Bull.* **1901**, *12*, 333–337.
3. Sadick, H.; Sadick, M.; Gotte, K.; Naim, R.; Riedel, F.; Bran, G.; Hormann, K. Hereditary hemorrhagic telangiectasia: An update on clinical manifestations and diagnostic measures. *Wien. Klin. Wochenschr.* **2006**, *118*, 72–80. [CrossRef] [PubMed]
4. Geirdal, A.O.; Dheyauldeen, S.; Bachmann-Harildstad, G.; Heimdal, K. Quality of life in patients with hereditary hemorrhagic telangiectasia in Norway: A population based study. *Am. J. Med. Genet. A* **2012**, *158A*, 1269–1278. [CrossRef]
5. Geisthoff, U.W.; Heckmann, K.; D'Amelio, R.; Grunewald, S.; Knobber, D.; Falkai, P.; Konig, J. Health-related quality of life in hereditary hemorrhagic telangiectasia. *Otolaryngol. Head Neck Surg.* **2007**, *136*, 726–733; discussion 734–735. [CrossRef]
6. Lennox, P.A.; Hitchings, A.E.; Lund, V.J.; Howard, D.J. The SF-36 health status questionnaire in assessing patients with epistaxis secondary to hereditary hemorrhagic telangiectasia. *Am. J. Rhinol.* **2005**, *19*, 71–74. [CrossRef]
7. Lenato, G.M.; Guanti, G. Hereditary Haemorrhagic Telangiectasia (HHT): Genetic and molecular aspects. *Curr. Pharm. Des.* **2006**, *12*, 1173–1193. [CrossRef]
8. McDonald, J.E.; Miller, F.J.; Hallam, S.E.; Nelson, L.; Marchuk, D.A.; Ward, K.J. Clinical manifestations in a large hereditary hemorrhagic telangiectasia (HHT) type 2 kindred. *Am. J. Med. Genet.* **2000**, *93*, 320–327. [CrossRef]
9. Lesca, G.; Olivieri, C.; Burnichon, N.; Pagella, F.; Carette, M.F.; Gilbert-Dussardier, B.; Goizet, C.; Roume, J.; Rabilloud, M.; Saurin, J.C.; et al. Genotype-phenotype correlations in hereditary hemorrhagic telangiectasia: Data from the French-Italian HHT network. *Genet. Med.* **2007**, *9*, 14–22. [CrossRef]
10. Park, S.O.; Wankhede, M.; Lee, Y.J.; Choi, E.J.; Fliess, N.; Choe, S.W.; Oh, S.H.; Walter, G.; Raizada, M.K.; Sorg, B.S.; et al. Real-time imaging of de novo arteriovenous malformation in a mouse model of hereditary hemorrhagic telangiectasia. *J. Clin. Investig.* **2009**, *119*, 3487–3496. [CrossRef]
11. Baeyens, N.; Larrivee, B.; Ola, R.; Hayward-Piatkowskyi, B.; Dubrac, A.; Huang, B.; Ross, T.D.; Coon, B.G.; Min, E.; Tsarfati, M.; et al. Defective fluid shear stress mechanotransduction mediates hereditary hemorrhagic telangiectasia. *J. Cell Biol.* **2016**, *214*, 807–816. [CrossRef] [PubMed]

12. Plauchu, H.; de Chadarevian, J.P.; Bideau, A.; Robert, J.M. Age-related clinical profile of hereditary hemorrhagic telangiectasia in an epidemiologically recruited population. *Am. J. Med. Genet.* **1989**, *32*, 291–297. [CrossRef] [PubMed]

13. Gonzalez, C.D.; Cipriano, S.D.; Topham, C.A.; Stevenson, D.A.; Whitehead, K.J.; Vanderhooft, S.; Presson, A.P.; McDonald, J. Localization and age distribution of telangiectases in children and adolescents with hereditary hemorrhagic telangiectasia: A retrospective cohort study. *J. Am. Acad. Dermatol.* **2019**, *81*, 950–955. [CrossRef] [PubMed]

14. Hodgson, C.H.; Burchell, H.B.; Good, C.A.; Clagett, O.T. Hereditary hemorrhagic telangiectasia and pulmonary arteriovenous fistula: Survey of a large family. *N. Engl. J. Med.* **1959**, *261*, 625–636. [CrossRef]

15. McAllister, K.A.; Grogg, K.M.; Johnson, D.W.; Gallione, C.J.; Baldwin, M.A.; Jackson, C.E.; Helmbold, E.A.; Markel, D.S.; McKinnon, W.C.; Murrell, J.; et al. Endoglin, a TGF-beta binding protein of endothelial cells, is the gene for hereditary haemorrhagic telangiectasia type 1. *Nat. Genet.* **1994**, *8*, 345–351. [CrossRef]

16. Johnson, D.W.; Berg, J.N.; Baldwin, M.A.; Gallione, C.J.; Marondel, I.; Yoon, S.J.; Stenzel, T.T.; Speer, M.; Pericak-Vance, M.A.; Diamond, A.; et al. Mutations in the activin receptor-like kinase 1 gene in hereditary haemorrhagic telangiectasia type 2. *Nat. Genet.* **1996**, *13*, 189–195. [CrossRef]

17. El-Harith el, H.A.; Kuhnau, W.; Schmidtke, J.; Gadzicki, D.; Ahmed, M.; Krawczak, M.; Stuhrmann, M. Hereditary hemorrhagic telangiectasia is caused by the Q490X mutation of the ACVRL1 gene in a large Arab family: Support of homozygous lethality. *Eur. J. Med. Genet.* **2006**, *49*, 323–330. [CrossRef]

18. Bourdeau, A.; Dumont, D.J.; Letarte, M. A murine model of hereditary hemorrhagic telangiectasia. *J. Clin. Investig.* **1999**, *104*, 1343–1351. [CrossRef]

19. Urness, L.D.; Sorensen, L.K.; Li, D.Y. Arteriovenous malformations in mice lacking activin receptor-like kinase-1. *Nat. Genet.* **2000**, *26*, 328–331. [CrossRef]

20. Pagenstecher, A.; Stahl, S.; Sure, U.; Felbor, U. A two-hit mechanism causes cerebral cavernous malformations: Complete inactivation of CCM1, CCM2 or CCM3 in affected endothelial cells. *Hum. Mol. Genet.* **2009**, *18*, 911–918. [CrossRef]

21. Amyere, M.; Aerts, V.; Brouillard, P.; McIntyre, B.A.; Duhoux, F.P.; Wassef, M.; Enjolras, O.; Mulliken, J.B.; Devuyst, O.; Antoine-Poirel, H.; et al. Somatic uniparental isodisomy explains multifocality of glomuvenous malformations. *Am. J. Hum. Genet.* **2013**, *92*, 188–196. [CrossRef] [PubMed]

22. Akers, A.L.; Johnson, E.; Steinberg, G.K.; Zabramski, J.M.; Marchuk, D.A. Biallelic somatic and germline mutations in cerebral cavernous malformations (CCMs): Evidence for a two-hit mechanism of CCM pathogenesis. *Hum. Mol. Genet.* **2009**, *18*, 919–930. [CrossRef] [PubMed]

23. Snellings, D.A.; Gallione, C.J.; Clark, D.S.; Vozoris, N.T.; Faughnan, M.E.; Marchuk, D.A. Somatic mutations in vascular malformations of hereditary hemorrhagic telangiectasia result in Bi-allelic loss of ENG or ACVRL1. *Am. J. Hum. Genet.* **2019**, *105*, 894–906. [CrossRef] [PubMed]

24. Choi, E.J.; Walker, E.J.; Degos, V.; Jun, K.; Kuo, R.; Pile-Spellman, J.; Su, H.; Young, W.L. Endoglin deficiency in bone marrow is sufficient to cause cerebrovascular dysplasia in the adult mouse after vascular endothelial growth factor stimulation. *Stroke* **2013**, *44*, 795–798. [CrossRef] [PubMed]

25. Choi, E.J.; Walker, E.J.; Shen, F.; Oh, S.P.; Arthur, H.M.; Young, W.L.; Su, H. Minimal homozygous endothelial deletion of Eng with VEGF stimulation is sufficient to cause cerebrovascular dysplasia in the adult mouse. *Cerebrovasc. Dis.* **2012**, *33*, 540–547. [CrossRef] [PubMed]

26. Chen, W.; Guo, Y.; Walker, E.J.; Shen, F.; Jun, K.; Oh, S.P.; Degos, V.; Lawton, M.T.; Tihan, T.; Davalos, D.; et al. Reduced mural cell coverage and impaired vessel integrity after angiogenic stimulation in the Alk1-deficient brain. *Arterioscler. Thromb. Vasc. Biol.* **2013**, *33*, 305–310. [CrossRef]

27. Garrido-Martin, E.M.; Nguyen, H.L.; Cunningham, T.A.; Choe, S.W.; Jiang, Z.; Arthur, H.M.; Lee, Y.J.; Oh, S.P. Common and distinctive pathogenetic features of arteriovenous malformations in hereditary hemorrhagic telangiectasia 1 and hereditary hemorrhagic telangiectasia 2 animal models—Brief report. *Arterioscler. Thromb. Vasc. Biol.* **2014**, *34*, 2232–2236. [CrossRef]

28. Han, C.; Choe, S.W.; Kim, Y.H.; Acharya, A.P.; Keselowsky, B.G.; Sorg, B.S.; Lee, Y.J.; Oh, S.P. VEGF neutralization can prevent and normalize arteriovenous malformations in an animal model for hereditary hemorrhagic telangiectasia 2. *Angiogenesis* **2014**, *17*, 823–830. [CrossRef]

29. Hiepen, C.; Jatzlau, J.; Knaus, P. Biomechanical stress provides a second hit in the establishment of BMP/TGFbeta-related vascular disorders. *Cell Stress* **2020**, *4*, 44–47. [CrossRef]

30. Crist, A.M.; Lee, A.R.; Patel, N.R.; Westhoff, D.E.; Meadows, S.M. Vascular deficiency of Smad4 causes arteriovenous malformations: A mouse model of Hereditary Hemorrhagic Telangiectasia. *Angiogenesis* **2018**, *21*, 363–380. [CrossRef]

31. Kim, Y.H.; Choe, S.W.; Chae, M.Y.; Hong, S.; Oh, S.P. SMAD4 Deficiency leads to development of arteriovenous malformations in neonatal and adult mice. *J. Am. Heart Assoc.* **2018**, *7*, e009514. [CrossRef] [PubMed]

32. Ruiz-Llorente, L.; Gallardo-Vara, E.; Rossi, E.; Smadja, D.M.; Botella, L.M.; Bernabeu, C. Endoglin and alk1 as therapeutic targets for hereditary hemorrhagic telangiectasia. *Expert Opin. Ther. Targets* **2017**, *21*, 933–947. [CrossRef] [PubMed]

33. Shovlin, C.L. Hereditary haemorrhagic telangiectasia: Pathophysiology, diagnosis and treatment. *Blood Rev.* **2010**, *24*, 203–219. [CrossRef] [PubMed]

34. Chen, J.Y.; Wang, W.C.; Chen, Y.K.; Lin, L.M. A retrospective study of trauma-associated oral and maxillofacial lesions in a population from southern Taiwan. *J. Appl. Oral Sci.* **2010**, *18*, 5–9. [CrossRef]

35. Meltem Koray, T.T. Oral mucosal trauma and injuries. In *Trauma in Dentistry*; Gözler, S., Ed.; IntechOpen: London, UK, 2019. [CrossRef]

36. Maruccia, M.; Onesti, M.G.; Parisi, P.; Cigna, E.; Troccola, A.; Scuderi, N. Lip cancer: A 10-year retrospective epidemiological study. *Anticancer Res.* **2012**, *32*, 1543–1546.

37. Sawyer, A.R.; See, M.; Nduka, C. 3D stereophotogrammetry quantitative lip analysis. *Aesthetic Plast Surg.* **2009**, *33*, 497–504. [CrossRef]

38. Papadopoulos, O.; Konofaos, P.; Tsantoulas, Z.; Chrisostomidis, C.; Frangoulis, M.; Karakitsos, P. Lip defects due to tumor excision: Apropos of 899 cases. *Oral Oncol.* **2007**, *43*, 204–212. [CrossRef]

39. Montes, D.M.; Ghali, G.E. Lip cancer. In *Peterson's Principles of Oral and Maxillofacial Surgery*, 3rd ed.; Miloro, M., Ghali, G.E., Larsen, P.E., Waite, P., Eds.; People's Medical Publishing House: Shelton, CO, USA, 2011; p. 727.

40. Halachmi, S.; Israeli, H.; Ben-Amitai, D.; Lapidoth, M. Treatment of the skin manifestations of hereditary hemorrhagic telangiectasia with pulsed dye laser. *Lasers Med. Sci.* **2014**, *29*, 321–324. [CrossRef]

41. Geisthoff, U.W.; Fiorella, M.L.; Fiorella, R. Treatment of recurrent epistaxis in HHT. *Curr. Pharm. Des.* **2006**, *12*, 1237–1242. [CrossRef]

42. Faughnan, M.E.; Palda, V.A.; Garcia-Tsao, G.; Geisthoff, U.W.; McDonald, J.; Proctor, D.D.; Spears, J.; Brown, D.H.; Buscarini, E.; Chesnutt, M.S.; et al. International guidelines for the diagnosis and management of hereditary haemorrhagic telangiectasia. *J. Med. Genet.* **2011**, *48*, 73–87. [CrossRef]

43. Jorgensen, G.; Lange, B.; Wanscher, J.H.; Kjeldsen, A.D. Efficiency of laser treatment in patients with hereditary hemorrhagic telangiectasia. *Eur. Arch. Otorhinolaryngol.* **2011**, *268*, 1765–1770. [CrossRef] [PubMed]

44. Abiri, A.; Goshtasbi, K.; Maducdoc, M.; Sahyouni, R.; Wang, M.B.; Kuan, E.C. Laser-assisted control of epistaxis in hereditary hemorrhagic telangiectasia: A systematic review. *Lasers Surg. Med.* **2019**. [CrossRef] [PubMed]

45. Sexton, A.; Gargan, B.; Taylor, J.; Bogwitz, M.; Winship, I. Living with Hereditary Haemorrhagic Telangiectasia: Stigma, coping with unpredictable symptoms, and self-advocacy. *Psychol. Health* **2019**, *34*, 1141–1160. [CrossRef] [PubMed]

46. Werner, J.A.; Lippert, B.M.; Geisthoff, U.W.; Rudert, H. Nd:YAG laser therapy of recurrent epistaxis in hereditary hemorrhagic telangiectasia. *Laryngorhinootologie* **1997**, *76*, 495–501. [CrossRef]

47. Barolet, D.; Christiaens, F.; Hamblin, M.R. Infrared and skin: Friend or foe. *J. Photochem. Photobiol. B* **2016**, *155*, 78–85. [CrossRef]

48. Werner, J.A.; Geisthoff, U.W.; Lippert, B.M.; Rudert, H. Treatment of recurrent epistaxis in Rendu-Osler-Weber disease. *HNO* **1997**, *45*, 673–681. [CrossRef]

49. Fernandez, L.A.; Garrido-Martin, E.M.; Sanz-Rodriguez, F.; Ramirez, J.R.; Morales-Angulo, C.; Zarrabeitia, R.; Perez-Molino, A.; Bernabeu, C.; Botella, L.M. Therapeutic action of tranexamic acid in hereditary haemorrhagic telangiectasia (HHT): Regulation of ALK-1/endoglin pathway in endothelial cells. *Thromb. Haemost.* **2007**, *97*, 254–262. [CrossRef]

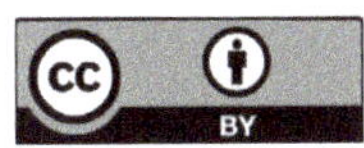

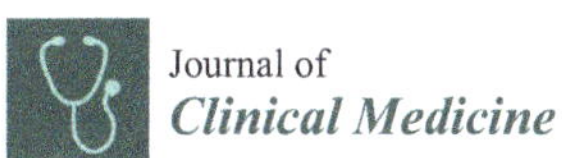

Journal of
Clinical Medicine

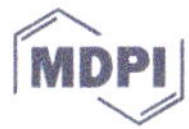

Review

Non-Coding RNAs and Hereditary Hemorrhagic Telangiectasia

Anthony Cannavicci [1,2], Qiuwang Zhang [2] and Michael J. B. Kutryk [1,2,*]

[1] Institute of Medical Science, University of Toronto, Toronto, ON M5S 1A8, Canada;
a.cannavicci@mail.utoronto.ca

[2] Division of Cardiology, Keenan Research Center for Biomedical Sciences, St. Michael's Hospital,
Unity Health Toronto, University of Toronto, Toronto, ON M5B 1T8, Canada;
Qiuwang.Zhang@unityhealth.to

* Correspondence: Michael.Kutryk@unityhealth.to; Tel.: +1-(416)-360-4000 (ext. 6155)

Received: 14 September 2020; Accepted: 15 October 2020; Published: 17 October 2020

Abstract: Non-coding RNAs (ncRNAs) are functional ribonucleic acid (RNA) species that include microRNAs (miRs), a class of short non-coding RNAs (~21–25 nucleotides), and long non-coding RNAs (lncRNAs) consisting of more than 200 nucleotides. They regulate gene expression post-transcriptionally and are involved in a wide range of pathophysiological processes. Hereditary hemorrhagic telangiectasia (HHT) is a rare disorder inherited in an autosomal dominant fashion characterized by vascular dysplasia. Patients can develop life-threatening vascular malformations and experience severe hemorrhaging. Effective pharmacological therapies are limited. The study of ncRNAs in HHT is an emerging field with great promise. This review will explore the current literature on the involvement of ncRNAs in HHT as diagnostic and pathogenic factors.

Keywords: non-coding RNAs; microRNAs; long non-coding RNAs; hereditary hemorrhagic telangiectasia; biomarkers; endothelial cells; angiogenesis

---

1. Introduction

Hereditary hemorrhagic telangiectasia (HHT) is a rare genetic vascular disorder inherited in an autosomal dominant fashion. On average, approximately one in 5000 to 8000 people are affected, while the founder effect has contributed to a higher prevalence in certain regions, such as the Netherlands Antilles, Jura in France and Funen in Denmark [1]. Vascular malformations in HHT include skin and mucocutaneous telangiectasias, and pulmonary, cerebral, hepatic and spinal arteriovenous malformations (AVMs) [2,3], all of which are susceptible to rupture with resultant spontaneous hemorrhage. Epistaxis is the most common symptom and is present in approximately 95% of patients [4,5]. HHT is a progressive disorder with significant morbidities and mortality, and lacks a universally effective pharmacological therapy [2].

HHT is caused by heterozygous mutations in at least three known genes: endoglin (*ENG*, chromosomal locus 9q34) [6], activin receptor-like kinase 1 (*ACVRL1*, also known as *ALK1*, chromosomal locus 12q1) [7] and mothers against decapentaplegic homolog 4 (*SMAD4*, chromosomal locus 18q21) [8]. Each gene encodes for a protein in the transforming growth factor beta (TGFβ)/bone morphogenetic protein (BMP) signaling pathway. This pathway is responsible for many cellular functions, including growth, differentiation and apoptosis, and is critical in angiogenesis and normal endothelial cell (EC) function [9]. The pathogenic role of these genes has been demonstrated in the adult mouse where the homozygous knockout of *ENG*, *ACVRL1* or *SMAD4* resulted in various vascular defects, including AVMs [10,11]. *ENG* encodes for a TGFβ co-receptor that enhances the affinity of ligand binding to TGFβI and II receptors. This co-receptor is predominately expressed on the endothelium, activated monocytes and macrophages [2]. *ACVRL1* encodes for a TGFβ1 receptor that is predominately expressed on endothelial, lung and placental cells [2]. Mutations in *ENG* and *ACVRL1* result in HHT1 and HHT2, respectively, and on average display distinct clinical manifestations, but overlap is not uncommon. Sabbà et al. demonstrated a higher prevalence of pulmonary (75.5% vs. 44.1%) and cerebral AVMs (20.9% vs. 0%) in HHT1, while liver manifestations were higher in HHT2 (83.1% vs. 60%) [12]. SMAD4 is a signal transducer in the TGFβ signaling pathway that directly regulates gene expression. Mutations in *SMAD4* not only result in HHT, but juvenile polyposis (JP), culminating in a combined syndrome designated as JP/HHT [8]. *ENG* and *ACVRL1* mutations are responsible for 90% of HHT cases, while *SMAD4* contributes to only 2% [13,14]. A small percentage of cases have been attributed to novel disease loci, HHT 3 (chromosomal locus 5q31) [15] and HHT 4 (chromosomal locus 7p14) [16], but these genes have yet to be identified. Over 700 pathogenic mutations have been identified in *ENG* and *ACVRL1* patients (https://arup.utah.edu/database/HHT/, access date: 20/04/2020), comprising single base pair changes, large deletions, duplications, substitutions and missense mutations [13,17]. Interestingly, disease severity and the presentation of clinical manifestations vary drastically between patients and this is further demonstrated in affected family members. This discrepancy suggests that the genetic mutations alone are not entirely responsible for disease characteristics and raises the question: what other biological factors could be at play?

Non-coding RNAs (ncRNAs) are functional ribonucleic acid (RNA) sequences that are transcribed from DNA, but not translated into protein. NcRNAs can be divided into three categories based on their length: (1) ncRNAs longer than 200 nucleotides (nts), including ribosomal RNA (rRNA), long non-coding RNA (lncRNA) and circular RNA (circRNA); (2) ncRNAs shorter than 200 nts, but longer than 40 nts, such as transfer RNA (tRNA), small nucleolar RNA (snoRNA), Ro-associated Y RNA (YRNA) and small nuclear ribonucleic acid RNA (snRNA); and (3) ncRNA shorter than 40 nts like microRNA (miRNA), piwi-interacting RNA (piRNA), short interfering RNA (siRNA) and tRNA-derived small RNA (tsRNA) [18]. NcRNAs regulate gene expression at the transcriptional and post-transcriptional levels, and are involved in a wide array of cellular processes. In particular, snRNAs and snoRNAs are involved in mRNA maturation; rRNAs and tRNAs are important components for protein translation and miRNAs, piRNAs and lncRNAs are involved in the regulation of target gene expression.

MiRNAs (miRs) are the best studied group of noncoding RNAs. They were first described in 1993 by the Ambros and Ruvkun groups and have since caused a paradigm shift in how we understand biological processes [19,20]. Over 2000 miRs have been identified and it has been postulated that they regulate 30% of known genes [20,21]. Processed by endonucleases, the single-stranded miRs bind to cognate mRNAs to induce translational silencing by altering transcript stability or impacting mRNA translation. A single miR can have multiple mRNA targets. MiRs are involved in almost every cellular process [22] and play a role in a wide range of human diseases [22,23]. They have been proven to have reliable diagnostic and prognostic attributes [24], especially in oncology, and are being pursued as potential therapeutic targets [25,26]. A growing class of miRs known as "angio-miRs" have also been shown to contribute to vascular diseases [27]. Given that HHT is a disorder characterized by vascular dysfunction, it is possible that "angio-miRs" play a role in HHT pathogenesis. However, the exact role of any class of miR has yet to be fully characterized in HHT. In this review, we discuss our current understanding of the involvement of ncRNAs in HHT as circulating biomarkers, pathogenic factors and the potential for ncRNAs as therapeutic targets.

2. MiR Biogenesis and Mechanisms of Action

Nearly half of all identified miRs are expressed from specific genes with their own promoters, with the remainder from protein-coding genes [28,29]. Additionally, multiple miRs may be expressed as a single transcript, defined as families or clusters, and share similar target homology [30]. Canonical miR biogenesis is initiated with miR gene transcription by an RNA polymerase II [31]. The result is an ~80 nucleotide stem–loop structure called a primary miR (pri-miR) [32]. The pri-miR is further processed by an RNase III enzyme and a double-stranded RNA-binding protein (dsRBP), called Drosha and DGCR8, respectively [32]. This complex shortens the pri-miR to ~70 nts to generate the pre-miR. The pre-miR is exported from the nucleus to the cytoplasm where it is once again processed by an RNase III enzyme and dsRBP, Dicer and transactivation-responsive (TAR) RNA-binding protein (TRBP), respectively, effectively removing the hairpin to produce a miR–miR duplex [32,33]. The duplex comprises a passenger strand and a guide strand. The passenger strand is degraded, while the guide strand is incorporated into the RNA-induced silencing complex (RISC). Strand incorporation is dependent on the thermodynamic stability of the 5′ end of the miR–miR duplex, where the less stable strand is incorporated [34]. RISC contains an RNA binding protein responsible for miR silencing activity, Argonaute 2 (AGO2). AGO2 has potent RNase-H-like endonuclease activity and is capable of cleaving mRNAs [35].

MiRs guide the RISC–AGO complex to target mRNAs by recognizing the miR response element (MRE) in the 3′ untranslated region (UTR) [36,37]. Alterative binding sites have been identified in the 5′ UTR, coding sequences and within promoter regions [37]. Base pair complementarity between miRs and MREs dictates the mode of gene silencing. Perfect complementarity activates AGO2′s endonuclease activity, resulting in the cleavage and subsequent degradation of target mRNAs [35]. However, in metazoans, this rarely occurs and the majority of miR–MRE interactions are not perfectly complementary [38]. In this scenario, translational inhibition can occur where the miR–RISC–AGO complex likely blocks translational machinery from binding. Alternatively, proteins in complex with AGO2 can recruit poly(A)-deadenylases to elicit mRNA degradation [38]. In this way, miRs can regulate the expression of tens to hundreds of mRNAs. Bioinformatic analyses can use algorithms to predict complementarity for the identification of hundreds of mRNA targets per miR, but realistically only a small subset are experimentally validated [21]. It is important to note that individual miR activity is dependent on several factors, including miR tissue expression profiles (tissue-specific vs. housekeeping) and miR expression levels. Typically, higher miR expression will have a more robust effect on target mRNAs.

3. Circulating MiR Biomarkers in HHT

The discovery of circulating miRs was achieved by several groups [39–41], most notably by Chim et al. who identified that stable plasma miRs could distinguish between pregnant and non-pregnant women [42]. Since then, circulating miRs have been established as stable and sensitive candidate biomarkers for various diseases, including cancers, cardiovascular diseases and neurological disorders [43–46]. The stability of circulating miRs can be attributed to their association with proteins such as AGO2 [47] and lipoproteins [48] or their containment in extracellular vesicles [49]. In this way, miRs are shielded from RNase enzymes and are stable in blood for up to 24 h [50]. Changes in circulating miR levels have been shown to be extremely sensitive to disease conditions and can outperform conventional biomarkers. For example, changes in circulating miR levels in response to disease states have been shown to be more rapid than those of mRNAs or proteins [46,51]. Oerlemans et al. demonstrated that changes in circulating miRs were detected earlier compared with that of troponin for the diagnosis and management of acute coronary syndrome [52].

HHT is diagnosed in combination by a clinical criteria known as the Curaçao criteria [53] and the molecular detection of known genetic mutations. Due to loci heterogeneity, technical challenges of molecular diagnostic techniques and de novo mutations, a clinical diagnosis is always required [53]. Additional biomarkers would greatly improve the diagnostic process as HHT is actually underdiagnosed [54]; they could also aid in the detection and management of clinical manifestations. The detection of AVMs is critical for the management of patient well-being. Approximately 50% of patients develop pulmonary AVMs (PAVMs), 80% develop hepatic AVMs (HAVMs), 10% develop cerebral AVMs (CAVMs) and 1% develop spinal AVMs (SAVMs) [2,55]. All AVMs are susceptible to rupture that can cause numerous life-threatening complications, including hemorrhagic and ischemic stroke, air embolism, congestive heart failure, cerebral abscess and seizure [55,56]. The timely detection of AVMs is critical to prevent serious and life-threatening complications, but current diagnostic screens are costly, relatively inaccessible and expose patients to unhealthy doses of radiation [57]. Circulating miRs could potentially provide a rapid, inexpensive, safe and relatively non-invasive screening test for the diagnosis of AVMs.

3.1. Elevated Circulating MiR-210 and PAVMs in HHT

A previous study from our laboratory identified a candidate circulating miR biomarker for the detection of PAVMs in HHT patients. Plasma miRs from HHT patients with PAVMs and healthy controls were profiled with a microarray analysis and a total of eight miRs were found to be dysregulated [58]. Select miRs identified by the array were validated with a reverse transcription quantitative polymerase chain reaction (RT-qPCR) and miR-210 was found to be significantly upregulated in plasma from HHT patients with PAVMs [58]. Additionally, miR-210 is a well characterized "hypoximir" that is robustly expressed in ECs under hypoxia [59,60]. The increased levels of circulating miR-210 identified in our study may be a result of PAVM-induced hypoxemia. It is also possible that this phenomenon may be a compensatory mechanism since EC overexpression of miR-210 has been shown to augment angiogenesis and tube formation [61]. Our study successfully identified a novel circulating miR biomarker that can potentially detect HHT patients only with PAVMs. However, it is necessary to improve the validity of this biomarker with a more clinically relevant sample size. Future work will aim to measure circulating miR-210 levels in HHT patients with treated PAVMs. Presumably, once an AVM is treated, typically by coil embolization, associated symptoms like hypoxemia should disappear. If miR-210 is in fact induced by hypoxia, then its levels should return to baseline once a PAVM has been treated. If this is the case, miR-210 stands to be an extremely sensitive and reliable biomarker for the detection of PAVMs in HHT.

3.2. Dysregulated Levels of Circulating MiR-205 and MiR-27a in HHT

Tabruyn et al. were the second to identify circulating miR dysregulation in HHT [62]. They conducted a miR microarray analysis on plasma from four HHT patients (two HHT1 and two HHT2) and identified 34 dysregulated miRs; 32 were upregulated, while two were downregulated. MiR-205 and miR-27a were selected for RT-qPCR validation in 24 HHT patients (11 HHT1 vs. 13 HHT2) and 16 controls. It was found that miR-205 was significantly decreased and miR-27a was significantly increased in HHT patient plasma. There were no significant differences between the expression of these miRs between HHT1 and HHT2 patients. This consistency highlights the potential of miRs as ideal candidates for the diagnosis of HHT.

MiR-27a is relatively well characterized and has been implicated in EC function [62,63], angiogenesis [63,64] and cancer [65]. Interestingly, a recent study has shown that miR-27a is hypoxia inducible [66]. Therefore, it is possible that the observed increase may be a result of HHT-related hypoxemia. However, Tabruyn et al. did not describe the clinical characteristics of enrolled patients. It would be interesting to explore the role hypoxia may play with regard to increased levels of miR-27a. Additionally, miR-27a has many putative targets in the TGFβ pathway, including SMADs (1/4/5/2), TGFβRI, ZEB2 and SP1 [67,68] (Figure 1). Future research should experimentally validate these targets in ECs. The involvement of miR-205 in angiogenesis and EC function is not well characterized; one study demonstrated that miR-205 regulates the expression of integrin β4, a major component of EC gap junctions [69]. Additionally, miR-205 has been shown to be involved in TGFβ signaling where it targets downstream transcription factors ZEB2 and SIP1 [70]. MiR-205 was shown to negatively respond to TGFβ1 stimulation in epithelial cells [71]. Tabruyn et al. further characterized the role of miR-205 in human umbilical vein endothelial cells (HUVECs). Overexpression of miR-205 in HUVECs decreased proliferation, migration and tube formation, while inhibition resulted in the opposite. Additionally, they described a role of miR-205 as a regulator of TGFβ signaling by targeting SMAD4 and SMAD1. They also demonstrated that miR-205 overexpression led to a significant increase in PAI-1 and a significant reduction in ID-1 mRNA levels. TGFβ signaling can be transduced by ALK1 and ALK5 pathways, where the former leads to EC activation, and the latter, EC quiescence. The effects of ALK1 and ALK5 signaling can predominately be attributed to the expression of PAI-1 and ID-1, respectively. They postulated that the observed reduction of circulating miR-205 levels is a result of reduced ALK1 signaling. They further suggested that the observed increase in circulating miR-27a is due to an increase in ALK5 signaling. This is based on the notion that an increase in ALK5 signaling is due to the reduction of ALK1 signaling in HHT. However, it has been demonstrated that ALK1 and ALK5 signaling maintain a very fine balance; if one pathway was reduced, the other would be equally reduced [9]. This was demonstrated in ECs cultured from HHT patient blood, known as blood outgrowth endothelial cells (BOECs) [72], and in ENG heterozygous mouse embryonic stem cells [73]. Thus, it is possible that the observed decrease and elevation in circulating miR-205 and miR-27a, respectively, may be the result of an alternate mechanism.

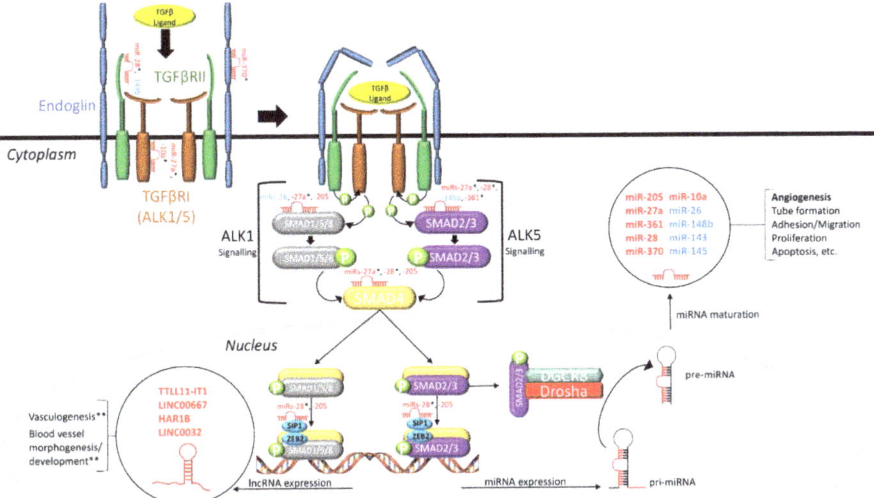

Figure 1. Interactions between non-coding RNAs and the TGFβ signaling pathway in hereditary hemorrhagic telangiectasia (HHT). As shown in this schematic diagram, dysregulated microRNAs (miRs) (in red) identified in HHT patients directly target a number of TGFβ signaling molecules, including SMADs and TGFβRs, and dysregulated lncRNAs (in red) found in HHT patients have a purported role in regulating vasculogenesis and vessel morphogenesis and development. SMAD2/3 can alternatively incorporate with the microprocessor complex to regulate the processing of pri-miRNA to pre-miRNA. Aberrant TGFβ signaling has been found to result in the altered expression of various miRs (in blue) that are involved in angiogenesis. The interaction between non-coding RNAs and TGFβ signaling establishes a narrative for their involvement in HHT pathogenesis. TGFβ: transforming growth factor beta; TGFβRI/II: TGFβ receptor I/II; ALK1/5: activin receptor-like kinase 1/5; miRNA: microRNA; lncRNA: long non-coding RNA; SMAD1/2/3/4/5/8: mothers against decapentaplegic homolog 1/2/3/4/5/8; SIP1: Smad interacting protein 1; ZEB2: zinc finger e-box binding homeobox 2; DGCR8: DiGeorge syndrome critical region gene 8; pri-miRNA: primary miRNA; pre-miRNA: precursor miRNA; "P": phosphoryl group (* putative targets, ** predicted by bioinformatics).

3.3. Dysregulated Circulating MiR-370 and MiR-10a in HHT1 and HHT2

Recently, Ruiz-Llorente et al. further identified dysregulated circulating miRs in HHT patient plasma [74]. In this study, the authors employed a miR-target prediction algorithm to specifically identify miRs that target ENG and/or ALK1. From the analysis, miR-370 and miR-10a were highly predicted to target ENG and ALK1, respectively, and miR-214 was highly predicted to target both ENG and ALK1. These miRs were selected for RT-qPCR validation in 34 HHT patients (17 HHT1 vs. 17 HHT2) and 16 controls. It was found that miR-370 was significantly decreased only in HHT1 patients compared with HHT2 patients and controls, while miR-10a was significantly increased only in HHT2 patients compared with HHT1 patients and controls. MiR-214 was not found to be significantly dysregulated.

MiR-370 has been experimentally validated to target ENG in ovarian cancer cells [75], yet its role in EC function and angiogenesis is unclear, as multiple reports have demonstrated conflicting evidence. Overexpression of miR-370 inhibited proliferation, migration and tube formation in human dermal microvascular ECs, retinal capillary ECs and HUVECs [76,77]. In contrast, miR-370 overexpression was shown to promote HUVEC proliferation, migration and tube formation to facilitate healing after finger amputation [78]. Additionally, miR-370 suppression by circular RNA circ_0003204 inhibited the proliferation, migration and tube formation of human aortic ECs [79]. It is unclear why this discrepancy exists, but suggests a far more complex role of miR-370 in EC function. MiR-10a has been shown to have anti-angiogenic effects in mouse umbilical vein ECs by targeting β-catenin [80]. It has also been shown to regulate VCAM1 expression in ECs under hemodynamic force by targeting GATA6 [81]. Therefore, an exact functional role in HHT pathogenesis remains unclear, but their potential as diagnostic biomarkers in HHT shows great promise. The ability of these miRs to distinguish between HHT1 or HHT2 patients could greatly improve the diagnostic process, as a number of HHT patients are asymptomatic or lack a known genetic mutation. Further research is required to validate these miRs in a more clinically relevant sample size and to directly confirm that these miRs indeed target ENG and ALK1 in ECs.

4. MiRs as Pathogenic Factors in HHT

MiRs have been demonstrated to play a pathogenic role in a variety of human diseases, including cancer, cardiovascular disease, autoimmune diseases and inflammatory diseases [22,23]. MiR profiling analyses have identified a plethora of up- and downregulated miRs in numerous types of cancers [24]. It has been shown that overexpressed miRs can act as "oncomiRs" by targeting tumor suppressors or by promoting proliferation and inhibiting apoptosis [82]. Additionally, the downregulation of certain "tumor suppressor" miRs, such as let-7, can also contribute to cancer pathogenesis [83,84]. A growing class of miRs known as "angio-miRs", predominately expressed in ECs and responsible for the regulation of angiogenic processes, have also been shown to contribute to cancer and cardiovascular disease [27]. Given that HHT is a disorder characterized by angiogenic and EC dysfunction, it would not be surprising if dysregulated "angio-miRs" played a role in disease pathogenesis. There are numerous studies that have identified the involvement of miRs in TGFβ signaling. They have demonstrated that various components of the TGFβ pathway are targeted by miRs and that the pathway itself regulates miR biogenesis [85].

4.1. Canonical TGFβ Signaling in HHT

The TGFβ signaling cascade is initiated with the TGFβ superfamily of ligands (TGFβ1/3, BMPs, activin) binding in complex to two cell surface receptors; Type I (RI), such as ALK1/5, and Type II (RII) [86] (Figure 1). Upon ligand binding, these receptors form a heteromeric complex, activating their serine/threonine kinase activity [86]. Endoglin is an auxiliary co-receptor that can interact with the RI–RII–ligand complex to enhance ligand affinity [87]. Subsequently, RII will trans-phosphorylate RI, which in turn will phosphorylate the family of receptor-regulated SMADs (R-SMAD 1/2/3/5/8) [88]. The TGFβ pathway can propagate the signal through two cascades: SMAD1/5/8 or SMAD2/3. ALK1 signals through SMAD1/5/8, leading to EC activation [9,13]. ALK5 propagates the signal through SMAD2/3, leading to EC quiescence [9,13]. It has been shown that endoglin enhances the SMAD1/5/8 pathway and inhibits the SMAD2/3 pathway. Cascade selection is determined by the combination of ligand and receptors. Regardless of the selected cascade, both groups of R-SMADs interact with a common partner SMAD (Co-SMAD) known as SMAD4 [88]. This complex of R- and Co-SMADs translocates to the nucleus where it regulates the transcription of target genes [88].

4.2. Drosha and HHT Pathogenesis

Drosha is part of a protein complex called the microprocessor that is responsible for the cleavage of pri-miR into pre-miR [89]. The silencing of Drosha in HeLa cells results in the aggregation of pri-miRs and a decrease in pre-miRs [90]. Drosha is fundamental in the biogenesis of almost all miRs, but has also been shown to be involved in the regulation of mRNAs [90]. A few studies have demonstrated that Drosha can bind and cleave mRNAs, and can also associate with promoter regions to regulate specific genes [91–93]. In the TGFβ pathway, SMAD2/3 has been shown to incorporate with the microprocessor complex to regulate target miR genes [82,91] (Figure 1).

Kuehbacher et al. demonstrated that the knockdown of Drosha in HUVECs had a minimal effect on EC migration, viability and tube formation [94]. In vivo analysis of Drosha knockdown in a matrigel plug did not reveal significant effects on sprouting angiogenesis [94]. Even though Drosha knockdown had an insignificant effect on angiogenesis and EC function it reduced the expression of 29 miRs by 30% [94]. It is possible that the knockdown of Drosha activated compensatory mechanisms that mitigated its effects on EC function and angiogenesis. An inducible EC-specific knockout mouse model of Drosha would certainly provide a more robust analysis.

A study by Jiang et al. identified a higher prevalence of Drosha mutations in an HHT population and generated robust Drosha knockout animal models. Exome sequencing was performed on a total of 98 individuals; 23 confirmed HHT patients and 75 probands suspected to have HHT who lacked known pathogenic mutations [95]. Three heterozygous Drosha mutations (P32L, P100L and K226E) were detected in seven of the 98 individuals (~7%) compared with 0.04% in the general population [93]. An additional Drosha mutant (R279L) was found in a separate HHT family [93]. These Drosha mutants were analyzed in mouse embryonic fibroblasts (MEFs); interestingly, only the P100L and R279L mutants were shown to reduce expression of specific miRs, by approximately 17% and 35%, respectively, compared to wild type (WT) [95]. P100L and R279L were introduced into zebrafish embryos to investigate their angiogenic functions. Zebrafish with these two mutants developed vascular defects, including vascular permeability and a reduction of vascular density [95]. An EC-specific inducible knockout Drosha mouse model also demonstrated vascular permeability, disorganized vasculature and, interestingly, intestinal bleeding [95]. However, no AVMs were detected in either animal model [95].

The presence of Drosha mutations in HHT populations may contribute to disease pathogenesis and the observed clinical spectrum. BOECs derived from HHT patients with Drosha mutations may be a robust cellular model to profile and characterize affected miRs and mRNAs. Drosha itself has also been shown to regulate gene expression directly [90]. It would be interesting to identify Drosha-targeted genes and elucidate how they may contribute to HHT pathogenesis.

4.3. MiRs and HHT Pathogenesis

Few studies have characterized the role of miRs in HHT pathogenesis. However, numerous miRs have been identified to be regulated by and target components of the TGFβ pathway in a variety of tissues and disease conditions [85]. MiR-26 has recently been shown to be involved in vascular stability, where its knockdown in zebrafish led to vascular hemorrhage [96]. MiR-26 from ECs can regulate vascular smooth muscle cell (VSMC) differentiation in a paracrine manner [96]. It was shown that a decrease in miR-26 leads to an increase in its target, SMAD1, resulting in VSMC dysregulation and hemorrhage [96]. Another study demonstrated that the overexpression of miR-148b can improve migration, proliferation and angiogenesis in HUVECs by targeting SMAD2 and TGFβRII [97]. Subsequently, wound vascularization and healing were greatly augmented by a miR-148b mimic in a wound-healing mouse model [97]. MiR-148b inhibition greatly impaired wound healing, which was rescued by silencing SMAD2 [97]. A separate study demonstrated that VSMCs could regulate EC function via TGFβ-mediated secretion of miRs-143/145 [98]. Co-culture of VSMCs overexpressing miRs-143/145 with ECs greatly impaired EC function, while inhibition of the TGFβ pathway reversed this effect [98]. This study demonstrates how VSMCs can regulate EC activation/quiescence through the secretion of miRs in a TGFβ-dependent manner [98].

A previous study from our laboratory identified significantly decreased levels of miR-361-3p and miR-28-5p in peripheral blood mononuclear cells (PBMCs) derived from HHT patients [99]. PBMCs are mostly comprise lymphocytes and monocytes [100]. The pathogenic potential of PBMCs has been demonstrated in HHT1 mouse models. It has been shown that dysregulated TGFβ signaling adversely affects PBMC migratory capacity, which contributes to vascular dysplasia and prolonged inflammation [101,102]. The mRNA level of insulin-like growth factor 1 (IGF1), a putative target of miR-28-5p and miR-361-3p, was shown to be significantly upregulated in HHT patient-derived PBMCs. However, IGF1 plasma protein levels were not significantly different between patients and controls. It is possible that IGF1 could be overexpressed at angiogenic or inflammatory sites rather than systemically, contributing to the development of vascular dysplasia. IGF1 has been shown to play a significant role in augmenting angiogenesis in vitro and in vivo [103]. A previous study demonstrated that miR-361-3p is involved in the function of proangiogenic Tie2-expressing monocytes by targeting IGF1 [104]. MiR-28-5p has been shown to directly target IGF1 in hepatocellular carcinomas [105] and liver cancer stem cells [106]. Additionally, miR-28-5p and miR-361-3p have multiple putative targets in the TGFβ pathway, including SMADs, TGFβRII and SP1 [66,67] (Figure 1). It is possible that the observed decrease in miR-28-5p and miR-361-3p and increase in IGF1 may be a compensatory mechanism in response to reduced TGFβ signaling. Further research is required to understand the role these miRs play in PBMC dysfunction and ultimately HHT pathogenesis.

5. LncRNAs and HHT

LncRNAs are non-coding RNA species that are greater than 200 nucleotides in length and regulate gene expression post-transcriptionally [18]. LncRNAs can be divided into two functional groups based on their sub-cellular localization: (1) nuclear and (2) cytoplasmic. Nuclear lncRNAs can influence gene expression via various mechanisms, including chromatin remodeling, protein sequestration and the enhancement or dampening of promoter activity [107]. One of the ways that cytoplasmic lncRNAs can influence gene expression is by regulating the availability and stability of miRs by acting as miR "sponges" [107]. Although lncRNA mechanisms have been well characterized, evidence suggests that most lncRNAs are non-functional [107]. Nonetheless, a few lncRNAs have been implicated in vascular and endothelial cell biology. For example, the lncRNA MALAT1 was shown to promote EC proliferation and migration under hypoxic conditions [108]. Conversely, MEG3 was demonstrated to inhibit EC proliferation, survival and tube formation [108]. Singh et al. were the first to identify differential expression of lncRNAs in TGFβ1-stimulated HUVECs [109]. They demonstrated that 2051 and 2393 lncRNAs were significantly upregulated and downregulated, respectively. Of these, MALAT1 was upregulated the most (~220-fold), contributing to its role in EC biology. Given the functional relevance of lncRNAs in EC biology, one would assume that they may play a role in HHT. Indeed, Tørring et al. sought to profile lncRNAs from nasal mucosa telangiectasias of HHT1 and HHT2 patients [110], and identified 42 lncRNAs that were significantly dysregulated ($p < 0.001$), including TTLL11-IT1, LINC00667, HAR1B and LINC0032, compared to non-telangiectasial nasal mucosa from the same HHT patients. However, none of the dysregulated lncRNAs have been characterized. Bioinformatic analysis revealed that these lncRNAs were enriched in HHT-related pathways, including vasculogenesis and blood vessel morphogenesis and development (Figure 1). Further research is required to characterize the role these dysregulated lncRNAs may play in HHT pathogenesis.

6. Conclusions and Future Research

The observation of ncRNA dysregulation in ECs and PBMCs from patients with HHT suggests that they may play a role in the pathogenesis of HHT. Further characterization of ncRNAs in other cell types involved in HHT, including VSMCs, pericytes and mononuclear cells is necessary to more fully understand the pathogenetic mechanisms controlling the disease and its progression.

To date, the targets and functions of only a small fraction of ncRNAs identified in humans have been rigorously explored. With further research, ncRNAs may prove to have both diagnostic and therapeutic applications for those with HHT.

Funding: Our HHT research was funded in part as a pilot project of the Brain Vascular Malformation Consortium (BVMC). The BVMC is supported by National Institutes of Health (NIH) grant U54 NS065705. The BVMC is part of the NIH Rare Disease Clinical Research Network (RDCRN), supported through collaboration between the NIH Office of Rare Diseases Research (ORDR) at the National Center for Advancing Translational Science (NCATS), and the National Institute of Neurological Disorders and Stroke (NINDS).

Acknowledgments: The authors would like to thank the staff at the Toronto HHT Centre at St. Michael's Hospital for their help in patient recruitment, and Si-Cheng Dai and Daniel Han from Western University and the University of Toronto, respectively, for editing.

Conflicts of Interest: The authors declare no conflict of interest.

References

1. Zarrabeitia, R.; Albiñana, V.; Salcedo, M.; Señaris-Gonzalez, B.; Fernandez-Forcelledo, J.-L.; Botella, L.-M. A review on clinical management and pharmacological therapy on hereditary haemorrhagic telangiectasia (HHT). *Curr. Vasc. Pharmacol.* **2010**, *8*, 473–481. [CrossRef] [PubMed]

2. McDonald, J.; Bayrak-Toydemir, P.; Pyeritz, R.E. Hereditary hemorrhagic telangiectasia: An overview of diagnosis, management, and pathogenesis. *Genet. Med.* **2011**, *13*, 607–616. [CrossRef] [PubMed]

3. Bayrak-Toydemir, P.; Mao, R.; Lewin, S.; McDonald, J. Hereditary hemorrhagic telangiectasia: An overview of diagnosis and management in the molecular era for clinicians. *Genet. Med.* **2004**, *6*, 175–191. [CrossRef] [PubMed]

4. Puente, R.Z.; Bueno, J.; Salcedo, M. Epidemiology of Hereditary Haemorrhagic Telangiectasia (HHT) in Spain. *Hered. Genet.* **2016**, *05*, 173. [CrossRef]

5. Clark, M.; Berry, P.; Martin, S.; Harris, N.; Sprecher, D.; Olitsky, S.; Hoag, J.B. Nosebleeds in hereditary hemorrhagic telangiectasia: Development of a patient-completed daily eDiary. *Laryngoscope Investig. Otolaryngol.* **2018**, *3*, 439–445. [CrossRef]

6. McAllister, K.A.; Grogg, K.M.; Johnson, D.W.; Gallione, C.J.; Baldwin, M.A.; Jackson, C.E.; Helmbold, E.A.; Markel, D.S.; McKinnon, W.C.; Murrell, J. Endoglin, a TGF-beta binding protein of endothelial cells, is the gene for hereditary haemorrhagic telangiectasia type 1. *Nat. Genet.* **1994**, *8*, 345–351. [CrossRef]

7. Johnson, D.W.; Berg, J.N.; Baldwin, M.A.; Gallione, C.J.; Marondel, I.; Yoon, S.J.; Stenzel, T.T.; Speer, M.; Pericak-Vance, M.A.; Diamond, A.; et al. Mutations in the Activin Receptor-Like Kinase 1 Gene in Hereditary Haemorrhagic Telangiectasia Type 2. *Nat. Genet.* **1996**, *13*, 189–195. [CrossRef]

8. Gallione, C.J.; Repetto, G.M.; Legius, E.; Rustgi, A.K.; Schelley, S.L.; Tejpar, S.; Mitchell, G.; Drouin, É.; Westermann, C.J.J.; Marchuk, D.A. A Combined Syndrome of Juvenile Polyposis and Hereditary Haemorrhagic Telangiectasia Associated with Mutations in MADH4 (SMAD4). *Lancet* **2004**, *363*, 852–859. [CrossRef]

9. Fernández-L, A.; Sanz-Rodriguez, F.; Blanco, F.J.; Bernabéu, C.; Botella, L.M. Hereditary hemorrhagic telangiectasia, a vascular dysplasia affecting the TGF-beta signaling pathway. *Clin. Med. Res.* **2006**, *4*, 66–78. [CrossRef]

10. Tual-Chalot, S.; Oh, S.P.; Arthur, H.M. Mouse models of hereditary hemorrhagic telangiectasia: Recent advances and future challenges. *Front. Genet.* **2015**, *6*, 1–25. [CrossRef]

11. Crist, A.M.; Lee, A.R.; Patel, N.R.; Westhoff, D.E.; Meadows, S.M. Vascular deficiency of Smad4 causes arteriovenous malformations: A mouse model of Hereditary Hemorrhagic Telangiectasia. *Angiogenesis* **2018**, *21*, 363–380. [CrossRef] [PubMed]

12. Sabbà, C.; Pasculli, G.; Lenato, G.M.; Suppressa, P.; Lastella, P.; Memeo, M.; Dicuonzo, F.; Guanti, G. Hereditary hemorrhagic telangiectasia: Clinical features in ENG and ALK1 mutation carriers. *J. Thromb. Haemost.* **2007**, *5*, 1149–1157. [CrossRef]

13. Bernabéu, C.; Blanco, F.J.; Langa, C.; Garrido-Martin, E.M.; Botella, L.M. Involvement of the TGF-β superfamily signalling pathway in hereditary haemorrhagic telangiectasia. *J. Appl. Biomed.* **2010**, *8*, 169–177. [CrossRef]

14. Gallione, C.J.; Richards, J.A.; Letteboer, T.G.W.; Rushlow, D.; Prigoda, N.L.; Leedom, T.P.; Ganguly, A.; Castells, A.; Ploos van Amstel, J.K.; Westermann, C.J.J.; et al. SMAD4 mutations found in unselected HHT patients. *J. Med. Genet.* **2006**, *43*, 793–797. [CrossRef]

15. Cole, S.G.; Begbie, M.E.; Wallace, G.M.F.; Shovlin, C.L. A new locus for hereditary haemorrhagic telangiectasia (HHT3) maps to chromosome 5. *J. Med. Genet.* **2005**, *42*, 577–582. [CrossRef] [PubMed]

16. Bayrak-Toydemir, P.; McDonald, J.; Akarsu, N.; Toydemir, R.M.; Calderon, F.; Tuncali, T.; Tang, W.; Miller, F.; Mao, R. A fourth locus for hereditary hemorrhagic telangiectasia maps to chromosome 7. *Am. J. Med. Genet. Part A* **2006**, *140A*, 2155–2162. [CrossRef]

17. Albiñana, V.; Zafra, M.P.; Colau, J.; Zarrabeitia, R.; Recio-Poveda, L.; Olavarrieta, L.; Pérez-Pérez, J.; Botella, L.M. Mutation affecting the proximal promoter of Endoglin as the origin of hereditary hemorrhagic telangiectasia type 1. *BMC Med. Genet.* **2017**, *18*, 20. [CrossRef]

18. Kapranov, P.; Cheng, J.; Dike, S.; Nix, D.A.; Duttagupta, R.; Willingham, A.T.; Stadler, P.F.; Hertel, J.; Hackermuller, J.; Hofacker, I.L.; et al. RNA Maps Reveal New RNA Classes and a Possible Function for Pervasive Transcription. *Science* **2007**, *316*, 1484–1488. [CrossRef]

19. Lee, R.C.; Feinbaum, R.L.; Ambros, V. The C. elegans heterochronic gene lin-4 encodes small RNAs with antisense complementarity to lin-14. *Cell* **1993**, *75*, 843–854. [CrossRef]

20. Wightman, B.; Ha, I.; Ruvkun, G. Posttranscriptional Regulation of the Heterochronic Gene lin-14 by lin-4 Mediates Temporal Pattern Formation in C. Elegans. *Cell* **1993**, *75*, 855–862. [CrossRef]

21. Hammond, S.M. An overview of microRNAs. *Adv. Drug Deliv. Rev.* **2015**, *87*, 3–14. [CrossRef] [PubMed]

22. Bushati, N.; Cohen, S.M. microRNA Functions. *Annu. Rev. Cell Dev. Biol.* **2007**, *23*, 175–205. [CrossRef] [PubMed]

23. Ardekani, A.M.; Naeini, M.M. The Role of MicroRNAs in Human Diseases. *Avicenna J. Med. Biotechnol.* **2010**, *2*, 161–179. [CrossRef] [PubMed]

24. Ha, T.-Y. MicroRNAs in Human Diseases: From Cancer to Cardiovascular Disease. *Immune Netw.* **2011**, *11*, 135. [CrossRef]

25. Wang, H.; Peng, R.; Wang, J.; Qin, Z.; Xue, L. Circulating microRNAs as potential cancer biomarkers: The advantage and disadvantage. *Clin. Epigenetics* **2018**, *10*, 1–10. [CrossRef]

26. Dwivedi, S.; Purohit, P.; Sharma, P. MicroRNAs and Diseases: Promising Biomarkers for Diagnosis and Therapeutics. *Indian J. Clin. Biochem.* **2019**, *34*, 243–245. [CrossRef]

27. Salinas-Vera, Y.M.; Marchat, L.A.; Gallardo-Rincón, D.; Ruiz-García, E.; Astudillo-De la Vega, H.; Echavarría-Zepeda, R.; López-Camarillo, C. AngiomiRs: MicroRNAs driving angiogenesis in cancer (Review). *Int. J. Mol. Med.* **2019**, *43*, 657–670. [CrossRef]

28. De Rie, D.; Abugessaisa, I.; Alam, T.; Arner, E.; Arner, P.; Ashoor, H.; Åström, G.; Babina, M.; Bertin, N.; Burroughs, A.M.; et al. An integrated expression atlas of miRNAs and their promoters in human and mouse. *Nat. Biotechnol.* **2017**, *35*, 872–878. [CrossRef]

29. Kim, Y.K.; Kim, V.N. Processing of intronic microRNAs. *EMBO J.* **2007**, *26*, 775–783. [CrossRef]

30. Tanzer, A.; Stadler, P.F. Molecular evolution of a microRNA cluster. *J. Mol. Biol.* **2004**, *339*, 327–335. [CrossRef]

31. Ha, M.; Kim, V.N. Regulation of microRNA biogenesis. *Nat. Rev. Mol. Cell Biol.* **2014**, *15*, 509–524. [CrossRef] [PubMed]

32. Denli, A.M.; Tops, B.B.J.; Plasterk, R.H.A.; Ketting, R.F.; Hannon, G.J. Processing of primary microRNAs by the Microprocessor complex. *Nature* **2004**, *432*, 231–235. [CrossRef] [PubMed]

33. Zhang, H.; Kolb, F.A.; Jaskiewicz, L.; Westhof, E.; Filipowicz, W. Single processing center models for human Dicer and bacterial RNase III. *Cell* **2004**, *118*, 57–68. [CrossRef] [PubMed]

34. Khvorova, A.; Reynolds, A.; Jayasena, S.D. Erratum: Functional siRNAs and miRNAs Exhibit Strand Bias (Cell 115 (209-216)). *Cell* **2003**, *115*, 209–216. [CrossRef]

35. Jo, M.H.; Shin, S.; Jung, S.R.; Kim, E.; Song, J.J.; Hohng, S. Human Argonaute 2 Has Diverse Reaction Pathways on Target RNAs. *Mol. Cell* **2015**, *59*, 117–124. [CrossRef]

36. Ipsaro, J.J.; Joshua-Tor, L. From guide to target: Molecular insights into eukaryotic RNA-interference machinery. *Nat. Struct. Mol. Biol.* **2015**, *22*, 20–28. [CrossRef]

37. Xu, W.; Lucas, A.S.; Wang, Z.; Liu, Y. Identifying microRNA targets in different gene regions. *BMC Bioinformatics* **2014**, *15*, S4. [CrossRef]

38. Jonas, S.; Izaurralde, E. Towards a molecular understanding of microRNA-mediated gene silencing. *Nat. Rev. Genet.* **2015**, *16*, 421–433. [CrossRef]

39. Chen, X.; Ba, Y.; Ma, L.; Cai, X.; Yin, Y.; Wang, K.; Guo, J.; Zhang, Y.; Chen, J.; Guo, X.; et al. Characterization of microRNAs in serum: A novel class of biomarkers for diagnosis of cancer and other diseases. *Cell Res.* **2008**, *18*, 997–1006. [CrossRef]

40. Hunter, M.P.; Ismail, N.; Zhang, X.; Aguda, B.D.; Lee, E.J.; Yu, L.; Xiao, T.; Schafer, J.; Lee, M.-L.T.; Schmittgen, T.D.; et al. Correction: Detection of microRNA Expression in Human Peripheral Blood Microvesicles. *PLoS ONE* **2010**, *5*. [CrossRef]

41. Mitchell, P.S.; Parkin, R.K.; Kroh, E.M.; Fritz, B.R.; Wyman, S.K.; Pogosova-Agadjanyan, E.L.; Peterson, A.; Noteboom, J.; O'Briant, K.C.; Allen, A.; et al. Circulating microRNAs as stable blood-based markers for cancer detection. *Proc. Natl. Acad. Sci. USA* **2008**, *105*, 10513–10518. [CrossRef] [PubMed]

42. Chim, S.S.C.; Shing, T.K.F.; Hung, E.C.W.; Leung, T.Y.; Lau, T.K.; Chiu, R.W.K.; Lo, Y.M.D. Detection and characterization of placental microRNAs in maternal plasma. *Clin. Chem.* **2008**, *54*, 482–490. [CrossRef] [PubMed]

43. Maqbool, R.; Hussain, M.U. MicroRNAs and human diseases: Diagnostic and therapeutic potential. *Cell Tissue Res.* **2014**, *358*, 1–15. [CrossRef]

44. Sohel, M.M.H. Circulating microRNAs as biomarkers in cancer diagnosis. *Life Sci.* **2020**, *248*, 117473. [CrossRef]

45. Khoury, S.; Tran, N. Circulating microRNAs: Potential biomarkers for common malignancies. *Biomark. Med.* **2015**, *9*, 131–151. [CrossRef] [PubMed]

46. Wang, J.; Chen, J.; Sen, S. MicroRNA as Biomarkers and Diagnostics. *J. Cell. Physiol.* **2016**, *231*, 25–30. [CrossRef]

47. Arroyo, J.D.; Chevillet, J.R.; Kroh, E.M.; Ruf, I.K.; Pritchard, C.C.; Gibson, D.F.; Mitchell, P.S.; Bennett, C.F.; Pogosova-Agadjanyan, E.L.; Stirewalt, D.L.; et al. Argonaute2 complexes carry a population of circulating microRNAs independent of vesicles in human plasma. *Proc. Natl. Acad. Sci. USA* **2011**, *108*, 5003–5008. [CrossRef]

48. Vickers, K.C.; Palmisano, B.T.; Shoucri, B.M.; Shamburek, R.D.; Remaley, A.T. MicroRNAs are transported in plasma and delivered to recipient cells by high-density lipoproteins. *Nat. Cell Biol.* **2011**, *13*, 423–435. [CrossRef]

49. Ismail, N.; Wang, Y.; Dakhlallah, D.; Moldovan, L.; Agarwal, K.; Batte, K.; Shah, P.; Wisler, J.; Eubank, T.D.; Tridandapani, S.; et al. Macrophage microvesicles induce macrophage differentiation and miR-223 transfer. *Blood* **2013**, *121*, 984–995. [CrossRef]

50. Glinge, C.; Clauss, S.; Boddum, K.; Jabbari, R.; Jabbari, J.; Risgaard, B.; Tomsits, P.; Hildebrand, B.; Kääb, S.; Wakili, R.; et al. Stability of Circulating Blood-Based MicroRNAs – Pre-Analytic Methodological Considerations. *PLoS ONE* **2017**, *12*, e0167969. [CrossRef]

51. Moldovan, L.; Batte, K.E.; Trgovcich, J.; Wisler, J.; Marsh, C.B.; Piper, M. Methodological challenges in utilizing miRNAs as circulating biomarkers. *J. Cell. Mol. Med.* **2014**, *18*, 371–390. [CrossRef] [PubMed]

52. Oerlemans, M.I.F.J.; Mosterd, A.; Dekker, M.S.; de Vrey, E.A.; van Mil, A.; Pasterkamp, G.; Doevendans, P.A.; Hoes, A.W.; Sluijter, J.P.G. Early assessment of acute coronary syndromes in the emergency department: The potential diagnostic value of circulating microRNAs. *EMBO Mol. Med.* **2012**, *4*, 1176–1185. [CrossRef] [PubMed]

53. Shovlin, C.L.; Guttmacher, A.E.; Buscarini, E.; Faughnan, M.E.; Hyland, R.H.; Westermann, C.J.J.; Kjeldsen, A.D.; Plauchu, H. Diagnostic criteria for hereditary hemorrhagic telangiectasia (Rendu-Osler-Weber syndrome). *Am. J. Med. Genet.* **2000**, *91*, 66–67. [CrossRef]

54. Latino, G.A.; Brown, D.; Glazier, R.H.; Weyman, J.T.; Faughnan, M.E. Targeting under-diagnosis in hereditary hemorrhagic telangiectasia: A model approach for rare diseases? *Orphanet J. Rare Dis.* **2014**, *9*, 1–10. [CrossRef]

55. Lupa, M.D.; Wise, S.K. Comprehensive management of hereditary hemorrhagic telangiectasia. *Curr. Opin. Otolaryngol. Head Neck Surg.* **2016**, *25*, 64–68. [CrossRef]

56. Dupuis-Girod, S.; Bailly, S.; Plauchu, H. Hereditary Hemorrhagic Telangiectasia: From Molecular Biology to Patient Care. *J. Thromb. Haemost.* **2010**, *8*, 1447–1456. [CrossRef]

57. Hanneman, K.; Faughnan, M.E.; Prabhudesai, V. Cumulative radiation dose in patients with hereditary hemorrhagic telangiectasia and pulmonary arteriovenous malformations. *Can. Assoc. Radiol. J.* **2014**, *65*, 135–140. [CrossRef]

58. Zhang, Q.; Kandic, I.; Faughnan, M.E.; Kutryk, M.J. Elevated circulating microRNA-210 levels in patients with hereditary hemorrhagic telangiectasia and pulmonary arteriovenous malformations: A potential new biomarker. *Biomarkers* **2013**, *18*, 23–29. [CrossRef]

59. Chan, S.Y.; Loscalzo, J. MicroRNA-210: A unique and pleiotropic hypoxamir. *Cell Cycle* **2010**, *9*, 1072–1083. [CrossRef]

60. Bavelloni, A.; Ramazzotti, G.; Poli, A.; Piazzi, M.; Focaccia, E.; Blalock, W.; Faenza, I. Mirna-210: A current overview. *Anticancer Res.* **2017**, *37*, 6511–6521.

61. Fasanaro, P.; D'Alessandra, Y.; Di Stefano, V.; Melchionna, R.; Romani, S.; Pompilio, G.; Capogrossi, M.C.; Martelli, F. MicroRNA-210 modulates endothelial cell response to hypoxia and inhibits the receptor tyrosine kinase ligand ephrin-A3. *J. Biol. Chem.* **2008**, *283*, 15878–15883. [CrossRef] [PubMed]

62. Tabruyn, S.P.; Hansen, S.; Ojeda-Fernández, M.L.; Bovy, N.; Zarrabeitia, R.; Recio-Poveda, L.; Bernabéu, C.; Martial, J.A.; Botella, L.M.; Struman, I. MiR-205 is downregulated in hereditary hemorrhagic telangiectasia and impairs TGF-beta signaling pathways in endothelial cells. *Angiogenesis* **2013**, *16*, 877–887. [CrossRef]

63. Sun, Y.; Xiao, Y.; Sun, H.; Zhao, Z.; Zhu, J.; Zhang, L.; Dong, J.; Han, T.; Jing, Q.; Zhou, J.; et al. MiR-27a regulates vascular remodeling by targeting endothelial cells' apoptosis and interaction with vascular smooth muscle cells in aortic dissection. *Theranostics* **2019**, *9*, 7961–7975. [CrossRef]

64. Urbich, C.; Kaluza, D.; Frömel, T.; Knau, A.; Bennewitz, K.; Boon, R.A.; Bonauer, A.; Doebele, C.; Boeckel, J.N.; Hergenreider, E.; et al. MicroRNA-27a/b controls endothelial cell repulsion and angiogenesis by targeting semaphorin 6A. *Blood* **2012**, *119*, 1607–1618. [CrossRef] [PubMed]

65. Wang, Y.L.; Gong, W.G.; Yuan, Q.L. Effects of miR-27a upregulation on thyroid cancer cells migration, invasion, and angiogenesis. *Genet. Mol. Res.* **2016**, *15*, 1–10. [CrossRef] [PubMed]

66. Feng, L.; Shen, F.; Zhou, J.; Li, Y.; Jiang, R.; Chen, Y. Hypoxia-induced up-regulation of miR-27a promotes paclitaxel resistance in ovarian cancer. *Biosci. Rep.* **2020**, *40*. [CrossRef]

67. Tokar, T.; Pastrello, C.; Rossos, A.E.M.; Abovsky, M.; Hauschild, A.C.; Tsay, M.; Lu, R.; Jurisica, I. MirDIP 4.1-Integrative database of human microRNA target predictions. *Nucleic Acids Res.* **2018**, *46*, D360–D370. [CrossRef]

68. Shirdel, E.A.; Xie, W.; Mak, T.W.; Jurisica, I. NAViGaTing the micronome using multiple microRNA prediction databases to identify signalling pathway-associated microRNAs. *PLoS ONE* **2011**, *6*. [CrossRef]

69. Gandellini, P.; Profumo, V.; Casamichele, A.; Fenderico, N.; Borrelli, S.; Petrovich, G.; Santilli, G.; Callari, M.; Colecchia, M.; Pozzi, S.; et al. MiR-205 regulates basement membrane deposition in human prostate: Implications for cancer development. *Cell Death Differ.* **2012**, *19*, 1750–1760. [CrossRef]

70. Gregory, P.A.; Bert, A.G.; Paterson, E.L.; Barry, S.C.; Tsykin, A.; Farshid, G.; Vadas, M.A.; Khew-Goodall, Y.; Goodall, G.J. The miR-200 family and miR-205 regulate epithelial to mesenchymal transition by targeting ZEB1 and SIP1. *Nat. Cell Biol.* **2008**, *10*, 593–601. [CrossRef]

71. Wang, B.; Koh, P.; Winbanks, C.; Coughlan, M.T.; McClelland, A.; Watson, A.; Jandeleit-Dahm, K.; Burns, W.C.; Thomas, M.C.; Cooper, M.E.; et al. MiR-200a prevents renal fibrogenesis through repression of TGF-β2 expression. *Diabetes* **2011**, *60*, 280–287. [CrossRef] [PubMed]

72. Fernandez-L, A.; Sanz-Rodriguez, F.; Zarrabeitia, R.; Pérez-Molino, A.; Hebbel, R.P.; Nguyen, J.; Bernabéu, C.; Botella, L.M. Blood outgrowth endothelial cells from Hereditary Haemorrhagic Telangiectasia patients reveal abnormalities compatible with vascular lesions. *Cardiovasc. Res.* **2005**, *68*, 235–248. [CrossRef] [PubMed]

73. Lebrin, F.; Goumans, M.-J.; Jonker, L.; Carvalho, R.L.C.; Valdimarsdottir, G.; Thorikay, M.; Mummery, C.; Arthur, H.M.; ten Dijke, P. Endoglin Promotes Endothelial Cell Proliferation and TGF-β/ALK1 Signal Transduction. *EMBO J.* **2004**, *23*, 4018–4028. [CrossRef]

74. Ruiz-Llorente, L.; Albiñana, V.; Botella, L.M.; Bernabeu, C. Differential Expression of Circulating Plasma miRNA-370 and miRNA-10a from Patients with Hereditary Hemorrhagic Telangiectasia. *J. Clin. Med.* **2020**, *9*, 2855. [CrossRef] [PubMed]

75. Chen, X.P.; Chen, Y.G.; Lan, J.Y.; Shen, Z.J. MicroRNA-370 suppresses proliferation and promotes endometrioid ovarian cancer chemosensitivity to cDDP by negatively regulating ENG. *Cancer Lett.* **2014**, *353*, 201–210. [CrossRef]

76. Gu, Y.; Becker, V.; Zhao, Y.; Menger, M.D.; Laschke, M.W. miR-370 inhibits the angiogenic activity of endothelial cells by targeting smoothened (SMO) and bone morphogenetic protein (BMP)-2. *FASEB J.* **2019**, *33*, 7213–7224. [CrossRef]

77. Wang, X.H.; Chen, L. MicroRNA-370 suppresses the retinal capillary endothelial cell growth by targeting KDR gene. *Bratislava Med. J.* **2017**, *118*, 202–207. [CrossRef]

78. Zhang, H.; Sun, X.; Hao, D. Upregulation of microRNA-370 facilitates the repair of amputated fingers through targeting forkhead box protein O1. *Exp. Biol. Med.* **2016**, *241*, 282–289. [CrossRef]

79. Zhang, S.; Song, G.; Yuan, J.; Qiao, S.; Xu, S.; Si, Z.; Yang, Y.; Xu, X.; Wang, A. Circular RNA circ_0003204 inhibits proliferation, migration and tube formation of endothelial cell in atherosclerosis via miR-370-3p/TGFβR2/phosph-SMAD3 axis. *J. Biomed. Sci.* **2020**, *27*, 1–17. [CrossRef]

80. Li, J.; Zhang, Y.; Zhao, Q.; Wang, J.; He, X. MicroRNA-10a influences osteoblast differentiation and angiogenesis by regulating β-catenin expression. *Cell. Physiol. Biochem.* **2015**, *37*, 2194–2208. [CrossRef]

81. Lee, D.Y.; Lin, T.E.; Lee, C.I.; Zhou, J.; Huang, Y.H.; Lee, P.L.; Shih, Y.T.; Chien, S.; Chiu, J.J. MicroRNA-10a is crucial for endothelial response to different flow patterns via interaction of retinoid acid receptors and histone deacetylases. *Proc. Natl. Acad. Sci. USA* **2017**, *114*, 2072–2077. [CrossRef] [PubMed]

82. Ors-Kumoglu, G.; Gulce-Iz, S.; Biray-Avci, C. Therapeutic microRNAs in human cancer. *Cytotechnology* **2019**, *71*, 411–425. [CrossRef]

83. Yang, G.; Zhang, W.; Yu, C.; Ren, J.; An, Z. MicroRNA let-7: Regulation, single nucleotide polymorphism, and therapy in lung cancer. *J. Cancer Res. Ther.* **2015**, *11*, C1–C6.

84. Castro, D.; Moreira, M.; Gouveia, A.M.; Pozza, D.H.; De Mello, R.A. MicroRNAs in lung cancer. *Oncotarget* **2017**, *8*, 81679–81685. [CrossRef] [PubMed]

85. Butz, H.; Rácz, K.; Hunyady, L.; Patócs, A. Crosstalk between TGF-B signaling and the microRNA machinery. *Trends Pharmacol. Sci.* **2012**, *33*, 382–393. [CrossRef]

86. Gordon, K.J.; Blobe, G.C. Role of transforming growth factor-β superfamily signaling pathways in human disease. *Biochim. Biophys. Acta Mol. Basis Dis.* **2008**, *1782*, 197–228. [CrossRef]

87. Guerrero-Esteo, M.; Sanchez-Elsner, T.; Letamendia, A.; Bernabeu, C. Extracellular and cytoplasmic domains of endoglin interact with the transforming growth factor-beta receptors I and II. *J. Biol. Chem.* **2002**, *277*, 29197–29209. [CrossRef]

88. Goumans, M.-J.; Liu, Z.; ten Dijke, P. TGF-β Signaling in Vascular Biology and Dysfunction. *Cell Res.* **2009**, *19*, 116–127. [CrossRef] [PubMed]

89. Hata, A.; Lagna, G. Deregulation of Drosha in the pathogenesis of hereditary hemorrhagic telangiectasia. *Curr. Opin. Hematol.* **2019**, *26*, 161–169. [CrossRef] [PubMed]

90. Lee, Y.; Ahn, C.; Han, J.; Choi, H.; Kim, J.; Yim, J.; Lee, J.; Provost, P.; Rådmark, O.; Kim, S.; et al. The nuclear RNase III Drosha initiates microRNA processing. *Nature* **2003**, *425*, 415–419. [CrossRef] [PubMed]

91. Han, J.; Pedersen, J.S.; Kwon, S.C.; Belair, C.D.; Kim, Y.K.; Yeom, K.H.; Yang, W.Y.; Haussler, D.; Blelloch, R.; Kim, V.N. Posttranscriptional Crossregulation between Drosha and DGCR8. *Cell* **2009**, *136*, 75–84. [CrossRef] [PubMed]

92. Rolando, C.; Erni, A.; Grison, A.; Beattie, R.; Engler, A.; Gokhale, P.J.; Milo, M.; Wegleiter, T.; Jessberger, S.; Taylor, V. Multipotency of Adult Hippocampal NSCs In Vivo Is Restricted by Drosha/NFIB. *Cell Stem Cell* **2016**, *19*, 653–662. [CrossRef] [PubMed]

93. Gromak, N.; Dienstbier, M.; Macias, S.; Plass, M.; Eyras, E.; Cáceres, J.F.; Proudfoot, N.J. Drosha regulates gene expression independently of RNA cleavage function. *Cell Rep.* **2013**, *5*, 1499–1510. [CrossRef]

94. Kuehbacher, A.; Urbich, C.; Zeiher, A.M.; Dimmeler, S. Role of Dicer and Drosha for endothelial microRNA expression and angiogenesis. *Circ. Res.* **2007**, *101*, 59–68. [CrossRef] [PubMed]

95. Jiang, X.; Wooderchak-Donahue, W.L.; McDonald, J.; Ghatpande, P.; Baalbaki, M.; Sandoval, M.; Hart, D.; Clay, H.; Coughlin, S.; Lagna, G.; et al. Inactivating mutations in drosha mediate vascular abnormalities similar to hereditary hemorrhagic telangiectasia. *Sci. Signal.* **2018**, *11*. [CrossRef]

96. Watterston, C.; Zeng, L.; Onabadejo, A.; Childs, S.J. MicroRNA26 attenuates vascular smooth muscle maturation via endothelial bmp signalling. *PLoS Genet.* **2019**, *15*. [CrossRef]

97. Miscianinov, V.; Martello, A.; Rose, L.; Parish, E.; Cathcart, B.; Mitić, T.; Gray, G.A.; Meloni, M.; Al Haj Zen, A.; Caporali, A. MicroRNA-148b Targets the TGF-β Pathway to Regulate Angiogenesis and Endothelial-to-Mesenchymal Transition during Skin Wound Healing. *Mol. Ther.* **2018**, *26*, 1996–2007. [CrossRef]

98. Climent, M.; Quintavalle, M.; Miragoli, M.; Chen, J.; Condorelli, G.; Elia, L. TGFβ triggers miR-143/145 transfer from smooth muscle cells to endothelial cells, thereby modulating vessel stabilization. *Circ. Res.* **2015**, *116*, 1753–1764. [CrossRef]

99. Cannavicci, A.; Zhang, Q.; Dai, S.-C.; Faughnan, M.E.; Kutryk, M.J.B. Decreased levels of miR-28-5p and miR-361-3p and increased levels of insulin-like growth factor 1 mRNA in mononuclear cells from patients with hereditary hemorrhagic telangiectasia. *Can. J. Physiol. Pharmacol.* **2019**, *97*, 562–569. [CrossRef]

100. Verhoeckx, K.; Cotter, P.; López-Expósito, I.; Kleiveland, C.; Lea, T.; Mackie, A.; Requena, T.; Swiatecka, D.; Wichers, H. *The Impact of Food Bioactives on Health*; Verhoeckx, K., Cotter, P., López-Expósito, I., Kleiveland, C., Lea, T., Mackie, A., Requena, T., Swiatecka, D., Wichers, H., Eds.; Springer International Publishing: Cham, Switzerland, 2015; ISBN 978-3-319-15791-7.

101. Post, S.; Smits, A.M.; Van Den Broek, A.J.; Sluijter, J.P.G.; Hoefer, I.E.; Janssen, B.J.; Snijder, R.J.; Mager, J.J.; Pasterkamp, G.; Mummery, C.L.; et al. Impaired recruitment of HHT-1 mononuclear cells to the ischaemic heart is due to an altered CXCR4/CD26 balance. *Cardiovasc. Res.* **2010**, *85*, 494–502. [CrossRef]

102. Peter, M.R.; Jerkic, M.; Sotov, V.; Douda, D.N.; Ardelean, D.S.; Ghamami, N.; Lakschevitz, F.; Khan, M.A.; Robertson, S.J.; Glogauer, M.; et al. Impaired Resolution of Inflammation in the Endoglin Heterozygous Mouse Model of Chronic Colitis. *Mediators Inflamm.* **2014**, *2014*, 1–13. [CrossRef]

103. Friedrich, C.C.; Lin, Y.; Krannich, A.; Wu, Y.; Vacanti, J.P.; Neville, C.M. Enhancing engineered vascular networks in vitro and in vivo: The effects of IGF1 on vascular development and durability. *Cell Prolif.* **2018**, *51*, e12387. [CrossRef] [PubMed]

104. Wang, X.; Dai, Z.; Wu, X.; Wang, K.; Wang, X. Distinct RNA transcriptome patterns are potentially associated with angiogenesis in Tie2-expressing monocytes. *Gene* **2016**, *580*, 1–7. [CrossRef]

105. Shi, X.; Teng, F. Down-regulated miR-28-5p in human hepatocellular carcinoma correlated with tumor proliferation and migration by targeting insulin-like growth factor-1 (IGF-1). *Mol. Cell. Biochem.* **2015**, *408*, 283–293. [CrossRef]

106. Xia, Q.; Han, T.; Yang, P.; Wang, R.; Li, H.; Zhang, J.; Zhou, X. MicroRNA-28-5p Regulates Liver Cancer Stem Cell Expansion via IGF-1 Pathway. *Stem Cells Int.* **2019**, *2019*, 1–16. [CrossRef] [PubMed]

107. Tsagakis, I.; Douka, K.; Birds, I.; Aspden, J.L. Long non-coding RNAs in development and disease: Conservation to mechanisms. *J. Pathol.* **2020**, *250*, 480–495. [CrossRef]

108. Jaé, N.; Dimmeler, S. Noncoding RNAs in Vascular Diseases. *Circ. Res.* **2020**, *126*, 1127–1145. [CrossRef]

109. Singh, K.K.; Matkar, P.N.; Quan, A.; Mantella, L.-E.; Teoh, H.; Al-Omran, M.; Verma, S. Investigation of TGF β 1-Induced Long Noncoding RNAs in Endothelial Cells. *Int. J. Vasc. Med.* **2016**, *2016*, 1–12. [CrossRef]

110. Tørring, P.M.; Larsen, M.J.; Kjeldsen, A.D.; Ousager, L.B.; Tan, Q.; Brusgaard, K. Long non-coding RNA expression profiles in hereditary haemorrhagic telangiectasia. *PLoS ONE* **2014**, *9*, 90272. [CrossRef] [PubMed]

Publisher's Note: MDPI stays neutral with regard to jurisdictional claims in published maps and institutional affiliations.

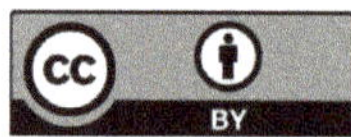

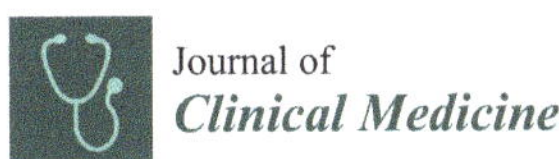 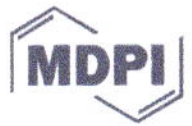

Journal of
Clinical Medicine

Article

Differential Expression of Circulating Plasma miRNA-370 and miRNA-10a from Patients with Hereditary Hemorrhagic Telangiectasia

Lidia Ruiz-Llorente [1,2], Virginia Albiñana [1], Luisa M. Botella [1] and Carmelo Bernabeu [1,*]

[1] Centro de Investigaciones Biológicas Margarita Salas, Consejo Superior de Investigaciones Científicas (CSIC) and Centro de Investigación Biomédica en Red de Enfermedades Raras (CIBERER), 28040 Madrid, Spain; lidia.ruizl@uah.es (L.R.-L.); vir_albi_di@yahoo.es (V.A.); cibluisa@cib.csic.es (L.M.B.)

[2] Department of Systems Biology, School of Medicine and Health Sciences, University of Alcalá, Alcalá de Henares, 28871 Madrid, Spain

* Correspondence: bernabeu.c@cib.csic.es

Received: 5 August 2020; Accepted: 31 August 2020; Published: 3 September 2020

Abstract: Hereditary hemorrhagic telangiectasia (HHT) is an autosomal dominant, vascular disorder that presents with telangiectases and arteriovenous malformations. HHT is a genetically heterogeneous disorder, involving mutations in endoglin (*ENG*; HHT1) and activin receptor-like kinase 1 (*ACVRL1/ALK1*; HHT2) genes that account for over 85% of all HHT patients. The current diagnosis of HHT patients remains at the clinical level, but many suspected patients do not have a clear HHT diagnosis or do not show pathogenic mutations in HHT genes. This situation has prompted the search for biomarkers to help in the early diagnosis of the disease. We have analyzed the plasma levels in HHT patients of selected micro-RNAs (miRNAs), small single-stranded RNAs that regulate gene expression at the transcriptional level by interacting with specific RNA targets. A total of 16 HHT1 and 17 HHT2 plasma samples from clinically confirmed patients and 16 controls were analyzed in this study. Total RNA was purified from plasma, and three selected miRNAs (miRNA-10a, miRNA-214, and miRNA-370), related to the pathobiology of cardiovascular diseases and potentially targeting *ENG* or *ALK1*, were measured by quantitative polymerase chain reaction. Compared with controls, levels of miRNA-370, whose putative target is *ENG*, were significantly downregulated in HHT1, but not in HHT2, whereas the levels of miRNA-10a, whose putative target is *ALK1*, were significantly upregulated in HHT2, but not in HHT1. In addition, the levels of miRNA-214, potentially targeting *ENG* and *ALK1*, did not change in either HHT1 or HHT2 patients versus control samples. While further studies are warranted, these results suggest that dysregulated plasma levels of miRNA-370 or miRNA-10a could help to identify undiagnosed HHT1 or HHT2 patients, respectively.

Keywords: microRNA; biomarker; hereditary hemorrhagic telangiectasia (HHT); plasma; telangiectases; arteriovenous malformations (AVMs); angiogenesis; endoglin; activin receptor-like kinase 1 (ALK1); transforming growth factor beta (TGF-β); bone morphogenetic protein (BMP)

---

1. Introduction

Hereditary hemorrhagic telangiectasia (HHT) is an autosomal dominant, vascular disorder with a prevalence of approximately 1 in 8000 people worldwide [1,2]. HHT is characterized by the presence of telangiectases in skin and mucocutaneous tissue and arteriovenous malformations (AVMs), direct connections between arteries and veins without capillary beds, in internal organs [1]. Over 90% of all HHT patients present chronic epistaxis due to nasal telangiectases, whereas chronic bleeding from gastrointestinal telangiectases develops in at least 20% of patients. The presence of pulmonary, hepatic, and cerebral AVMs in HHT patients suggests that they are at risk of life-threatening hemorrhage and complications involving shunting, leading to stroke, high-output cardiac failure, or brain abscess [3–5].

HHT is genetically heterogeneous with heterozygous mutations in at least three known genes including endoglin (*ENG*) causing HHT1 [6], activin receptor-like kinase 1 (*ACVRL1* or *ALK1*), causing HHT2 [7], and mothers against decapentaplegic homolog 4 (*MADH4* or *SMAD4*) causing familial juvenile polyposis associated with HHT (JP/HT) [8]. In addition, mutations in the *GDF2* gene, encoding bone morphogenetic protein 9 (BMP9), were described as the cause of an HHT-like syndrome [9]. *ENG* and *ACVRL1* are the predominant genes whose mutations account for over 85% of all HHT patients [10,11] and are considered potential therapeutic targets [12]. The phenotypes generated by either *ENG* or *ACVRL1* mutations (HHT1 or HHT2, respectively) generally display distinct clinical manifestations, but an overlap of their clinical symptoms commonly occurs. Interestingly, all the genes mutated in HHT encode proteins that are involved in the signaling pathway of transforming growth factor beta (TGF-β)/bone morphogenetic protein (BMP). Thus, the auxiliary receptor endoglin associates with the signaling serine/threonine receptor ALK1 and both proteins are able to bind ligands like BMP9, leading to the phosphorylation and nuclear translocation of a Smad protein complex that includes Smad4 [12–14]. Because endothelial cells are functional targets of circulating BMP9, and predominantly express endoglin and ALK1, these are widely accepted as the target cells in HHT.

A deficient expression of the HHT genes has been postulated to underlie the molecular basis of HHT pathogenesis. Mono-allelic loss of expression leading to haploinsufficiency of the respective HHT proteins has been shown to dysregulate TGF-β/BMP signaling in endothelial cells, negatively impacting in cell proliferation, migration, and recruitment during vascular remodeling and angiogenesis [11,12]. In addition, in mice, homozygous knockdown of *ENG* or *ACVRL1* leads to HHT phenotypes [15–17]. More recently, using next-generation sequencing, Marchuk et al. [18] have been able to demonstrate the presence of low-frequency somatic mutations in telangiectases of HHT1 and HHT2 patients, suggesting that the bi-allelic loss of *ENG* or *ACVRL1* may also contribute to the development of vascular lesions.

MicroRNAs (miRNAs) are small noncoding RNAs (about 22 nucleotides in length) able to post-transcriptionally regulate gene expression by RNA interference [19,20]. They act as guides in complementary miRNA–mRNA complexes that recruit enzymatic species to silence mRNAs by mRNA cleavage (perfect complementarity) or ribosome destabilization (nonperfect complementarity). In this process, Drosha is a ribonuclease that plays a key role for miRNA biogenesis and regulates the TGF-β/BMP pathway by interacting with the Smad protein family which, in turn, modulates gene expression via miRNAs [21]. Interestingly, mice lacking Drosha in the vascular endothelium develop a vascular phenotype resembling HHT including dilated and disorganized vasculature, AVMs, and hemorrhages [22]. In this regard, the emerging role of miRNAs in human diseases [23,24] has prompted a few studies searching for specific miRNAs in HHT patients [25–27]. However, the expression of miRNAs associated with HHT remains mostly unexplored. Our aim in this work was to identify dysregulated miRNAs in plasma samples from HHT patients through quantitative polymerase chain reaction compared with controls. We find i) a downregulation in HHT1, but not in HHT2, patients of miRNA-370, which is predicted to target *ENG*; and ii) an upregulation in HHT2, but not in HHT1, patients of miRNA-10a, whose putative target is *ALK1*. These results suggest that dysregulated plasma levels of miRNA-370 or miRNA-10a are potential biomarkers that could help to identify undiagnosed HHT1 or HHT2 patients, respectively. In addition, they also may contribute to a better understanding of the complex biological processes associated with the development of HHT.

2. Material and Methods

2.1. Algorithms for miRNA-target Predictions

Computational prediction of miRNA targets was carried out using three target prediction programs which use different algorithms: (i) microRNA (www.microRNA.org) [28]; (ii) Target Scan (http://www.targetscan.org/vert_72/) [29]; and (iii) MicroCosm (https://tools4mirs.org/software/mirna_databases/microcosm-targets/) [30]. The mirSVR score was used as a regression method for predicting likelihood of target mRNA downregulation from sequence and structure features in microRNA/mRNA predicted target sites.

2.2. Patients

A total of 34 HHT patient plasma samples were evaluated by quantitative reverse transcriptase–polymerase chain reaction (qRT-PCR). Seventeen of them were HHT1, and the remaining seventeen patients were HHT2. Plasma samples from 16 control healthy subjects were also assayed to establish the normal range of microRNAs (miRNAs). In all three groups, donors from different sex and age were included. Peripheral venous blood samples were collected with ethylenediamine tetra-acetic acid (EDTA) as anticoagulant. Blood samples were centrifuged at 15,000 g for 15 min, and the resulting plasma was stored at −80 °C until analysis. Written informed consent was obtained from all the participants, or their legally authorized representative, in this study, and the protocol was supervised and received full approval from our Institutional Review Board (IRB) of the Spanish National Research Council (CSIC) with the ethical code number 075/2017. All HHT patients included in the present study were clinically diagnosed following the Curaçao criteria [3], and their genetic mutations were identified by sequencing. Their genetic characteristics and clinical manifestations are summarized in Table 1.

Table 1. Summary of genotypes and mutations of hereditary hemorrhagic telangiectasia (HHT) of patients [1].

HHT Type	Patient#	Genotype	Mutation
HHT1	P#1.1	*ENG*	5′ UTR (gene promoter) c.-127 G>A
HHT1	P#1.2	*ENG*	5′ UTR (gene promoter) c.-127 G>A
HHT1	P#1.3	*ENG*	5′ UTR (gene promoter) c.-58 G>A
HHT1	P#1.4	*ENG*	5′ UTR (gene promoter) c.-58 G>A
HHT1	P#1.5	*ENG*	5′ UTR (gene promoter) c.-58 G>C
HHT1	P#1.6	*ENG*	Intron 1 c.68-2A>T
HHT1	P#1.7	*ENG*	Intron 1 c.68-2A>T
HHT1	P#1.8	*ENG*	Intron 1 c.68-2A>T
HHT1	P#1.9	*ENG*	Exon 4 c.392 C>T; p.Pro131Leu
HHT1	P#1.10	*ENG*	Exon 5 c.588 G>A; p.Trp196 *
HHT1	P#1.11	*ENG*	Exon 5 c.588 G>A; p.Trp196 *
HHT1	P#1.12	*ENG*	Exon 5 c.617delG; p.G206AfsX16
HHT1	P#1.13	*ENG*	Exon 5 c.617delG; p.G206AfsX16
HHT1	P#1.14	*ENG*	Exon 7 c.967_968del GT; p.V323fs *
HHT1	P#1.15	*ENG*	Exon 7 c.967_968delGT; p.V323fs *
HHT1	P#1.16	*ENG*	Exon 11 c.1434_1435 del AG p. R478fs *
HHT2	P#2.1	*ALK1*	Exon 6 c.673_674delAG; p.S225fs
HHT2	P#2.2	*ALK1*	Exon 6 c.673_674delAG; p.S225fs
HHT2	P#2.3	*ALK1*	Exon 6 c.635 G>A; p.R212H
HHT2	P#2.4	*ALK1*	Exon 7 c.889delC; H297fs *
HHT2	P#2.5	*ALK1*	Exon 7 c.921-927dupATGCGGC; p.L310fs
HHT2	P#2.6	*ALK1*	Exon 7 c. 926 G>A; p.G309A
HHT2	P#2.7	*ALK1*	Exon 7 c.941 A>C; p.His314Pro
HHT2	P#2.8	*ALK1*	Exon 7 c.988 G>T; p.D330Y
HHT2	P#2.9	*ALK1*	Exon 7 c.1027 C>T; p.Q374X
HHT2	P#2.10	*ALK1*	Exon 7 c.1027 C>T; p.Q374X
HHT2	P#2.11	*ALK1*	Exon 7 c.1027 C>T; p.Q374X
HHT2	P#2.12	*ALK1*	Exon 7 c.1030 C>T; p.C344R

Table 1. *Cont.*

HHT Type	Patient#	Genotype	Mutation
HHT2	P#2.13	*ALK1*	Exon 8 c.1120 C>T; p.R374W
HHT2	P#2.14	*ALK1*	Exon 8 c.1120 C>T; p.Arg374Trp
HHT2	P#2.15	*ALK1*	Exon 8 c.1232 G>A; p.Arg411Gln
HHT2	P#2.16	*ALK1*	Exon 10 c.1435 C>T; p.Arg479X

[1] A total of 33 HHT patients were included in this microRNA analyses. All HHT patients were clinically diagnosed following the Curaçao criteria [3]. Sixteen patients were genetically diagnosed as HHT1 as they harbor a mutation in *ENG*, whereas the remaining 17 patients were HHT2 with pathogenic mutations in *ALK1*; fs—frameshift mutation; Asterisks (*) represent stop codons.

2.3. Extraction of miRNAs from Plasma Samples

miRNAs were extracted with the miRNeasy Micro kit (Qiagen, Hilden, Germany; #217084) according to the manufacturer's instructions and following a previously described protocol [25,31]. Briefly, 50 µL plasma samples from HHT patients were homogenized with 1 mL QIAzol® Lysis Reagent and 6.25×10^{-3} fmol/µL of the spike-in control cel-miR-39-3p (5′ UCA CCG GGU GUA AAU CAG CUU G 3′). Next, the homogenate was incubated at room temperature for 5 min, and then 200 µL chloroform was added to each sample, followed by centrifugation at 12,000× g for 5 min at 4 °C. Equal volumes from the upper aqueous phase were transferred to new tubes and mixed by pipetting with 1.5 volumes of 100% ethanol; finally total miRNAs were eluted in 40 µL RNase-free water.

2.4. Quantitative Reverse Transcriptase–Polymerase Chain Reaction (qRT-PCR) Analysis of miRNAs

qRT-PCR was performed to validate selected miRNAs. They were reverse-transcribed into cDNA using TaqMan™ MicroRNA Reverse Transcription kit (Thermo Fisher Scientific, #4366596) following the manufacturer´s protocol. The reaction components were mixed with the corresponding reverse transcriptase (RT) primers of hsa-miR-370-3p, hsa-miR-214-3p, hsa-miR-10a-3p, hsa-miR-16-5p, and cel-miR-39-3p (Thermo Fisher Scientific, Waltham, MA, USA; #4427975; Assay ID 002275, 002306, 002288, 000391, and 000200, respectively). RT reaction was carried out as follows: 16 °C for 30 min, 42 °C for 30 min, 85 °C for 5 min, and 4 °C hold. The resulting cDNAs were used for quantitative real-time PCR experiments using Taqman Universal PCR Master Mix, no AmpErase® UNG (Thermo Fisher Scientific, Waltham, MA, USA; #4324018), and the specific PCR primers (references detailed above). Thermal cycling was performed on LightCycler® 96 detection system (Roche) as follows: 95 °C for 10 min, 40 cycles of 95 °C for 15s and 60 °C for 1 min. Relative quantification of individual miRNA expression was carried out with the 2-ΔΔCT method and normalized against two internal controls, miR-16-5p and the spike-in miRNA cel-miR-39-3p. In studies focused on cardiovascular disease, miR-16-5p is one of the miRNAs with the best performance as normalizer [32], whereas cel-miR-39-3p is one of the most used and reliable spike-in controls [25].

2.5. Statistical Analysis

HHT patient and control groups were compared using Kruskal–Wallis test. Subsequent Mann–Whitney U tests were run to test for pairwise comparisons in a post hoc fashion; significance values were adjusted by the Bonferroni correction for multiple tests. Statistical analyses were carried out with the IBM SPSS Statistics version 25 (Windows10 64-bit) software (IBM Corp., Armonk, NY, USA). Box Whisker plots show median (central line), upper and lower quartiles (box), and range excluding outliers (whiskers). Asterisks indicate statistically significant values between selected conditions (* $p < 0.05$; ** $p < 0.01$; ns, not significant).

3. Results

3.1. Identification of miRNA-10a, miRNA-214, and miRNA-370, Potentially Related to HHT, Using in Silico and Literature Data

Recently, studies on circulating miRNAs as potential biomarkers in different types of diseases [33], including HHT [21,27], have received increasing attention. In order to identify specific biomarkers of HHT, we searched for miRNAs involved in angiogenesis and vascular homeostasis and predicted to target *ENG* and/or *ALK1* using three robust target prediction programs which use different algorithms: (i) microRNA [28]; (ii) Target Scan [29]; and (iii) MicroCosm [30]. Using this stringent approach, we selected miRNA-370, miRNA-10a, and miRNA-214 for further analyses.

miRNA-370 was considered to be very relevant to endoglin function since it was the only miRNA predicted to target *ENG* with a good mirSVR score (−0.1740), according to the microRNA database (www.microRNA.org). This website also describes miRNA-370 as an evolutionary well-conserved miRNA because its alignment with *ENG* is found in other species as well. Likewise, algorithms from Target Scan and MicroCosm programs indicate that *ENG* is predicted to be targeted by miRNA-370. In fact, the negative regulation of *ENG* by miRNA-370 has been validated in ovarian cancer cells where miRNA-370 suppresses their proliferation and promotes chemosensitivity to cisplatin by negatively regulating *ENG* [34]. Based on predictions of microRNA webs, miRNA-370 not only regulates *ENG*, but also other gene products with essential roles in endothelial cell biology and angiogenesis, some of which have been already validated as targets in the literature. One of these proteins is TGF-β receptor type 2 (TGFBR2) that is negatively regulated by miRNA-370. By acting via TβRII, miRNA-370 plays a potential role in hepatic ischaemia-reperfusion injury and indeed, its inhibition efficiently attenuates liver damage [35]. In addition, upregulation of miRNA-370 might promote the repair of amputated fingers by regulating angiogenesis through targeting Forkhead box protein O1 (FOXO1) [36]. miRNA-370 can also induce growth and tube formation inhibition, and apoptosis in endothelial cells [37,38]. The miRNA-370-induced endothelial effects may explain its anti-angiogenic activity, as well as its developmental regulation of cerebral aneurysms [38–40]. Noteworthy, the effects miRNA-370 are mediated by targeting, at least, a receptor for vascular endothelial growth factor (VEGF), which is the major driver of angiogenesis [38,39].

We next focused our interest on miRNA-10a and miRNA-214 because both are predicted to target *ENG* or *ALK1*, and their dysregulated expression in HHT patients with pulmonary AVMs (pAVMs) has been reported [26] Thus, *ENG* has been revealed, by MicroCosm and Target Scan, as a confident target of miRNA-214. A search in microRNA.org revealed that miRNA-214 is also expected to bind ALK1 mRNA at two different sites with high mirSVR scores (−0.1277 and −0.5112), and ranks in the first position among all miRNAs potentially targeting ALK1. Moreover, by targeting matrix metalloproteinase 8 (MMP8), hepatoma-derived growth factor (HDGF), brain-specific angiogenesis inhibitors (BAIs), and other vascular-related genes, miRNA-214 contributes to the pathogenesis of various cardiovascular conditions, including ischaemic heart diseases, angiogenesis, and cardiac hypertrophy [41–43]. Of note, miRNA-214 is a response element to hypoxia in patients with pulmonary arterial hypertension (PHA), a complication of HHT. Moreover, inhibition of miRNA-214 can ameliorate the symptoms of PHA in animal models, suggesting its use for the prevention and treatment of PHA in humans [41].

Bioinformatics analysis of microRNA database showed that miRNA-10a does not target *ENG*, but appears to regulate *ALK1* with a good mirSVR score (−0.3837). In addition, miRNA-10a targets endothelial gene products such as VEGF receptor 1 (FLT1), β-catenin, GATA-binding factor 6 (GATA6), or mib-1, which may account for its active regulatory role in endothelial cell biology and angiogenesis [44–46].

3.2. Circulating Levels of miRNA-370, miRNA-10a, and miRNA-214 in HHT1 and HHT2 Patient Plasma

Taken together, the above studies suggest that miRNA-370, miRNA-10a, and miRNA-214 are predicted to target not only *ENG* and/or *ALK1*, but also other relevant gene products involved in vascular functions related to the pathophysiology of HHT. Therefore, the chosen miRNAs were next validated by qRT-PCR in the plasma samples from a cohort of HHT1 and HHT2 patients and healthy controls in order to assess their possible diagnostic or biomarker value.

3.2.1. Circulating Levels of miRNA-370 are Decreased in HHT1 Patient Plasma

The expression levels of miRNA-370, as measured by qRT-PCR, were found to be significantly lower in plasma samples from HHT1 patients (Figure 1), using miRNA-16 (Figure 1A; $p = 0.001$) or cel-miR-39-3p (Figure 1B; $p = 0.004$), as normalizers when compared with healthy controls. The levels of miRNA-370 in HHT1 patients were also significantly lower than those in HHT2 patients when using miR-16 as a normalizer (Figure 1A; $p = 0.019$), and showed a not significant but clear decreasing trend versus HHT2 samples when using cel-miR-39-3p as a normalizer (Figure 1B; $p = 0.116$). By contrast, the expression levels of miRNA-370 in HHT2 patients were not significantly affected compared with healthy control individuals. The specific downregulation in HHT1 patients suggests that the decreased levels of miRNA-370 may have potential diagnostic utility as an HHT1 biomarker. Interestingly, since miRNA-370 is predicted to target *ENG* to downregulate its expression [34] and a deficient *ENG* expression underlies the pathogenicity of HHT1, both results also suggest the existence of a common link between the expression levels of miRNA-370 and endoglin in HHT1 patients.

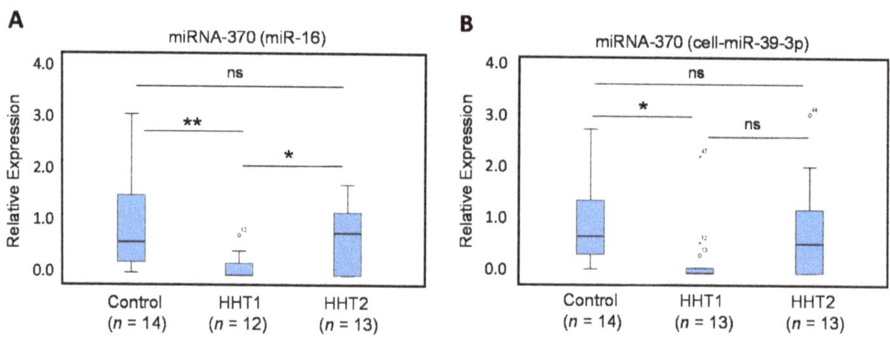

Figure 1. Quantitative Reverse Transcriptase–Polymerase Chain Reaction (qRT-PCR) of miRNA-370. Total plasma RNA was isolated from HHT1 and HHT2 patients and control subjects. Relative expression levels of miR-370 were measured by qRT-PCR using miR-16 (**A**) or cel-miR-39-3p (**B**) as normalizers. The number of samples analyzed is indicated in parentheses. Symbols outside the box plot represent extreme values (°) and outliers (*) with their corresponding sample numbers. Experiments were performed in triplicates. (* $p < 0.05$; ** $p < 0.01$; ns, not significant).

3.2.2. Circulating Levels of miRNA-10a, but not of miRNA-214, are Dysregulated in HHT2 Patient Plasma

As measured by qRT-PCR, the expression levels of miRNA-10a were significantly higher in plasma samples from HHT2 patients (Figure 2), using miRNA-16 (Figure 2A; $p = 0.026$) or cel-miR-39-3p (Figure 2B; $p = 0.024$), as normalizers, when compared with healthy controls. By contrast, the expression levels of miRNA-10a in HHT1 patients were not significantly affected compared with healthy control individuals. Even more, the levels of miRNA-10a in HHT2 patients were significantly higher than those in HHT1 patients when using miR-16 (Figure 2A; $p = 0.03$) or cel-miR-39-3p (Figure 2B; $p = 0.018$), as normalizers. The specific upregulation in HHT2 patients suggests that the increased levels of miRNA-10a may have potential diagnostic utility as an HHT2 biomarker. Interestingly, since miRNA-10 potentially targets ALK1 and a deficient ALK1 expression underlies the pathogenicity of HHT2, these results also suggest the existence of a common link between the expression levels of both miRNA-10a and ALK1 in HHT2 patients. Plasma levels of miRNA-214 were also measured by qRT-PCR, using miR-16 or cel-miR-39-3p as normalizers (Figure 2C,D). However, no statistically significant differences were found in the expression levels of miRNA-214 from either HHT1 or HHT2 patients, when compared with healthy controls, or between each other (Figure 2C,D).

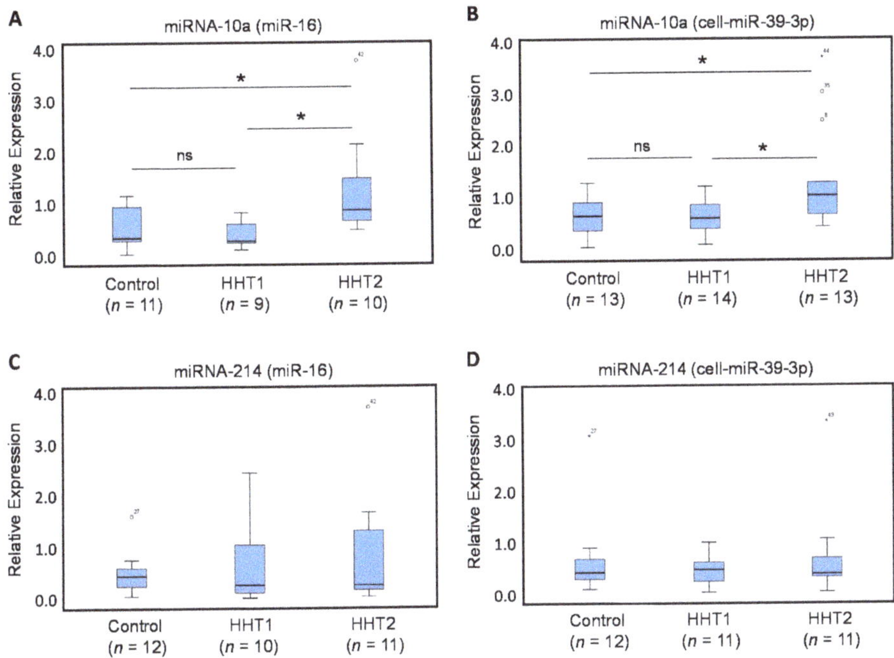

Figure 2. qRT-PCR of miRNA-10a and miRNA-214. Total plasma RNA was isolated from HHT1 and HHT2 patients and control subjects. Relative expression levels of miRNA-10a (**A,B**) and miRNA-214 (**C,D**), measured by qRT-PCR using miR-16 (**A,C**) or cel-miR-39-3p (**B,D**) as normalizers. Symbols outside the box plot represent extreme values (°) and outliers (*) with their corresponding sample numbers. The number of samples analyzed is indicated in parentheses. Experiments were performed in triplicates. (* $p < 0.05$; ns, not significant).

4. Discussion

Over 1900 miRNAs have been identified in humans and many of them have been reported to be involved in a variety of human diseases, biological functions, and signaling pathways, including the TGF-β/BMP route [23,24]. Among these, there are a growing number of miRNAs with high potential to be used as biomarkers in plasma and/or serum to clinically diagnose or provide accurate prognosis for survival in patients with cardiovascular diseases [47]. HHT is an autosomal dominant, genetic disorder in which patients develop hemorrhagic vascular lesions called telangiectases and AVMs. A few reports have previously searched for specific miRNAs in plasma [25,26] or peripheral mononuclear cells [27] from HHT patients. Recently, it has been reported that Drosha, a key enzyme in miRNA biogenesis, regulates vascular development and homeostasis via the TGFβ/BMP pathway, and rare missense mutations in the Drosha gene may predispose carriers to HHT [21,22]. These findings support the hypothesis that miRNAs play a functional role in HHT. However, the expression of miRNAs and their potential application as biomarkers in HHT remains mostly unexplored. In addition, how miRNAs might be involved in HHT development is not fully understood. Our goal was to measure several miRNAs in HHT patient-derived plasma as in previous studies [25,26], but with the novel strategy of selecting miRNAs potentially targeting the predominant HHT genes. We report here for the first time that plasma miRNA-370 levels are downregulated in HHT1, but not in HHT2, patients; while plasma miRNA-10a levels are increased in HHT2, but not in HHT1, patients. While further studies in a large cohort of patients are warranted, this finding suggests that miRNA-370 and miRNA-10a could be used as biomarkers with potential application in HHT diagnosis [48]. Actually, this possibility would be of great interest because there is a need to diagnose HHT in those individuals who do not present with all of the typical symptoms, such as in asymptomatic children and young adults [4,5]. When the HHT gene mutation of the family is known, the genetic testing is the choice option in children and teenagers; the genetic results being definite for either the positive diagnosis or exclusion [10,49]. However, in the absence of a known family mutation, genetic determinations imply the sequencing of at least *ENG* and *ACVRL1* genes, a process that is time-consuming and expensive. Even so, in 10–15% of the subjects, the mutation is not identified. Therefore, it would be useful to have alternative tools to ideally allow an earlier, faster, cheaper, and easier HHT diagnosis. In this sense, several potential biomarkers, including miRNAs, have been described in HHT [48]. Thus, the specific downregulation of miRNA-370 in HHT1 and upregulation of miRNA-10a in HHT2 can be added to the reported dysregulated expression of miRNA-27a, miRNA-205 [25], miRNA-210 [26], miRNA-28-5p, and miRNA-361-3p [27] in different HHT subsets, as shown in Table 2. Unfortunately, due to the different experimental approach and material source (plasma or peripheral mononuclear cells (PMNCs)) used in each of these studies, no comparative conclusions could be drawn. Regarding miRNA-10a and miRNA-214, a previous report has suggested their dysregulated expression using miRNA array analysis in a pool of genotyped and nongenotyped HHT patients with pAVMs [26]. However, to the best of our knowledge, no conclusive, quantitative measurements of these miRNAs have been made so far. In this work, we find that miR10a expression is specifically upregulated in HHT2, whereas the levels of miRNA-214 were unaffected in either HHT1 or HHT2 patients. Nonetheless, a direct comparison between the results by Zhang et al. (2013) and this work is not feasible since the HHT population analyzed in each case is different and pAVMs are present in up to 50% of the HHT population with a predominant association with HHT1 patients [5,50]. Future investigations should be addressed to unify the source of the patient samples and its methodological processing in order to identify miRNAs that could serve as reliable biomarkers in HHT.

Table 2. miRNAs associated with HHT [1].

miRNA	HHT1	HHT2	HHT (Pool)	Blood Sample	Reference
miRNA-370	↓	↔	ND	Plasma	Present work
miRNA-10a	↔	↑	ND	Plasma	Present work
miRNA-28-5p	ND	ND	↓	PMNCs	Cannavicci et al., 2019
miRNA-361-3p	ND	ND	↓	PMNCs	Cannavicci et al., 2019
miRNA-210	ND	ND	↑	Plasma	Zhang et al., 2013
miRNA-210	ND	ND	(with PAVMs)	Plasma	Zhang et al., 2013
miRNA-27a	↑	↑	↔	Plasma	Tabruyn et al., 2013
miRNA-205	↓	↓	(without PAVMs)	Plasma	Tabruyn et al., 2013

[1] Total RNA from either plasma or peripheral mononuclear cells (PMNCs) was isolated, and levels of specific miRNAs were quantified, as indicated in the corresponding references. Increased (↑), decreased (↓), or unaffected (↔) levels of miRNAs are shown. HHT, hereditary hemorrhagic telangiectasia. ND, not determined.

A good biomarker is a defined characteristic that is measured as an indicator of normal biological processes, pathogenic processes, or responses to an exposure or intervention [51,52]. This broad definition encompasses molecular characteristics such as the dysregulated expression of miRNA-370 and miRNA-10a presented in this work. Once a potential biomarker is identified, the next step is to assure that it can be measured reliably and precisely [51,52]. In this regard, further validation studies using a larger cohort of HHT patients are needed, including disease stratification analysis to assess the possible correlation between the levels of miRNA-370 and miRNA-10a and the severity of symptoms. In addition, it would be interesting to measure the circulating subsets of miRNA-370 and miRNA-10a such as those in plasma exosomes, plasma free miRNAs, or mononuclear cells from HHT patients.

To understand the value of a biomarker, it is necessary to know the pathophysiological relationship between the biomarker and the relevant clinical endpoint [51]. That miRNAs have a functional impact on HHT development is supported by recent next-generation sequencing studies of DROSHA, a key ribonuclease involved in miRNA biogenesis [21]. Thus, four rare variants of DROSHA, predicted to damage protein function (P32L, P100L, K226E, R279L), are present at a much higher frequency in HHT patients compared with healthy controls, suggesting that they may contribute to the HHT onset [22]. However, the function of miRNAs associated with HHT, such as miRNA-370 and miRNA-10a, remains to be elucidated. Both miRNA-370 and miRNA-10a regulate angiogenesis [36,38,53], a VEGF-dependent biological process involved in the pathophysiology and therapy of HHT [54,55], by targeting, at least, the VEGF receptors (VEGFR) KDR (kinase insert domain receptor) [38,39] and FLT1 (fms-related tyrosine kinase 1) [45], respectively. In addition, circulating VEGF levels are increased in HHT1 and HHT2 patients compared with the control population [48,56,57], and therapeutic antibodies to VEGF (bevacizumab) are currently used to alleviate HHT symptoms [55,58]. Interestingly, the VEGF/VEGFR pathway can be activated by endoglin or ALK1, thus promoting angiogenesis [59,60]. Therefore, by regulating VEGF-dependent angiogenesis, miRNA-370 and miRNA-10a may potentially impact the pathophysiology of HHT1 and HHT2. Of note, several experimental reports have already demonstrated the involvement of miRNA-370 in different functions of endothelial cells, the target cells in HHT where endoglin is predominantly expressed [38,40]. Thus, miRNA-370 suppresses retinal capillary endothelial cell growth and apoptosis [38], inhibits the angiogenic activity of endothelial cells, and reduces microvessel density and sprouting in vivo, whereas a miRNA-370 inhibitor promotes endothelial sprout formation [40]. The antiangiogenic activity of miRNA-370 is fully compatible with the key functional role of its putative target endoglin in endothelial cells, as endoglin promotes angiogenesis in vivo and in vitro, at least, by stimulating proliferation and anti-apoptotic activity of endothelial cells [61]. Noteworthy, miRNA-370 and miRNA-10a are predicted to target *ENG* and *ALK1*, respectively, thus inhibiting its expression. While targeting of *ENG* by miRNA-370 in nonendothelial cells has been previously validated [34], to the best of our knowledge, the validation of *ALK1* targeting by miRNA-10a has not been reported. One limitation of our study is that the predicted targeting of *ENG* and *ALK1* by miRNA-370 and miRNA-10a, respectively, has not been experimentally validated in human endothelial cells. Whether the altered levels of circulating miRNA-370 or miRNA-10a in HHT1 or HHT2 patients contribute to the regulated expression and function of endoglin or ALK1 in the endothelium remains an interesting avenue of research in the future. Because the levels of miRNA-370 or miRNA-10a are specifically dysregulated in patients who present a deficient expression of *ENG* (HHT1) or *ALK1* (HHT2), respectively, a possible link between the expression levels of the HHT genes and those miRNAs can be postulated (Figure 3). Since haploinsufficiency underlies the pathogenic mechanism in HHT1 and HHT2, it can be speculated that the dysregulated expression of miRNA-370 and miRNA-10a may affect HHT development by modulating the expression levels of *ENG* or *ALK1*. However, there is an opposite effect in the expression levels of miRNA-370 (upregulated) versus miRNA-10a (downregulated), suggesting a contrary effect on the expression levels of *ENG* or *ALK1*. Moreover, the expression levels of miRNA-214, which is predicted to target *ENG* and *ALK1*, are not significantly affected in our HHT population study. These apparent discrepancies are likely explained by the fact that the genes encoding miRNA-370 (MIR370; chromosome 14), miRNA-10a (MIR10A; chromosome 17), and miRNA-214 (MIR214; chromosome 1) are differentially regulated by distinct gene expression programs. Furthermore, miRNA-370 and miRNA-10a may target not only *ENG* or *ALK1*, but also the other genes, especially those relevant to vascular development, which may turn out be of greater relevance in the complex mechanism of lesion development in HHT.

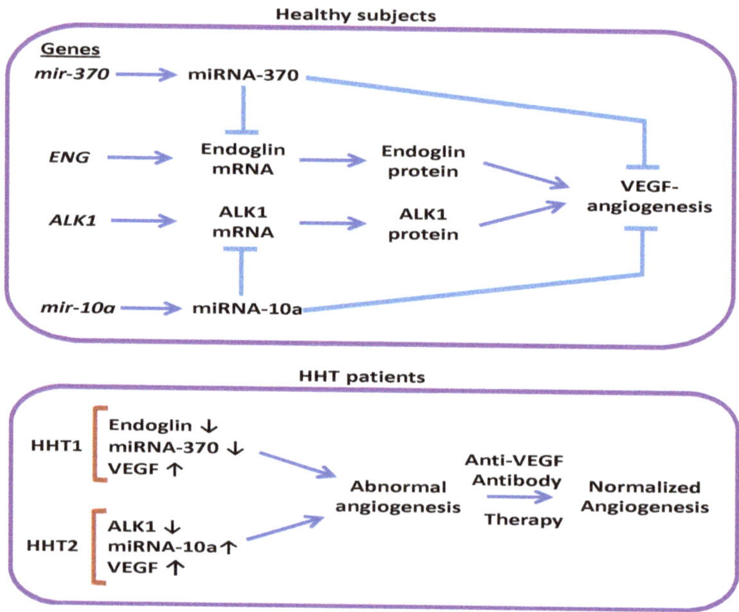

Figure 3. Hypothetical model for the involvement of miRNA-370 and miRNA-10a in HHT. Top, in healthy subjects, basal levels of miRNA-370 and miRNA-10a are predicted to target endoglin, ALK1, as well as the VEGF/VEGFR pathway, thus regulating angiogenesis. Bottom, in HHT patients, heterozygous mutations lead to a deficient expression of endoglin (HHT1) or ALK1 (HHT2), associated with increased levels of VEGF and the dysregulated expression of miRNA-370 and miRNA-10a, resulting in abnormal angiogenesis. Treatment with antibodies to VEGF (bevacizumab) contributes to angiogenesis normalization. ALK1: activin receptor-like kinase 1; VEGF: vascular endothelial growth factor; VEGFR: VEGF receptors.

5. Conclusions

In summary, here we find that decreased levels of miRNA-370 or increased levels of miRNA-10a in plasma from HHT patients represent novel biomarkers that could help to identify undiagnosed patients within the HHT1 or HHT2 subsets, respectively. Both miRNA-370 and miRNA-10a can regulate angiogenesis, a VEGF-dependent biological process involved in the pathophysiology and therapy of HHT, by targeting, at least, VEGF receptors. Additionally, miRNA-370 and miRNA-10a are predicted to target *ENG* and *ALK1* genes, respectively, whose deleterious mutations lead to HHT1 or HHT2, respectively. These findings open up a new research avenue to better understand the functional impact of dysregulated miRNAs in HHT development. Future independent studies remain to be performed in order to further validate the role of miRNA-370 and miRNA-10a as biomarkers in HHT, as well as to investigate the functional and pathophysiological significance of these newly discovered miRNA-370/HHT1 and miRNA-10a/ALK1 associations.

Author Contributions: Conceptualization, L.R.-L., L.M.B., and C.B.; methodology, L.R.-L., and V.A.; software, L.R.-L., and V.A.; validation, L.R.-L.; formal analysis, L.R.-L., V.A., L.M.B., and C.B.; investigation, L.R.-L.; resources, L.M.B. and C.B.; writing—original draft preparation, L.R.-L., and C.B.; writing—review and editing, L.R.-L., V.A., L.M.B., and C.B.; visualization, L.R.-L., and C.B.; supervision and project administration, C.B.; funding acquisition, C.B.; All authors have read and agreed to the published version of the manuscript.

Funding: This research was funded by grants from Ministerio de Ciencia, Innovación y Universidades of Spain (SAF2013-43421-R to CB), Centro de Investigación Biomédica en Red de Enfermedades Raras (CIBERER; ISCIII-CB06/07/0038 to CB), and Consejo Superior de Investigaciones Científicas (CSIC; 201920E022 to CB).

CIBERER is an initiative of the Instituto de Salud Carlos III (ISCIII) of Spain supported by European Regional Development (FEDER) funds.

Acknowledgments: We thank Laura Barrios (Statistics Department, Computing Center, CSIC, Madrid, Spain) for expert statistical analysis, and Carmen Langa, Elena de Blas and Lucia Recio-Poveda for technical support.

Conflicts of Interest: The authors declare no conflict of interest.

References

1. Shovlin, C.L. Hereditary haemorrhagic telangiectasia: Pathophysiology, diagnosis and treatment. *Blood Rev.* **2010**, *24*, 203–219. [CrossRef] [PubMed]
2. McDonald, J.; Bayrak-Toydemir, P.; Pyeritz, R.E. Hereditary hemorrhagic telangiectasia: An overview of diagnosis, management, and pathogenesis. *Genet. Med.* **2011**, *13*, 607–616. [CrossRef] [PubMed]
3. Shovlin, C.L.; Guttmacher, A.E.; Buscarini, E.; Faughnan, M.E.; Hyland, R.H.; Westermann, C.J.J.; Kjeldsen, A.D.; Plauchu, H. Diagnostic criteria for Hereditary Hemorrhagic Telangiectasia (Rendu-Osler-Weber Syndrome). *Am. J. Med. Genet.* **2000**, *91*, 66–67. [CrossRef]
4. Shovlin, C.L.; Buscarini, E.; Kjeldsen, A.D.; Mager, H.J.; Sabba, C.; Droege, F.; Geisthoff, U.; Ugolini, S.; Dupuis-Girod, S. European Reference Network for Rare Vascular Diseases (VASCERN) Outcome Measures for Hereditary Haemorrhagic Telangiectasia (HHT). *Orphanet. J. Rare. Dis.* **2018**, *13*, 136. [CrossRef]
5. Faughnan, M.E.; Palda, V.A.; Garcia-Tsao, G.; Geisthoff, U.W.; McDonald, J.; Proctor, D.D.; Spears, J.; Brown, D.H.; Buscarini, E.; Chesnutt, M.S.; et al. International guidelines for the diagnosis and management of hereditary haemorrhagic telangiectasia. *J. Med. Genet.* **2011**, *48*, 73–87. [CrossRef]
6. McAllister, K.A.; Grogg, K.M.; Johnson, D.W.; Gallione, C.J.; Baldwin, M.A.; Jackson, C.E.; Helmbold, E.A.; Markel, D.S.; McKinnon, W.C.; Murrel, J.; et al. Endoglin, a TGF-β binding protein of endothelial cells, is the gene for hereditary haemorrhagic telangiectasia type 1. *Nat. Genet.* **1994**, *8*, 345–351. [CrossRef]
7. Johnson, D.W.; Berg, J.N.; Baldwin, M.A.; Gallione, C.J.; Marondel, I.; Yoon, S.J.; Stenzel, T.T.; Speer, M.; Pericak-Vance, M.A.; Diamond, A.; et al. Mutations in the activin receptor-like kinase 1 gene in hereditary haemorrhagic telangiectasia type. *Nat. Genet.* **1996**, *13*, 189–195. [CrossRef]
8. Gallione, C.J.; Repetto, G.M.; Legius, E.; Rustgi, A.K.; Schelley, S.L.; Tejpar, S.; Mitchell, G.; Drouin, É.; Westermann, C.J.J.; Marchuk, D.A. A combined syndrome of juvenile polyposis and hereditary haemorrhagic telangiectasia associated with mutations in MADH4 (SMAD4). *Lancet* **2004**, *363*, 852–859. [CrossRef]
9. Wooderchak-Donahue, W.L.; McDonald, J.; O'Fallon, B.; Upton, P.D.; Li, W.; Roman, B.L.; Young, S.; Plant, P.; Fülöp, G.T.; Langa, C.; et al. BMP9 mutations cause a vascular-anomaly syndrome with phenotypic overlap with hereditary hemorrhagic telangiectasia. *Am. J. Hum. Genet.* **2013**, *93*, 530–537. [CrossRef]
10. McDonald, J.; Bayrak-Toydemir, P.; DeMille, D.; Wooderchak-Donahue, W.; Whitehead, K. Curaçao diagnostic criteria for hereditary hemorrhagic telangiectasia is highly predictive of a pathogenic variant in ENG or ACVRL1 (HHT1 and HHT2). *Genet. Med.* **2020**. [CrossRef]
11. Abdalla, S.A.; Letarte, M. Hereditary haemorrhagic telangiectasia: Current views on genetics and mechanisms of disease. *J. Med. Genet.* **2006**, *43*, 97–110. [CrossRef] [PubMed]
12. Ruiz-Llorente, L.; Gallardo-Vara, E.; Rossi, E.; Smadja, D.M.; Botella, L.M.; Bernabeu, C. Endoglin and alk1 as therapeutic targets for hereditary hemorrhagic telangiectasia. *Expert Opin. Ther. Targets* **2017**, *21*, 933–947. [CrossRef] [PubMed]
13. Roman, B.L.; Hinck, A.P. ALK1 signaling in development and disease: New paradigms. *Cell. Mol. Life Sci.* **2017**, *74*, 4539–4560. [CrossRef] [PubMed]
14. Wood, J.H.; Guo, J.; Morrell, N.W.; Li, W. Advances in the molecular regulation of endothelial BMP9 signalling complexes and implications for cardiovascular disease. *Biochem. Soc. Trans.* **2019**, *47*, 779–791. [CrossRef] [PubMed]
15. Park, S.O.; Wankhede, M.; Lee, Y.J.; Choi, E.-J.; Fliess, N.; Choe, S.-W.; Oh, S.-H.; Walter, G.; Raizada, M.; Sorg, B.; et al. Real-time imaging of de novo arteriovenous malformation in a mouse model of hereditary hemorrhagic telangiectasia. *J. Clin. Investig.* **2009**, *119*, 3487–3496. [CrossRef]
16. Choi, E.J.; Chen, W.; Jun, K.; Arthur, H.M.; Young, W.L.; Su, H. Novel brain arteriovenous malformation mouse models for type 1 hereditary hemorrhagic telangiectasia. *PLoS ONE* **2014**, *9*, e88511. [CrossRef]

17. Garrido-Martin, E.M.; Nguyen, H.L.; Cunningham, T.A.; Choe, S.W.; Jiang, Z.; Arthur, H.M.; Lee, Y.J.; Oh, S.P. Common and distinctive pathogenetic features of arteriovenous malformations in hereditary hemorrhagic telangiectasia 1 and hereditary hemorrhagic telangiectasia 2 animal models—Brief report. *Arterioscler. Thromb. Vasc. Biol.* **2014**, *34*, 2232–2236. [CrossRef]

18. Snellings, D.A.; Gallione, C.J.; Clark, D.S.; Vozoris, N.T.; Faughnan, M.E.; Marchuk, D.A. Somatic Mutations in Vascular Malformations of Hereditary Hemorrhagic Telangiectasia Result in Bi-allelic Loss of ENG or ACVRL1. *Am. J. Hum. Genet.* **2019**, *105*, 894–906. [CrossRef]

19. Bartel, D.P. Metazoan MicroRNAs. *Cell* **2018**, *173*, 20–51. [CrossRef]

20. Treiber, T.; Treiber, N.; Meister, G. Regulation of microRNA biogenesis and its crosstalk with other cellular pathways. *Nat. Rev. Mol. Cell Biol.* **2019**, *20*, 5–20. [CrossRef]

21. Hata, A.; Lagna, G. Deregulation of Drosha in the pathogenesis of hereditary hemorrhagic telangiectasia. *Curr. Opin. Hematol.* **2019**, *26*, 161–169. [CrossRef]

22. Jiang, X.; Wooderchak-Donahue, W.L.; McDonald, J.; Ghatpande, P.; Baalbaki, M.; Sandoval, M.; Hart, D.; Clay, H.; Coughlin, S.; Lagna, G.; et al. Inactivating mutations in drosha mediate vascular abnormalities similar to hereditary hemorrhagic telangiectasia. *Sci. Signal.* **2018**, *11*, eaan6831. [CrossRef] [PubMed]

23. Hammond, S.M. An overview of microRNAs. *Adv. Drug Deliv. Rev.* **2015**, *87*, 3–14. [CrossRef] [PubMed]

24. Matsuyama, H.; Suzuki, H.I. Systems and synthetic microRNA biology: From biogenesis to disease pathogenesis. *Int. J. Mol. Sci.* **2020**, *21*, 132. [CrossRef] [PubMed]

25. Tabruyn, S.P.; Hansen, S.; Ojeda-Fernández, M.L.; Bovy, N.; Zarrabeitia, R.; Recio-Poveda, L.; Bernabéu, C.; Martial, J.A.; Botella, L.M.; Struman, I. MiR-205 is downregulated in hereditary hemorrhagic telangiectasia and impairs TGF-beta signaling pathways in endothelial cells. *Angiogenesis* **2013**, *16*, 877–887. [CrossRef] [PubMed]

26. Zhang, Q.; Kandic, I.; Faughnan, M.E.; Kutryk, M.J. Elevated circulating microRNA-210 levels in patients with hereditary hemorrhagic telangiectasia and pulmonary arteriovenous malformations: A potential new biomarker. *Biomarkers* **2013**, *18*, 23–29. [CrossRef]

27. Cannavicci, A.; Zhang, Q.; Dai, S.C.; Faughnan, M.E.; Kutryk, M.J.B. Decreased levels of miR-28-5p and miR-361-3p and increased levels of insulin-like growth factor 1 mRNA in mononuclear cells from patients with hereditary hemorrhagic telangiectasia. *Can. J. Physiol. Pharmacol.* **2019**, *97*, 562–569. [CrossRef]

28. John, B.; Enright, A.J.; Aravin, A.; Tuschl, T.; Sander, C.; Marks, D.S. Human microRNA targets. *PLoS Biol.* **2004**, *2*, e363. [CrossRef]

29. Lewis, B.P.; Burge, C.B.; Bartel, D.P. Conserved seed pairing, often flanked by adenosines, indicates that thousands of human genes are microRNA targets. *Cell* **2005**, *120*, 15–20. [CrossRef]

30. Griffiths-Jones, S.; Hui, J.H.L.; Marco, A.; Ronshaugen, M. MicroRNA evolution by arm switching. *EMBO Rep.* **2011**, *12*, 172–177. [CrossRef]

31. Kroh, E.M.; Parkin, R.K.; Mitchell, P.S.; Tewari, M. Analysis of circulating microRNA biomarkers in plasma and serum using quantitative reverse transcription-PCR (qRT-PCR). *Methods* **2010**, *50*, 298–301. [CrossRef] [PubMed]

32. Wang, X.; Zhang, X.; Yuan, J.; Wu, J.; Deng, X.; Peng, J.; Wang, S.; Yang, C.; Ge, J.; Zou, Y. Evaluation of the performance of serum miRNAs as normalizers in microRNA studies focused on cardiovascular disease. *J. Thorac. Dis.* **2018**, *10*, 2599–2607. [CrossRef] [PubMed]

33. Gareev, I.; Beylerli, O.; Yang, G.; Sun, J.; Pavlov, V.; Izmailov, A.; Shi, H.; Zhao, S. The current state of MiRNAs as biomarkers and therapeutic tools. *Clin. Exp. Med.* **2020**. [CrossRef] [PubMed]

34. Chen, X.P.; Chen, Y.G.; Lan, J.Y.; Shen, Z.J. MicroRNA-370 suppresses proliferation and promotes endometrioid ovarian cancer chemosensitivity to cDDP by negatively regulating ENG. *Cancer Lett.* **2014**, *353*, 201–210. [CrossRef] [PubMed]

35. Li, L.; Li, G.; Yu, C.; Shen, Z.; Xu, C.; Feng, Z.; Zhang, X.; Li, Y. A role of microRNA-370 in hepatic ischaemia-reperfusion injury by targeting transforming growth factor-β receptor II. *Liver Int.* **2015**, *35*, 1124–1132. [CrossRef]

36. Zhang, H.; Sun, X.; Hao, D. Upregulation of microRNA-370 facilitates the repair of amputated fingers through targeting forkhead box protein O1. *Exp. Biol. Med.* **2016**, *241*, 282–289. [CrossRef]

37. Zhang, S.; Song, G.; Yuan, J.; Qiao, S.; Xu, S.; Si, Z.; Yang, Y.; Xu, X.; Wang, A. Circular RNA circ_0003204 inhibits proliferation, migration and tube formation of endothelial cell in atherosclerosis via miR-370-3p/TGFβR2/phosph-SMAD3 axis. *J. Biomed. Sci.* **2020**, *27*, 11. [CrossRef]

38. Wang, X.H.; Chen, L. MicroRNA-370 suppresses the retinal capillary endothelial cell growth by targeting KDR gene. *Bratislava Med. J.* **2017**, *118*, 202–207. [CrossRef]

39. Hou, W.Z.; Chen, X.L.; Wu, W.; Hang, C.H. MicroRNA-370-3p inhibits human vascular smooth muscle cell proliferation via targeting KDR/AKT signaling pathway in cerebral aneurysm. *Eur. Rev. Med. Pharmacol. Sci.* **2017**, *21*, 1080–1087.

40. Gu, Y.; Becker, V.; Zhao, Y.; Menger, M.D.; Laschke, M.W. miR-370 inhibits the angiogenic activity of endothelial cells by targeting smoothened (SMO) and bone morphogenetic protein (BMP)-2. *FASEB J.* **2019**, *33*, 7213–7224. [CrossRef]

41. Zhao, Y.; Ponnusamy, M.; Zhang, L.; Zhang, Y.; Liu, C.; Yu, W.; Wang, K.; Li, P. The role of miR-214 in cardiovascular diseases. *Eur. J. Pharmacol.* **2017**, *816*, 138–145. [CrossRef] [PubMed]

42. Shih, T.C.; Tien, Y.J.; Wen, C.J.; Yeh, T.S.; Yu, M.C.; Huang, C.H.; Lee, Y.S.; Yen, T.C.; Hsieh, S.Y. MicroRNA-214 downregulation contributes to tumor angiogenesis by inducing secretion of the hepatoma-derived growth factor in human hepatoma. *J. Hepatol.* **2012**, *57*, 584–591. [CrossRef] [PubMed]

43. Van Mil, A.; Grundmann, S.; Goumans, M.J.; Lei, Z.; Oerlemans, M.I.; Jaksani, S.; Doevendans, P.A.; Sluijter, J.P.G. MicroRNA-214 inhibits angiogenesis by targeting Quaking and reducing angiogenic growth factor release. *Cardiovasc. Res.* **2012**, *93*, 655–665. [CrossRef] [PubMed]

44. Li, J.; Zhang, Y.; Zhao, Q.; Wang, J.; He, X. MicroRNA-10a influences osteoblast differentiation and angiogenesis by regulating β-catenin expression. *Cell. Physiol. Biochem.* **2015**, *37*, 2194–2208. [CrossRef] [PubMed]

45. Wang, X.; Ling, C.C.; Li, L.; Qin, Y.; Qi, J.; Liu, X.; You, B.; Shi, Y.; Zhang, J.; Jiang, Q.; et al. MicroRNA-10a/10b represses a novel target gene mib1 to regulate angiogenesis. *Cardiovasc. Res.* **2016**, *110*, 140–150. [CrossRef]

46. Lee, D.Y.; Lin, T.E.; Lee, C.I.; Zhou, J.; Huang, Y.H.; Lee, P.L.; Shih, Y.T.; Chien, S.; Chiu, J.J. MicroRNA-10a is crucial for endothelial response to different flow patterns via interaction of retinoid acid receptors and histone deacetylases. *Proc. Natl. Acad. Sci. USA* **2017**, *114*, 2072–2077. [CrossRef]

47. Navickas, R.; Gal, D.; Laucevičius, A.; Taparauskaite, A.; Zdanyte, M.; Holvoet, P. Identifying circulating microRNAs as biomarkers of cardiovascular disease: A systematic review. *Cardiovasc. Res.* **2016**, *111*, 322–337. [CrossRef]

48. Botella, L.M.; Albiñana, V.; Ojeda-Fernandez, L.; Recio-Poveda, L.; Bernabéu, C. Research on potential biomarkers in hereditary hemorrhagic telangiectasia. *Front. Genet.* **2015**, *6*, 115. [CrossRef]

49. McDonald, J.; Wooderchak-Donahue, W.; VanSant Webb, C.; Whitehead, K.; Stevenson, D.A.; Bayrak-Toydemir, P. Hereditary hemorrhagic telangiectasia: Genetics and molecular diagnostics in a new era. *Front. Genet.* **2015**, *6*, 1. [CrossRef]

50. Majumdar, S.; McWilliams, J.P. Approach to Pulmonary Arteriovenous Malformations: A Comprehensive Update. *J. Clin. Med.* **2020**, *9*, 1927. [CrossRef]

51. Aronson, J.K.; Ferner, R.E. Biomarkers-A General Review. *Curr. Protoc. Pharmacol.* **2017**, *76*, 9.23.1–9.23.17. [CrossRef] [PubMed]

52. Califf, R.M. Biomarker definitions and their applications. *Exp. Biol. Med.* **2018**, *243*, 213–221. [CrossRef] [PubMed]

53. Hosseinpour, S.; He, Y.; Nanda, A.; Ye, Q. MicroRNAs Involved in the Regulation of Angiogenesis in Bone Regeneration. *Calcif. Tissue. Int.* **2019**, *105*, 223–238. [CrossRef] [PubMed]

54. Han, C.; Choe, S.W.; Kim, Y.H.; Acharya, A.P.; Keselowsky, B.G.; Sorg, B.S.; Lee, Y.J.; Oh, S.P. VEGF neutralization can prevent and normalize arteriovenous malformations in an animal model for hereditary hemorrhagic telangiectasia 2. *Angiogenesis* **2014**, *17*, 823–830. [CrossRef] [PubMed]

55. Albiñana, V.; Cuesta, A.M.; de Rojas-P., I.; Gallardo-Vara, E.; Recio-Poveda, L.; Bernabéu, C.; Botella, L.M. Review of Pharmacological Strategies with Repurposed Drugs for Hereditary Hemorrhagic Telangiectasia Related Bleeding. *J. Clin. Med.* **2020**, *9*, 1766.

56. Cirulli, A.; Liso, A.; D'Ovidio, F.; Mestice, A.; Pasculli, G.; Gallitelli, M.; Rizzi, R.; Specchia, G.; Sabbà, C. Vascular endothelial growth factor serum levels are elevated in patients with hereditary hemorrhagic telangiectasia. *Acta Haematol.* **2003**, *110*, 29–32. [CrossRef]

57. Sadick, H.; Riedel, F.; Naim, R.; Goessler, U.; Hörmann, K.; Hafner, M.; Lux, A. Patients with hereditary hemorrhagic telangiectasia have increased plasma levels of vascular endothelial growth factor and transforming growth factor-β1 as well as high ALK1 tissue expression. *Haematologica* **2005**, *90*, 818–828.

58. Buscarini, E.; Botella, L.M.; Geisthoff, U.; Kjeldsen, A.D.; Mager, H.J.; Pagella, F.; Suppressa, P.; Zarrabeitia, R.; Dupuis-Girod, S.; Shovlin, C.L.; et al. Safety of thalidomide and bevacizumab in patients with hereditary hemorrhagic telangiectasia. *Orphanet J. Rare Dis.* **2019**, *14*, 28. [CrossRef]
59. Shao, E.S.; Lin, L.; Yao, Y.; Boström, K.I. Expression of vascular endothelial growth factor is coordinately regulated by the activin-like kinase receptors 1 and 5 in endothelial cells. *Blood* **2009**, *114*, 2197–2206. [CrossRef]
60. Tian, H.; Huang, J.J.; Golzio, C.; Gao, X.; Hector-Greene, M.; Katsanis, N.; Blobe, G.C. Endoglin interacts with VEGFR2 to promote angiogenesis. *FASEB J.* **2018**, *32*, 2934–2949. [CrossRef]
61. López-Novoa, J.M.; Bernabeu, C. The physiological role of endoglin in the cardiovascular system. *Am. J. Physiol. Heart Circ. Physiol.* **2010**, *299*, H959–H974. [CrossRef]

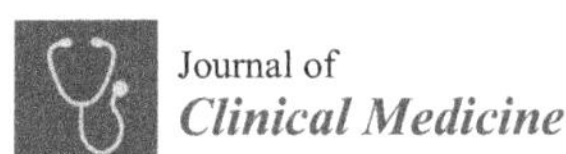
Journal of
Clinical Medicine

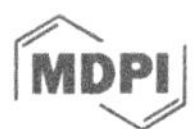

Article

Genotype–Phenotype Correlations in Children with HHT

Alexandra Kilian [1], Giuseppe A. Latino [1,2], Andrew J. White [3], Dewi Clark [1,4], Murali M. Chakinala [5], Felix Ratjen [6], Jamie McDonald [7], Kevin J. Whitehead [8,9], James R. Gossage [10], Doris Lin [11], Katharine Henderson [12], Jeffrey Pollak [12], Justin P. McWilliams [13], Helen Kim [14,15,16], Michael T. Lawton [17], Marie E. Faughnan [1,4,*] and the Brain Vascular Malformation Consortium HHT Investigator Group [†]

1   Toronto HHT Centre, St. Michael's Hospital and Li Ka Shing Knowledge Institute, Toronto, ON M5B 1W8, Canada; alexandra.kilian@mail.utoronto.ca (A.K.); Giuseppe.Latino@nygh.on.ca (G.A.L.); dewi.clark@unityhealth.to (D.C.)
2   Department of Pediatrics, North York General Hospital, University of Toronto, Toronto, ON M2K 1E1, Canada
3   Department of Pediatrics, Washington University School of Medicine, St Louis, MO 63110, USA; white_a@wustl.edu
4   Division of Respirology, Department of Medicine, University of Toronto, Toronto, ON M5S 3H2, Canada
5   Division of Pulmonary and Critical Care Medicine, Washington University School of Medicine, St Louis, MO 63110, USA; chakinalam@wustl.edu
6   Division of Respiratory Medicine and Translational Medicine, The Hospital for Sick Children, Toronto, ON M5G 1X8, Canada; felix.ratjen@sickkids.ca
7   Department of Pathology, University of Utah, Salt Lake City, UT 84132, USA; jamie.mcdonald@hsc.utah.edu
8   Department of Medicine, Division of Cardiovascular Medicine, University of Utah, Salt Lake City, UT 84132, USA; kevin.whitehead@hsc.utah.edu
9   Department of Pediatrics, Division of Pediatric Cardiology, University of Utah, Salt Lake City, UT 84132, USA
10   Department of Medicine, Augusta University, Augusta, GA 30912, USA; jgossage@augusta.edu
11   Department of Radiology, The Johns Hopkins University School of Medicine, Baltimore, MD 21205, USA; ddmlin@jhmi.edu
12   Department of Radiology and Biomedical Imaging, and HHT Program, Yale University School of Medicine, New Haven, CT 06510, USA; katharine.henderson@yale.edu (K.H.); jeffrey.pollak@yale.edu (J.P.)
13   Department of Interventional Radiology, University of California Los Angeles, Los Angeles, CA 90095, USA; jumcwilliams@mednet.ucla.edu
14   USA Center for Cerebrovascular Research, Department of Anesthesia and Perioperative Care, University of California San Francisco, San Francisco, CA 94110, USA; Helen.Kim2@ucsf.edu
15   Institute for Human Genetics, University of California San Francisco, San Francisco, CA 94143, USA
16   Department of Epidemiology and Biostatistics, University of California San Francisco, San Francisco, CA 94158, USA
17   Department of Neurosurgery, Barrow Neurological Institute, Phoenix, AZ 85013, USA; michael.lawton@barrowbrainandspine.com
*   Correspondence: Marie.Faughnan@unityhealth.to
†   For Collaborator Tab: Murali M. Chakinala, Marianne S Clancy, Marie E Faughnan, James R Gossage, Katharine Henderson, Vivek Iyer, Raj S Kasthuri, Helen Kim, Timo Krings, Michael T Lawton, Doris Lin, Johannes Jurgen Mager, Douglas A Marchuk, Justin P McWilliams, Jamie McDonald, Ludmila Pawlikowska, Jeffrey Pollak, Felix Ratjen, Karen Swanson, Dilini Vethanayagam, Andrew J White, Pearce Wilcox.

Received: 11 July 2020; Accepted: 19 August 2020; Published: 22 August 2020

Abstract: Hereditary hemorrhagic telangiectasia (HHT), a rare autosomal dominant disease mostly caused by mutations in three known genes (*ENG*, *ACVRL1*, and *SMAD4*), is characterized by the development of vascular malformations (VMs). Patients with HHT may present with mucocutaneous telangiectasia, as well as organ arteriovenous malformations (AVMs) of the central nervous system, lungs, and liver. Genotype–phenotype correlations have been well described in adults with

HHT. We aimed to investigate genotype–phenotype correlations among pediatric HHT patients. Demographic, clinical, and genetic data were collected and analyzed in 205 children enrolled in the multicenter Brain Vascular Malformation Consortium HHT Project. A chi-square test was used to determine the association between phenotypic presentations and genotype. Among 205 patients (age range: 0–18 years; mean: 11 years), *ENG* mutation was associated with the presence of pulmonary AVMs ($p < 0.001$) and brain VM ($p < 0.001$). The presence of a combined phenotype—defined as both pulmonary AVMs and brain VMs—was also associated with *ENG* mutation. Gastrointestinal bleeding was rare (4.4%), but was associated with *SMAD4* genotype ($p < 0.001$). We conclude that genotype–phenotype correlations among pediatric HHT patients are similar to those described among adults. Specifically, pediatric patients with *ENG* mutation have a greater prevalence of pulmonary AVMs, brain VMs, and a combined phenotype.

Keywords: Hereditary hemorrhagic telangiectasia; pediatrics; genotype–phenotype correlation; arteriovenous malformation; *ENG*; *ACVRL1*; *SMAD4*

---

1. Introduction

Hereditary hemorrhagic telangiectasia (HHT) is a rare autosomal dominant disease affecting approximately 1 in 5000 people [1–4]. HHT can be diagnosed clinically using the Curaçao clinical diagnostic criteria [5] or by genetic testing [6]. Mutations in the endoglin (*ENG*) and activin A receptor-like kinase 1 (*ACVRL1*) genes account for approximately 96% of cases, when the Curaçao clinical diagnostic criteria are strictly applied [7]. In addition, less than 2% of patients present with an HHT–Juvenile Polyposis (JP) overlap syndrome, caused by mutations in the *SMAD4* gene [7–9]. HHT is characterized by the development of arteriovenous malformations (AVMs) in visceral organs, including the brain, lungs, liver, and rarely the spine. AVMs carry risks of life-threatening complications, including hemorrhage and paradoxical embolisms [6,10,11]. Additionally, smaller vascular malformations—called telangiectases—occur on mucocutaneous surfaces [11]. Bleeding from telangiectases in the nasal mucosa results in spontaneous recurrent epistaxis. Additionally, patients can have chronic bleeding from telangiectases in the gastrointestinal (GI) mucosa, often complicated by secondary iron-deficiency anemia [12].

Genotype–phenotype correlations have been well described in adult cohorts [10,13–19]. Most conclusively, the *ENG* genotype (HHT1: OMIM# 18730) has been associated with the presence of pulmonary AVMs [10,13–15,17,19–21] and brain VMs [10,13–16,21] in adults. While there are multiple brain VM subtypes seen in HHT, including arteriovenous fistulas (AVFs), nidus-type AVMs, and capillary vascular malformations, no correlations between brain VM subtype and genotype have been described [22]. The *ACVRL1* mutation (HHT2: OMIM# 600376) has been associated with the presence of liver VMs [10,13,14,20,21]. However, there is a relative paucity of literature regarding genotype–phenotype correlations, as well as HHT manifestations and complications in pediatric patients. Smaller pediatric cohorts have demonstrated that the *ENG* genotype is correlated with pulmonary AVMs and brain VMs [23–25]. The visible features of HHT—mucocutaneous telangiectases and spontaneous recurrent epistaxis—increase with age [26–28]. This, combined with the rarity of the disease, can result in delayed presentation and diagnosis in children [5,6,29,30]. Thus, a more robust understanding of genotype–phenotype correlations will have implications for diagnosis of HHT and organ screening in children. Accordingly, we aimed to report data from a large pediatric cohort of patients with HHT and describe the genotype-phenotype correlations.

2. Materials and Methods

2.1. Cohort

Demographic, clinical, and genetic data were collected from 205 pediatric patients (age at recruitment ≤18) enrolled in the Brain Vascular Malformation Consortium (BVMC) HHT Project. The BVMC HHT Project includes 1679 HHT patients with a definite clinical or genetic diagnosis of HHT, enrolled at multiple recruiting centers in the US, Canada, and the Netherlands between 2010 and 2019. Cohort recruitment has been previously described [18,31]. The 205 pediatric patients in this study were recruited from nine of the BVMC recruiting centers. Informed written consent was obtained from all patients to be included in all BVMC related projects. The study protocol was approved by the institutional review board at each recruiting center (SMH REB#09-212 for lead site at St. Michael's Hospital). Patients were screened for organ VMs and other clinical features according to standard clinical practice (not as study procedure) and International HHT Guidelines [6]. Organ VM screening typically included: comprehensive history, physical exam, and routine investigations; pulmonary AVMs screening with contrast echocardiography or positional oximetry (protocols varied by center); brain VM screening by magnetic resonance imaging (MRI); clinical screening for liver VMs (chronic right upper quadrant pain, portal hypertension, high-output heart failure, liver bruit on examination); clinical screening for recurrent spontaneous epistaxis (>1 episode per month for >1 year); and screening for HHT-related GI bleeding (history of anemia, iron deficiency, known GI telangiectases on endoscopy, melena, rectal bleeding). If screening was positive for pulmonary AVM or brain VM, patients underwent confirmatory diagnostic imaging and treatment where appropriate. If clinical assessment was suggestive of symptomatic liver VM, diagnostic imaging was recommended and therapy was initiated where appropriate. Finally, if the initial clinical assessment was suggestive of GI bleeding, diagnostic endoscopy was recommended and endoscopic, medical, and supportive therapies were undertaken on a case-by-case basis. The BVMC HHT cohort targets 25% of brain VM-positive patients, while other characteristics are similar to other cohorts [13,16].

2.2. Analysis

We tested whether HHT genotype (*ACVRL1*, *ENG*, *SMAD4*) was associated with clinical features including the presence of epistaxis, typical mucocutaneous telangiectasia, anemia, pulmonary AVMs, brain VMs, GI bleeding, and symptomatic liver VMs. For the purposes of our analysis, patients with micro-pulmonary AVMs were considered to be negative for pulmonary AVMs. All brain VM subtypes met the criteria for the brain VM phenotype. A combined phenotype was defined as the presence of both pulmonary AVM(s) and brain VM(s). Statistical analysis was conducted using the SPSS version 21.0.0. All *p*-values calculated were two-sided and significance was defined at $p < 0.05$. The Kruskal–Wallis test was used to compare the association between continuous variables (age) and genotype. To determine the association between clinical features and genotype (*ACVRL1*, *ENG*, *SMAD4*), a chi-square test was used.

3. Results

Table 1 shows demographic and clinical characteristics of the 205 pediatric HHT patients comprising our cohort, as well as the phenotype characteristics by genotype. Our cohort was 47% female with an average age of 9.9 years. There was no significant difference in the distribution of age or sex between the three genotypes. Among the 205 patients, 176 (85.9%) had epistaxis, 107 (52.2%) had typical mucocutaneous telangiectases, 62 (30.2%) had at least one pulmonary AVM, seven (3.4%) had symptomatic liver VMs, and 70 (34.1%) had one or more brain VM. There was evidence of GI bleeding in nine patients (4.4%) and 30 patients (14.6%) were anemic.

3.1. Genotype

A total of 171 (83.4%) patients in our cohort had a known genetic mutation, confirmed by genetic testing of the patient (156/171 (91.2%)) or a family member (15/171 (8.8%)). The *ENG* genotype was the most common in our cohort, present in 101 of 171 patients (59.1%) with a known mutation. In our cohort, 6/162 (3.7%) patients who underwent genetic testing did not have an identifiable mutation.

3.2. Epistaxis

The most common clinical manifestation of HHT in pediatric patients was spontaneous recurrent epistaxis, present among 172/205 (83.9%) of our patients. There was no significant association between genotype and the presence of epistaxis ($p = 0.865$).

Table 1. Demographic and clinical characteristics of pediatric HHT patients.

Characteristic	All Patients $n = 205$	ENG (101/171, 59%)	ACVRL1 (59/171, 35%)	SMAD4 (11/171, 6%)	p-Value
Female Sex (%)	97 (47%)	51/101 (50.5%)	28/59 (47.5%)	2/11 (18.2%)	0.125
Mean Age (yrs) (±Standard Deviation (years))	9.9 (±6.5)	9.4 (±5.4)	9.2 (±5.5)	11.27 (±4.9)	0.430
Age range	1 month–18 years	1 month–18 years	1 month–18 years	4–17 years	–
Epistaxis	172/205 (83.9%)	86/101 (85.1%)	51/59 (86.4%)	10/11 (90.9%)	0.865
Telangiectasia	104/205(50.7%)	47/101 (46.5%)	28/59 (47.5%)	4/11 (36.4%)	0.790
Pulmonary AVM	62/205 (30.2%)	44/101 (43.6%)	4/59 (6.8%)	1/11 (9.1%)	<0.001
Brain VM	70/205 (34.1%)	45/101 (44.6%)	10/59 (17.0%)	0/11 (0%)	<0.001
GI bleeding	9/205 (4.4%)	2/101 (1.8%)	1/59 (1.7%)	5/11 (45.5%)	<0.001
Anemia	28/205 (13.7%)	13/101 (12.9%)	10/59 (17.0%)	2/11 (18.2%)	0.735
Liver VM	7/205 (3.4%)	1/101 (0.9%)	4/59 (6.8%)	0/11 (0%)	0.093
Any VM	103/205 (50.2%)	65/101 (64.4%)	17/59 (28.8%)	1/11 (0.9%)	<0.001
Combined phenotype [1]	33/205 (16.1%)	24/101 (23.8%)	2/59 (3.4%)	0/10 (0%)	0.001

[1] Combined phenotype: combined presence of both pulmonary AVM(s) and brain VM(s). HHT: hereditary hemorrhagic Telangiectasia; VM: vascular malformation; AVM: Arteriovenous malformation; GI: gastrointestinal.

3.3. Mucocutaneous Telangiectases

Approximately half (50.7%) of patients in our cohort had typical mucocutaneous telangiectases. The prevalence by genotype was almost equivalent between patients with *ENG* and *ACVRL1* mutations at 46.5% and 47.5%, respectively. Four (36.4%) patients with a *SMAD4* mutation had typical mucocutaneous telangiectases. There was no significant association between genotype and the presence of telangiectasia ($p = 0.790$).

3.4. GI Bleeding

A history of GI bleeding was reported in 9/205 (4.4%) patients. Patients with a *SMAD4* mutation were significantly more likely to experience GI bleeding ($p < 0.001$), compared to patients with *ENG* or *ACVRL1* mutations. Clinical and endoscopic data was available in 7/9 (77.8%) patients with GI bleeding. All 7/7 (100%) had lower GI bleeding; none reported upper GI bleeding. In 5/7 (71.4%) patients, polyps were identified as the cause of GI bleeding. No cause was identified in the remaining 2/7 (28.6%) patients with GI bleeding and GI bleeding resolved spontaneously

3.5. Anemia

A history of anemia was reported in 28/205 (13.7%) patients. No genotype was significantly associated with current or historical anemia ($p = 0.735$). Notably, history of anemia was not significantly associated with epistaxis or GI bleeding.

3.6. Organ Vascular Malformations

Pulmonary AVMs were reported in 62/205 (30.2%) patients in our cohort. Brain VMs were reported in 70/205 (34.1%) patients. Pediatric patients with an *ENG* mutation were significantly more likely to have pulmonary AVMs ($p < 0.001$) and brain VMs ($p < 0.001$). Patients with an *ENG* mutation were also more likely to have any organ VM (pulmonary, brain, liver) compared to patients with *ACVRL1* or *SMAD4* mutations ($p < 0.001$). While a higher proportion of patients with an *ACVRL1* mutation had liver VMs compared to patients with an *ENG* gene mutation, this was not statistically significant ($p = 0.093$).

3.7. Combined Phenotype

Thirty-three (16.1%) of patients in our cohort had a combined phenotype, characterized by the presence of both pulmonary AVM(s) and brain VM(s). The majority (72.7%) of the patients with this combined phenotype had an *ENG* mutation and this association was found to be statistically significant ($p < 0.001$). Notably, sex was not a risk factor for the combined phenotype; 17/33 patients (51.5%) with a combined phenotype were male.

4. Discussion

Here, we report data from a large pediatric cohort of patients with HHT and describe genotype–phenotype correlations. Most significantly, our data demonstrate that in pediatric patients, pulmonary AVMs and brain VMs are more frequent in patients with an *ENG* mutation, as reported in adult studies [10,13–15,17,19–21]. Moreover, the *ENG* genotype is associated with a combined phenotype, characterized by the presence of both pulmonary AVM(s) and brain VM(s), in pediatric patients. Finally, while GI bleeding is rare in pediatric HHT patients, it is associated with an *SMAD4* mutation and seen commonly in patients with this genotype.

In our cohort, *ENG* mutation was associated with increased prevalence of brain VMs and pulmonary AVMs. This is consistent with previous literature describing genotype–phenotype correlations in adults, in which the *ENG* genotype was associated with the presence of pulmonary AVMs [10,13–15,17,19–21] and with the presence of brain VMs [10,13–16,21]. Our results also confirm those of previous smaller pediatric series reported by Giordano et al. [23] and A-Saleh et al. [24], comprised of 44 and 61 patients, respectively. While certain clinical features of HHT are age-dependent, including telangiectasia and epistaxis, a similar prevalence of pulmonary AVMs in children as in adults has been reported [25]. This suggests that the pulmonary AVM phenotype is consistent across age groups and may not be age dependent [25].

These observations may have important implications for clinical care and diagnostics in HHT. First, given the similarities in genotype–phenotype correlations, children, like adults, are at risk of complications from organ VMs. Thus, organ screening should be considered. The rationale for pulmonary AVM screening is to identify children at risk of serious complications and who might benefit from preventative management with transcatheter embolization. The rationale for brain VM screening is similar; screening allows for the identification of children at risk of life-threatening and debilitating complications and allows for the consideration of preventative management. The decision to treat brain VMs is typically made on a case-by-case basis, with an expert neurovascular team, balancing the risks of the brain VM with those of the treatment. There is some controversy internationally regarding the role for brain VM screening, resulting in regional practice variation. In North America, the current standard of practice is to screen for brain VMs at the time of diagnosis using MRI. Currently, if initial screening for brain VMs is negative, in childhood, some centers repeat screening every five years or at least once in early adulthood [32].

Second, while children with an *ENG* mutation are at greater risk of having pulmonary AVMs, this feature is present across all genotypes, as in adults. There is, therefore, no evidence to support genotype based pulmonary screening recommendations. Similarly, while the literature suggests increased prevalence of brain VMs in adult patients with an *ENG* mutation [10,13–16,21], brain VMs have been described across all genotypes in adult patients [16]. Our observations are consistent with this; while an *ENG* mutation is associated with brain VM in children, brain VMs are also reported in children with an *ACVRL1* mutation. Although we reported no brain VMs in children with an *SMAD4* mutation, this may have been due to small numbers in this group. Notably, the presence of brain VMs in 34% of patients in our series is higher than previous adult and pediatric reports. Giordano et al. reported brain VM presence in 7/44 (15.9%) children [23]. In adult patients with HHT, the current data suggests that approximately 23% will have a brain VM [33–35]. The increased representation in our cohort was expected due to the explicit recruitment strategy of the BVMC HHT project, which targets recruiting HHT patients but with a 25% recruitment target for patients with brain VMs [31]. Third, as organ VMs are common in children, testing for their presence may be helpful in confirming the clinical diagnosis of HHT in children of families where genetics are not informative.

We also demonstrated that, overall, GI bleeding was a rare clinical manifestation in children with HHT, but was frequent in children with an *SMAD4* mutation. This is not surprising given the known overlap between HHT and Juvenile Polyposis (OMIM# 175050) in patients with *SMAD4* mutations [8,9]. The overall low prevalence of GI bleeding in our pediatric cohort is consistent with previous literature demonstrating later-life onset of GI bleeding in HHT patients [1,28,36]. In fact, Plauchu et al. reported that only 1.5% of patients had GI bleeding at ages younger than 30 [28]. In adults, anemia is a typical complication of chronic GI bleeding in HHT [6,36–38], and Kasthuri et al. described GI bleeding as an independent predictor of anemia in adult HHT patients [12]. Given the typically later-life onset of GI bleeding, the current HHT guidelines [6] recommend monitoring hemoglobin and hematocrit after the age of 35, as a marker of GI bleeding. Our data corroborates the appropriateness of delayed screening for GI bleeding in children with an *ENG* or *ACVRL1* mutation until adulthood. However, children with an *SMAD4* mutation should be considered at risk for earlier GI bleeding and secondary anemia.

Children with an *ENG* gene mutation are at higher risk of a combined phenotype, with the presence of both brain VM(s) and pulmonary AVM(s). The *ENG* genotype has been previously implicated in this combined phenotype in adults [13]. In our cohort, two patients with an *ACVRL1* mutation demonstrated a combined phenotype presentation. Additionally, a causative mutation was unknown in over 20% of cases. The frequency of the combined phenotype in our cohort (16.1%) is higher than the prevalence of 8.7% reported by Letteboer et al. in an adult population [13] and higher than the prevalence of 11.4% reported by Giordano et al. in a pediatric population [23]. Though our prevalence of the combined phenotype may have been overestimated due to selection bias, the association with an *ENG* mutation is highly significant and clinically important. In addition, the presence of the combined phenotype in non-HHT1 children was also an important observation, which once again suggests that organ VM screening in children with HHT should not be reserved for children with *ENG* mutations only. This is in line with the recommendations made by the International HHT guidelines, that genotype should not guide screening practices [6].

We believe our results can be generalized to children with HHT for several reasons. The clinical characteristics of the children in our cohort are similar to other previously published pediatric cohorts. In addition, the multi-center nature of the data supports generalizability. The *ENG* and *ACVRL1* genotype distribution in our data set—59% of patients with an *ENG* mutation, 35% of patients with an *ACVRL1* gene mutation—are in the usual range for North American and some European HHT populations [10,39,40]. In addition, our results align with genotype–phenotype correlations from earlier smaller pediatric cohorts [20,23–25], as well as the previously described trends in the adult population [10,13–16,21].

There are several limitations to our study that warrant discussion. Firstly, the prevalence of brain VMs in our cohort was intentionally enriched in the recruitment design. The BVMC HHT Project aims for 25% of patients with brain VMs. Thus, our cohort likely over represents the brain VM prevalence. Moreover, given that our cohort consisted of patients that were ≤18 years of age at the time of recruitment, we did not include patients diagnosed in childhood, but recruited in adulthood. Additionally, the data collection in the BVMC HHT project is retrospective. While we did not distinguish between brain VM subtypes, this is a topic of interest for future research. Finally, we collected and reported on the presence of anemia based on patient reports and chart review, but we did not collect laboratory data for confirmation or to classify type of anemia. Though this may have led us to underestimate the prevalence of anemia in the cohort, our observed low prevalence of anemia in children with HHT is in keeping with clinical experience [41]. Despite these limitations, the results remain robust and clinically important given the larger size of the patient cohort, the statistical significance of the genotype–phenotype correlations and the consistency of the results with adult observations in HHT.

5. Conclusions

From the largest genotype–phenotype cohort of pediatric patients with HHT to date, we demonstrate that organ involvement and associated genotype-phenotype correlations in children with HHT are similar to those previously described in the adult population. Specifically, the *ENG* genotype is associated with pulmonary AVMs and brain VMs in children with HHT. Moreover, pediatric patients can present with a combined phenotype, with both pulmonary AVM and brain VM, which is also associated with the *ENG* genotype. Our results highlight the importance of organ VM screening in pediatric patients with HHT.

Author Contributions: Conceptualization, A.K., G.A.L., A.J.W., D.C., and M.E.F.; Data curation, The Brain Vascular Malformation Consortium HHT Investigator Group; Formal analysis, A.K. and M.E.F.; Investigation, A.K., G.A.L., A.J.W., D.C., M.M.C., F.R., J.M., K.W., J.R.G., D.L., K.H., J.P., J.P.M., H.K., M.T.L., and M.E.F.; Methodology, A.K., G.A.L., and M.E.F.; Project administration, H.K., M.T.L., and M.E.F.; Supervision, M.F.; Writing—original draft, A.K., G.A.L., A.J.W., D.C., and M.F.; Writing—review and editing, A.K. and M.E.F. All authors have read and agreed to the published version of the manuscript.

Funding: The Brain Vascular Malformation Consortium (U54NS065705) is a part of the NCATS Rare Diseases Clinical Research Network (RDCRN) and is supported by the RDCRN Data Management and Coordinating Center (DMCC) (U2CTR002818). RDCRN is an initiative of the Office of Rare Diseases Research (ORDR), NCATS, funded through a collaboration between NCATS and NINDS. M.E.F. was also supported by the Nelson Arthur Hyland Foundation and Li Ka Shing Knowledge Institute.

References

1. Kjeldsen, A.D.; Vase, P.; Green, A. Hereditary haemorrhagic telangiectasia: A population-based study of prevalence and mortality in Danish patients. *J. Intern. Med.* **1999**, *245*, 31–39. [CrossRef] [PubMed]

2. Donaldson, J.; McKeever, T.M.; Hall, I.P.; Hubbard, R.; Fogarty, A.W. The UK prevalence of hereditary haemorrhagic telangiectasia and its association with sex, socioeconomic status and region of residence: A population-based study. *Thorax* **2014**, *69*, 161–167. [CrossRef] [PubMed]

3. Sabba, C.; Pasculli, G.; Cirulli, A.; Gallitelli, M.; Virgilio, G.; Resta, F.; Guastamacchia, E.; Palasciano, G. Hereditary hemorrhagic teleangiectasia (Rendu-Osler-Weber disease). *Minerva Cardioangiol.* **2002**, *50*, 221–238. [PubMed]

4. Dakeishi, M.; Shioya, T.; Wada, Y.; Shindo, T.; Otaka, K.; Manabe, M.; Nozaki, J.-I.; Inoue, S.; Koizumi, A. Genetic epidemiology of hereditary hemorrhagic telangiectasia in a local community in the northern part of Japan. *Hum. Mutat.* **2002**, *19*, 140–148. [CrossRef] [PubMed]

5. Shovlin, C.L.; Guttmacher, A.E.; Buscarini, E.; Faughnan, M.E.; Hyland, R.H.; Westermann, C.J.; Kjeldsen, A.D.; Plauchu, H. Diagnostic criteria for hereditary hemorrhagic telangiectasia (Rendu-Osler-Weber syndrome). *Am. J. Med. Genet. A* **2000**, *91*, 66–67. [CrossRef]

6. Faughnan, M.; Palda, V.; Garcia-Tsao, G.; Geisthoff, U.; McDonald, J.; Proctor, D.; Spears, J.; Brown, D.; Buscarini, E.; Chesnutt, M. International guidelines for the diagnosis and management of hereditary haemorrhagic telangiectasia. *J. Med. Genet.* **2011**, *48*, 73–87. [CrossRef]

7. McDonald, J.; Bayrak-Toydemir, P.; DeMille, D.; Wooderchak-Donahue, W.; Whitehead, K. Curaçao diagnostic criteria for hereditary hemorrhagic telangiectasia is highly predictive of a pathogenic variant in ENG or ACVRL1 (HHT1 and HHT2). *Genet. Med.* **2020**, 1–5. [CrossRef]

8. Gallione, C.J.; Richards, J.A.; Letteboer, T.; Rushlow, D.; Prigoda, N.L.; Leedom, T.P.; Ganguly, A.; Castells, A.; Van Amstel, J.P.; Westermann, C. SMAD4 mutations found in unselected HHT patients. *J. Med. Genet.* **2006**, *43*, 793–797. [CrossRef]

9. Gallione, C.; Aylsworth, A.S.; Beis, J.; Berk, T.; Bernhardt, B.; Clark, R.D.; Clericuzio, C.; Danesino, C.; Drautz, J.; Fahl, J. Overlapping spectra of SMAD4 mutations in juvenile polyposis (JP) and JP–HHT syndrome. *Am. J. Med. Genet. A* **2010**, *152*, 333–339. [CrossRef]

10. Bayrak-Toydemir, P.; McDonald, J.; Markewitz, B.; Lewin, S.; Miller, F.; Chou, L.S.; Gedge, F.; Tang, W.; Coon, H.; Mao, R. Genotype–phenotype correlation in hereditary hemorrhagic telangiectasia: Mutations and manifestations. *Am. J. Med. Genet. A* **2006**, *140*, 463–470. [CrossRef]

11. Guttmacher, A.E.; Marchuk, D.A.; White, R.I., Jr. Hereditary hemorrhagic telangiectasia. *N. Engl. J. Med.* **1995**, *333*, 918–924. [CrossRef] [PubMed]

12. Kasthuri, R.S.; Montifar, M.; Nelson, J.; Kim, H.; Lawton, M.T.; Faughnan, M.E.; Brain Vascular Malformation Consortium HHT Investigator Group. Prevalence and predictors of anemia in hereditary hemorrhagic telangiectasia. *Am. J. Hematol.* **2017**. [CrossRef] [PubMed]

13. Letteboer, T.G.; Mager, J.; Snijder, R.J.; Koeleman, B.P.; Lindhout, D.; Van Amstel, J.P.; Westermann, C. Genotype-phenotype relationship in hereditary haemorrhagic telangiectasia. *J. Med. Genet.* **2006**, *43*, 371–377. [CrossRef] [PubMed]

14. Sabba, C.; Pasculli, G.; Lenato, G.; Suppressa, P.; Lastella, P.; Memeo, M.; Dicuonzo, F.; Guanti, G. Hereditary hemorrhagic telangiectasia: Clinical features in ENG and ALK1 mutation carriers. *J. Thromb. Haemost.* **2007**, *5*, 1149–1157. [CrossRef]

15. Berg, J.; Porteous, M.; Reinhardt, D.; Gallione, C.; Holloway, S.; Umasunthar, T.; Lux, A.; McKinnon, W.; Marchuk, D.; Guttmacher, A. Hereditary haemorrhagic telangiectasia: A questionnaire based study to delineate the different phenotypes caused by endoglin and ALK1 mutations. *J. Med. Genet.* **2003**, *40*, 585–590. [CrossRef]

16. Nishida, T.; Faughnan, M.E.; Krings, T.; Chakinala, M.; Gossage, J.R.; Young, W.L.; Kim, H.; Pourmohamad, T.; Henderson, K.J.; Schrum, S.D.; et al. Brain arteriovenous malformations associated with hereditary hemorrhagic telangiectasia: Genotype-phenotype correlations. *Am. J. Med. Genet. A* **2012**, *158A*, 2829–2834. [CrossRef]

17. Pawlikowska, L.; Nelson, J.; Guo, D.E.; McCulloch, C.E.; Lawton, M.T.; Kim, H.; Faughnan, M.E.; Brain Vascular Malformation Consortium HHT Investigator Group; Chakinala, M.; Clancy, M. Association of common candidate variants with vascular malformations and intracranial hemorrhage in hereditary hemorrhagic telangiectasia. *Mol. Genet. Genom. Med.* **2018**, *6*, 350–356. [CrossRef]

18. Pawlikowska, L.; Nelson, J.; Guo, D.E.; McCulloch, C.E.; Lawton, M.T.; Young, W.L.; Kim, H.; Faughnan, M.E. The ACVRL1 c.314-35A>G polymorphism is associated with organ vascular malformations in hereditary hemorrhagic telangiectasia patients with ENG mutations, but not in patients with ACVRL1 mutations. *Am. J. Med. Genet. A* **2015**, *167*, 1262–1267. [CrossRef]

19. Kjeldsen, A.D.; Møller, T.; Brusgaard, K.; Vase, P.; Andersen, P.E. Clinical symptoms according to genotype amongst patients with hereditary haemorrhagic telangiectasia. *J. Intern. Med.* **2005**, *258*, 349–355. [CrossRef]

20. Lesca, G.; Olivieri, C.; Burnichon, N.; Pagella, F.; Carette, M.-F.; Gilbert-Dussardier, B.; Goizet, C.; Roume, J.; Rabilloud, M.; Saurin, J.-C. Genotype-phenotype correlations in hereditary hemorrhagic telangiectasia: Data from the French-Italian HHT network. *Genet. Med.* **2007**, *9*, 14–22. [CrossRef]

21. Sánchez-Martínez, R.; Iriarte, A.; Mora-Luján, J.M.; Patier, J.L.; López-Wolf, D.; Ojeda, A.; Torralba, M.A.; Juyol, M.C.; Gil, R.; Añón, S. Current HHT genetic overview in Spain and its phenotypic correlation: Data from RiHHTa registry. *J. Rare Disord.* **2020**, *15*, 1–8. [CrossRef] [PubMed]

22. Krings, T.; Kim, H.; Power, S.; Nelson, J.; Faughnan, M.; Young, W.L.; Brain Vascular Malformation Consortium HHT Investigator Group. Neurovascular manifestations in hereditary hemorrhagic telangiectasia: Imaging features and genotype-phenotype correlations. *AJNR Am. J. Neuroradiol.* **2015**, *36*, 863–870. [CrossRef] [PubMed]

23. Giordano, P.; Lenato, G.M.; Suppressa, P.; Lastella, P.; Dicuonzo, F.; Chiumarulo, L.; Sangerardi, M.; Piccarreta, P.; Valerio, R.; Scardapane, A. Hereditary hemorrhagic telangiectasia: Arteriovenous malformations in children. *Pediatrics* **2013**, *163*, 179–186.e3. [CrossRef] [PubMed]

24. Al-Saleh, S.; Mei-Zahav, M.; Faughnan, M.; MacLusky, I.; Carpenter, S.; Letarte, M.; Ratjen, F. Screening for pulmonary and cerebral arteriovenous malformations in children with hereditary haemorrhagic telangiectasia. *Eur. Respir. J.* **2009**, *34*, 875–881. [CrossRef]

25. Latino, G.A.; Al-Saleh, S.; Alharbi, N.; Edwards, C.; Faughnan, M.E.; Ratjen, F. Prevalence of pulmonary arteriovenous malformations in children versus adults with hereditary hemorrhagic telangiectasia. *Pediatrics* **2013**, *163*, 282–284. [CrossRef]

26. Krings, T.; Ozanne, A.; Chng, S.; Alvarez, H.; Rodesch, G.; Lasjaunias, P. Neurovascular phenotypes in hereditary haemorrhagic telangiectasia patients according to age. *Neuroradiology* **2005**, *47*, 711–720. [CrossRef]

27. Pasculli, G.; Resta, F.; Guastamacchia, E.; Suppressa, P.; Sabbà, C. Health-related quality of life in a rare disease: Hereditary hemorrhagic telangiectasia (HHT) or Rendu–Osler–Weber Disease. *Qual. Life Res.* **2004**, *13*, 1715–1723. [CrossRef]

28. Plauchu, H.; De Chadarévian, J.P.; Bideau, A.; Robert, J.M. Age—Related clinical profile of hereditary hemorrhagic telangiectasia in an epidemiologically recruited population. *Am. J. Med. Genet.* **1989**, *32*, 291–297. [CrossRef] [PubMed]

29. Pierucci, P.; Lenato, G.M.; Suppressa, P.; Lastella, P.; Triggiani, V.; Valerio, R.; Comelli, M.; Salvante, D.; Stella, A.; Resta, N. A long diagnostic delay in patients with Hereditary Haemorrhagic Telangiectasia: A questionnaire-based retrospective study. *J. Rare Disord.* **2012**, *7*, 33. [CrossRef]

30. Pahl, K.S.; Choudhury, A.; Wusik, K.; Hammill, A.; White, A.; Henderson, K.; Pollak, J.; Kasthuri, R.S. Applicability of the Curaçao criteria for the diagnosis of hereditary hemorrhagic telangiectasia in the pediatric population. *Pediatrics* **2018**, *197*, 207–213. [CrossRef]

31. Akers, A.L.; Ball, K.L.; Clancy, M.; Comi, A.M.; Faughnan, M.E.; Gopal-Srivastava, R.; Jacobs, T.P.; Kim, H.; Krischer, J.; Marchuk, D.A.; et al. Brain Vascular Malformation Consortium: Overview, progress and future directions. *J. Rare Disord.* **2013**, *1*, 5. [PubMed]

32. Pahl, K.; Kasthuri, R.S. 11—Hereditary Hemorrhagic Telangiectasia. In *Consultative Hemostasis and Thrombosis*, 4th ed.; Kitchens, C.S., Kessler, C.M., Konkle, B.A., Streiff, M.B., Garcia, D.A., Eds.; Elsevier: Philadelphia, PA, USA, 2019; pp. 190–206.

33. Morgan, M.; Zurin, A.; Harrington, T.; Little, N. Changing role for preoperative embolisation in the management of arteriovenous malformations of the brain. *J. Clin. Neurosci.* **2000**, *7*, 527–530. [CrossRef] [PubMed]

34. Fulbright, R.K.; Chaloupka, J.C.; Putman, C.M.; Sze, G.K.; Merriam, M.M.; Lee, G.K.; Fayad, P.B.; Awad, I.A.; White, R.I. MR of hereditary hemorrhagic telangiectasia: Prevalence and spectrum of cerebrovascular malformations. *AJNR Am. J. Neuroradiol.* **1998**, *19*, 477–484.

35. Maher, C.O.; Piepgras, D.G.; Brown, R.D., Jr.; Friedman, J.A.; Pollock, B.E. Cerebrovascular manifestations in 321 cases of hereditary hemorrhagic telangiectasia. *Stroke* **2001**, *32*, 877–882. [CrossRef] [PubMed]

36. Vase, P.; Grove, O. Gastrointestinal lesions in hereditary hemorrhagic telangiectasia. *Gastroenterology* **1986**, *91*, 1079–1083. [CrossRef]

37. Jelsig, A.M.; Tørring, P.M.; Kjeldsen, A.; Qvist, N.; Bojesen, A.; Jensen, U.; Andersen, M.K.; Gerdes, A.-M.; Brusgaard, K.; Ousager, L.B. JP–HHT phenotype in Danish patients with SMAD4 mutations. *Clin. Genet.* **2016**, *90*, 55–62. [CrossRef]

38. Mora-Luján, J.M.; Iriarte, A.; Alba, E.; Sánchez-Corral, M.Á.; Berrozpe, A.; Cerdà, P.; Cruellas, F.; Ribas, J.; Castellote, J.; Riera-Mestre, A. Gastrointestinal Bleeding in Patients with Hereditary Hemorrhagic Telangiectasia: Risk Factors and Endoscopic Findings. *J. Clin. Med.* **2020**, *9*, 82. [CrossRef]

39. Letteboer, T.; Zewald, R.; Kamping, E.; De Haas, G.; Mager, J.; Snijder, R.; Lindhout, D.; Hennekam, F.; Westermann, C.; van Amstel, J.P. Hereditary hemorrhagic telangiectasia: ENG and ALK-1 mutations in Dutch patients. *Hum. Genet.* **2005**, *116*, 8–16. [CrossRef]

40. Lesca, G.; Burnichon, N.; Raux, G.; Tosi, M.; Pinson, S.; Marion, M.J.; Babin, E.; Gilbert–Dussardier, B.; Rivière, S.; Goizet, C. Distribution of ENG and ACVRL1 (ALK1) mutations in French HHT patients. *Hum. Mutat.* **2006**, *27*, 598. [CrossRef]

41. Gonzalez, C.; Mcdonald, J.; Stevenson, D.; Whitehead, K.; Petersen, M.; Presson, A.; Ding, Q.; Wilson, K. Epistaxis in Children and Adolescents with Hereditary Hemorrhagic Telangiectasia. *Laryngoscope* **2017**, *128*, 1714–1719. [CrossRef]

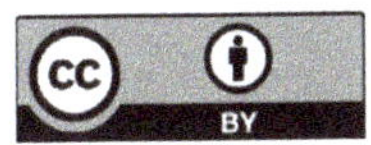

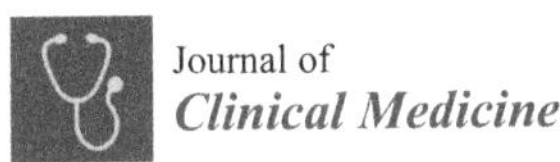

Journal of
Clinical Medicine

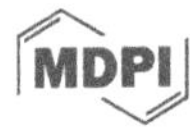

Article

Comparison of Contrast Enhanced Magnetic Resonance Angiography to Computed Tomography in Detecting Pulmonary Arteriovenous Malformations

Daniel A.F. van den Heuvel [1,*], Marco C. Post [2,3], Ward Koot [1], Johannes C. Kelder [2], Hendrik W. van Es [1], Repke J. Snijder [4], Jan-Albert Vos [1] and Johannes J. Mager [4]

[1] Department of Radiology, St. Antonius Hospital, 3435 CM Nieuwegein, The Netherlands; w.koot@antoniusziekenhuis.nl (W.K.); h.es@antoniusziekenhuis.nl (H.W.v.E.); j.a.vos@antoniusziekenhuis.nl (J.-A.V.)

[2] Department of Cardiology, St Antonius Hospital, 3435 CM Nieuwegein, The Netherlands; m.post@antoniusziekenhuis.nl (M.C.P.); keld01@antoniusziekenhuis.nl (J.C.K.)

[3] Department of Cardiology, University Medical Center Utrecht, 3584 CX Utrecht, The Netherlands

[4] Department of Pulmonology, St Antonius Hospital, 3435 CM Nieuwegein, The Netherlands; r.snijder@antoniusziekenhuis.nl (R.J.S.); j.mager@antoniusziekenhuis.nl (J.J.M.)

* Correspondence: d.van.den.heuvel@antoniusziekenhuis.nl; Tel.: +31-88-320-80-63

Received: 24 September 2020; Accepted: 12 November 2020; Published: 14 November 2020

Abstract: Background: Computed tomography (CT) is considered the imaging modality of choice to diagnose pulmonary arteriovenous malformations PAVMs. The drawback of this technique is that it requires ionizing radiation. Magnetic resonance (MR) imaging does not have the limitation, but little is known about the performance of MR compared to CT for the detection of PAVMs. The aim of this study is to investigate the sensitivity of contrast-enhanced MR angiography (CE-MRA) in the detection of PAVMs with feeding artery diameters (FAD) > 2 mm. Methods: Patients with a grade 2 or 3 shunt on screening transthoracic contrast echocardiography (TTCE) were asked to participate. Included patients underwent chest CT and CE-MRA. CT was considered the reference standard. CT and CE-MRA scans were anonymized and assessed for the presence of PAVMs with FAD > 2 mm by one and two readers respectively. Data analysis was performed on per patient and per PAVM basis. Results: Fifty-three patients were included. 105 PAVMs were detected on CT, 45 with a FAD ≥ 2 mm. In per patient analysis, sensitivity and specificity of CE-MRA were 92% and 97% respectively for reader 1 and 92% and 62% for reader 2. Negative and positive predictive value (NPV/PPV) were 93% and 96% for R1 and 90% and 67% for R2. In per PAVM analysis, sensitivity, specificity, NPV and PPV were 96%, 99%, 100% and 86% for R1 and 93%, 96%, 100% and 56% for R2, respectively. Conclusions: CE-MRA has excellent sensitivity and NPV for detection of PAVMs with FAD ≥ 2 mm and can therefore be used to detect these PAVMs. We are hopeful that future advancements in CE-MRA technology will reduce false positive rates and allow for more broad use of CE-MRA in PAVM diagnosis and management.

Keywords: pulmonary arteriovenous malformation; contrast enhanced magnetic resonance angiography; hereditary hemorrhagic telangiectasia

---

1. Introduction

Pulmonary arteriovenous malformations (PAVM) are vascular malformations frequently encountered in patients with hereditary hemorrhagic telangiectasia (HHT), also known as Rendu–Osler–Weber disease. In this type of vascular malformation, the normal capillary bed is absent and there is a direct connection between the pulmonary artery and vein. As a result, unfiltered and unsaturated blood enters the systemic circulation, which may cause hypoxemia and forms a potential conduit for paradoxical emboli. The latter may lead to serious clinical complications; the most feared are cerebral infarctions or cerebral abscesses [1,2]. Hence, it is important that these vascular malformations are detected and treated before they cause irreversible damage. In the 2011 International Guidelines for the Diagnosis and Management of HHT, it is recommended that all PAVMs with a feeding artery diameter (FAD) of 3 mm and, if feasible, >2 mm are treated [3]. Computed tomography (CT) is considered the imaging modality of choice to diagnose these PAVMs [3,4]. The drawback of this technique is that it requires ionizing radiation. This is important to realize because in this relatively young population CT investigations are used during long-term follow-up to assess PAVM persistence after embolotherapy and growth of untreated PAVMs [5–10]. Hanneman et al., reported an average of four chest CT scans (range 0–20) per patient and that 11% of their study cohort received a cumulative effective dose of >100 mSv at which patients are considered to be at risk for radiation induced harm [11]. Advancements in low-dose and ultra-low-dose (submillisievert) CT imaging have significantly lowered radiation burden [12]. This facilitates a more liberate use of CT in PAVM management, probably without increasing the radiation risks. However, the 'as low as reasonably achievable' principle still applies in radiology and technical developments in magnetic resonance imaging (MRI) offer the possibility of dynamic and functional imaging of PAVMs without radiation burden. It is therefore, interesting to investigate the role of MRI in PAVM management. A first prerequisite is that MRI can reliably detect PAVMs. Therefore, the aim of this study was to investigate the sensitivity of contrast-enhanced MR angiography (CE-MRA) compared to CT in the detection of PAVMs with a FAD > 2 mm.

2. Materials and Methods

All subjects gave their informed consent for inclusion before they participated in the study. The study was conducted in accordance with the Declaration of Helsinki and was approved by the institutional review board of our hospital (MEC-U NL39415.100.12).

2.1. Patient Population

Consecutive patients presenting at the HHT outpatient clinic (a tertiary referral center for HHT), suspected having untreated PAVMs based on a moderate or severe shunt (grade 2 or 3) diagnosed by transthoracic contrast echocardiography (TTCE), were asked to participate in the study. As part of our protocol, all patients with a moderate or severe shunt on TTCE undergo a chest CT scan to evaluate the presence of PAVMs. After signing informed consent, they also underwent a CE-MRA of the pulmonary arteries.

2.2. Trans Thoracic Contrast Echocardiography Protocol

A detailed description of the TTCE protocol can be found in the paper by Velthuis et al. [13]. The contrast agent, consisted of 8 mL of saline 0.9%, 1 mL of room air and 1 mL of blood, was administration through the right antecubital vein. The number of microbubbles in the left side of the heart was counted on one still frame. A moderate (grade 2) or large (grade 3) shunt was present if 30–100 or >100 microbubbles appeared in the left ventricle, respectively. All shunts visualized in the left atrium through a pulmonary vein or after at least four cardiac cycles were classified as a pulmonary shunt.

2.3. CT Acquisition Protocol

All CT scans were performed on a 256-slice scanner (Philips Brilliance iCT, Best, The Netherlands). Scan direction was from the lung bases to apices and in a single breath hold. Scan parameters were 100 kV, reference mAs 120, collimation 128 × 0.625, pitch 0.68. Images were reconstructed at 1 mm slice thickness. In case of a previous embolization procedure a contrast enhanced CT scan was performed. Scan parameters were identical to nonenhanced CT scans. Scan delay after administration of 80 mL Iobitridol (Xenetix® 300, Guerbet Laboratories, Roissy, France) was 30 s. A 40 mL saline flush was administered at the beginning of the scan.

2.4. CE-MRA Acquisition Protocol

CE-MRA was performed at 1.5 T (Philips Achieva, Best, The Netherlands) using a five-element cardiac coil. Time-resolved CE-MRA acquisition was with a T1 weighted fast field echo (FFE), repetition/echo time of 2.9/1.5 and a flip angle of 30 degrees. Field of view was 320×345 with a 200×200 matrix, 230 slices with slice oversampling factor of 1.1, slice thickness reconstruction 1.5 mm and $0.57 \times 0.57 \times 1.5$ voxel. The resulting sagittal 3D scan was repeated three times: noncontrast, arterial phase and venous phase. Contrast agent used is Dotarem (Guerbet 0.5 mmol/m; 30 mL flow 2.5 mL/sec followed by saline flush of 20 mL).

2.5. CT and CE-MRA Assessment

There were two readers in this study. Reader 1 (R1) with >10 years of experience in chest and interventional radiology was also involved in the development of the MRA protocol. Reader 2 (R2) was a resident in radiology and reviewed five learning cases in a session with R1 prior to study assessment. First, all CT scans were reviewed by R1. The CE-MRAs were independently and randomly reviewed by R1 and R2. To minimize recall bias, the time interval between the CT and the CE-MRA reviewing sessions was > four weeks for R1. All scans were assessed for the presence and location of PAVMs. Both readers scored the location per segment on CE-MRA to enable adequate correlation between the CT and MRA. For this the Jackson and Huber classification was used [14]. R1 measured the feeding artery diameter on CT within 1 cm of the sac. The 2011 guidelines recommend embolization of PAVMs with feeding artery diameter of 3 mm and if technically feasible also of PAVMs with feeding artery diameters of 2 mm [3]. In the current study, all PAVMs with a FAD of >2 mm were assessed. For the assessment of the CE-MRA the sagittal source images as well as axial 1 mm reconstructions and the sagittal and axial maximum intensity projections were used (Figure 1).

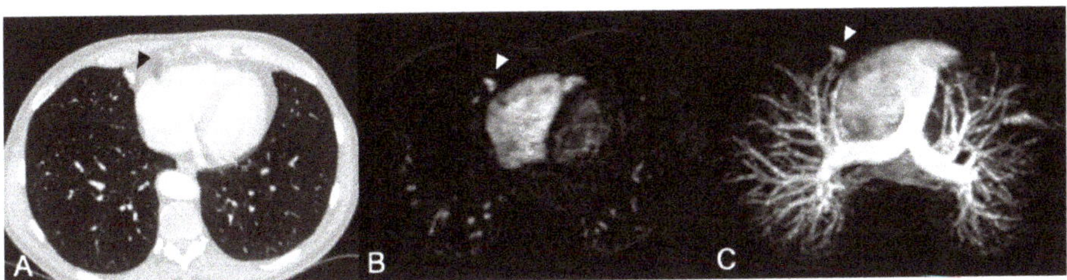

Figure 1. (**A**) Computed tomography (CT) scan 1.5 mm slice thickness with an inconspicuous PAVM (pulmonary arteriovenous malformation) in the medial segment of the middle lobe (arrow). (**B,C**) CE-MRA (contrast enhanced magnetic resonance angiography) axial reconstruction and axial MIP (maximum intensity projection) demonstrating the same PAVM.

2.6. Statistical Analysis

CT was considered the reference standard and the CE-MRA the index test. Per-patient and per-PAVM analysis were performed for both readers. The per-patient analysis was limited to distinguishing between the presence or absence of PAVMs with a feeding artery diameter of ≥ 2 mm in an individual. The per-PAVM analysis was focused on finding and correlating all PAVMs per segment. Sensitivity, specificity and negative predictive values (NPV) and positive predictive value (PPV) were calculated for the per-patient analysis. For the per-PAVM analysis the same test statistics were calculated taking into account that for each patient 18 segments were screened. With this approach it was also possible to determine the specificity and NPV for the per-PAVM analysis. Statistical analysis was performed with R version 3.6.3 [15].

3. Results

Fifty-five consecutive HHT patients with a pulmonary shunt (grade > 1) on TTCE were asked to participate. Two patients declined and therefore 53 patients were included in this study representing 105 PAVMs. Forty-five PAVMs had a feeding artery diameter of ≥2 mm (42.9%). Out of these, 11 PAVMs had a feeding artery diameter of ≥3 mm. The 45 PAVMs with a FAD ≥ 2 mm were present in 24 patients (45.3%). Patients' demographics are shown in Table 1.

Table 1. Baseline patient characteristics.

Total	**53**
Female	29 (55)
Male	24 (45)
Age (y)	47 ± 16
HHT	52 (98)
Eng	36 (68)
Alk	5 (9)
SMAD 4	3 (6)
Unknown *	8 (15)
Idiopathic	1 (2)
PAVMs per patient	
0	9 (17)
1	15 (28)
2–5	19 (36)
>5	10 (19)

Data are presented as number, (%) and mean ± SD; HHT = hereditary hemorrhagic telangiectasia; PAVM = pulmonary arteriovenous malformation; * diagnosis only based on Curacao criteria.

3.1. Per-Patient Analysis

With the threshold set at a diameter of the feeding artery of ≥2 mm, R1 correctly diagnosed PAVMs in 22 patients based on CE-MRA. The absence of PAVMs was correctly diagnosed in 28 patients; there were two false negative cases and one false positive case (sensitivity 92% (73–99%) and specificity 97% (82–100%)). Reader 2 also correctly diagnosed PAVMs in 22 patients. The absence of PAVMs was correctly diagnosed in 18. Similar to R1, R2 had two false negative cases, but 11 false positive cases (sensitivity 92% (73–99%) and specificity 62% (42–79%)). Both readers correctly diagnosed PAVMs in all patients when the threshold of ≥ 3 mm was applied. Results are presented in Tables 2 and 3.

Table 2. Contingency table of Reader 1 and 2 per-patient analysis.

Reader 1	**CT +**	**CT −**	**Total**
CE-MRA +	22	1	23
CE-MRA −	2	28	30
Total	24	29	53
Reader 2	CT +	CT −	Total
CE-MRA +	22	11	33
CE-MRA −	2	18	20
Total	24	29	53

3.2. Per-PAVM Analysis

One hundred and five PAVMs were identified in a total of 954 segments (53 patients × 18 segments per patient) on CT, of which 45 PAVMs had a feeding artery diameter of ≥2 mm. R1 correctly diagnosed 43 of 45 PAVMs and had seven false positives (sensitivity 96% (85–99%) and specificity 99% (98–100%)) on CE-MRA. R2 identified 42 of 45 PAVMs and had 33 false positives (sensitivity 93% (82–99%) and specificity 96% (95–97%)). As in the per-patient analysis, all PAVMs were identified by both readers when the threshold was set at ≥3 mm. Results are presented in Tables 3 and 4.

Table 3. Sensitivity, Specificity, NPV and PPV of CE-MRA.

	Per Patient Analysis		Per PAVM Analysis	
	CE-MRA Reader 1	**CE-MRA Reader 2**	**CE-MRA Reader 1**	**CE-MRA Reader 2**
Sensitivity	92 (73–99)	92 (73–99)	96 (85–99)	93 (82–99)
Specificity	97 (82–100)	62 (42–79)	99 (98–100)	96 (95–97)
NPV	93 (78–99)	90 (68–99)	100 (99–100)	100 (99–100)
PPV	96 (78–100)	67 (48–82)	86 (73–94)	56 (44–67)

Data are in percentages, data in parenthesis are 95% confidence intervals. PAVM = pulmonary arteriovenous malformation, CE-MRA = contrast enhanced magnetic resonance angiography, NPV = negative predictive value, PPV = positive predictive value.

Table 4. Contingency table of Reader 1 and 2 per-PAVM analysis (18-segment model).

Reader 1	**CT +**	**CT −**	**Total**
CE-MRA +	43	7	50
CE-MRA −	2	902	904
Total	45	909	954
Reader 2	CT +	CT −	Total
CE-MRA +	42	33	75
CE-MRA −	3	876	879
Total	45	909	954

4. Discussion

In this study, CE-MRA showed a high sensitivity and negative predictive value for the diagnosis of PAVMs with a FAD $\geq$ 2 mm in patients with PAVMs and a TTCE confirmed significant pulmonary shunt. PAVMs with a FAD $\geq$ 2 mm were diagnosed by chest CT in 45% of patients with at least a moderate pulmonary shunt on TTCE. PAVMs with a FAD $\geq$ 2 mm were found in 43% using CE-MRA, with a sensitivity of 92% and a NPV between 90 and 93%.

Earlier, we have shown that, in the presence of a moderate or severe shunt on TTCE, the chest CT is negative for PAVMs in 55% and 8%, respectively [13]. Chest CT has an important role in the detection and follow-up of PAVMs in HHT. Its high spatial resolution enables imaging of feeding arteries, sacs and draining veins and thereby is able to accurately diagnose and assess treatment effect of PAVMs. However, the use of chest CT comes at the expense of ionizing radiation, which is an important disadvantage in this cohort of HHT patients, who are generally young and are likely to require several follow-up CT scans during their lifetime. In addition, metal artifacts hamper evaluation of PAVMs with CT after coil embolization. MRA is not limited by radiation burden and also seems to perform well with respect to the evaluation of PAVM persistence.

In the last two decades, a handful of studies have been published reporting on the feasibility of MRI in the management of PAVMs. In 2008, Schneider et al. reported a study including 203 HHT patients evaluating CE-MRA as a screening procedure for the detection of PAVMs [16]. They showed that CE-MRA is more sensitive in detecting PAVMs compared to pulmonary angiography (PA), which was the reference standard. Overall, there were 40 patients identified in whom 119 PAVMs were found with screening and follow-up using CE-MRA. Interestingly, with PA only 92 PAVMs were found (77%). As pointed out by the authors, there were important limitations in this study. First, patients with a negative CE-MRA were not compared to the reference standard. Second, there was no comparison to chest CT as the most important diagnostic tool in current algorithms. A third limitation was that the lower threshold for detection was defined as a sac diameter of at least 5 mm instead of feeding artery diameter $\geq$ 2 mm which is advocated in the guidelines [3].

Although not the subject in our study, MRA could also have a role in the follow-up of embolized PAVMs. Several studies have demonstrated the feasibility of (CE)-MRA for detecting PAVM persistence [17–20]. Kawai et al. used time-resolved CE-MRA to assess PAVMs and correlated with the recanalization rate on chest CT and PA [18]. The sensitivity (96%) and specificity (96%) were excellent, with good interobserver agreement. Important limitations of this study were the low number of included PAVMs (n = 28) and that 3 PAVMs could not be imaged by CE-MRA because of field of view limitation. For the detection of PAVM perfusion after embolotherapy, Hamamoto et al. investigated the feasibility of time-spatial labeling inversion pulse MRA (time-SLIP MRA or arterial spin labeling), a cinematic MRI method in which the inversion pulse facilitates the determination of blood flow without a contrast medium [20]. In 11 patients, 38 PAVMs were imaged with the time-SLIP MRA technique that was compared to PA as reference standard. The sensitivity and specificity of time-SLIP MRA for detecting perfusion after embolization were both 100%, with an excellent inter-observer agreement. Although very promising, time-SLIP MRA is also limited by the relatively small field of view. In this small study, four PAVMs could not be imaged because of this.

MRA is a very promising imaging method for PAVMs but there are limitations. Our study and previous studies have shown that (CE)-MRA is a feasible method to detect PAVMs. It performs well compared to chest CT in the detection of PAVMs with a FAD $\geq$ 2 mm. However, the number of false positives needs to be improved. The experience of the operator seems to play an important role in this, as there is a large difference between both operators in the number of false positives. With respect to the detection of perfusion of embolized PAVMs, MRA seems to perform superior compared to CT because it is less influenced by the presence of micro coils [17,18]. This is attributable to the fact that micro coils are of platinum material which has few paramagnetic effects. MRA could therefore be feasible for the postembolization follow-up as well. As mentioned above, with CE-MRA and time-SLIP MRA, it is possible that the field of view is not large enough to cover the whole lung. The time-SLIP MRA technique often requires targeted imaging and thus knowledge of the location of the PAVM of interest. This means that either extra contrast administration during the MRA investigation or a chest CT scan prior to the MRA investigation will be necessary. Considering these limitations, the relative high costs and limited availability of MR imaging, it may be too early to use (CE)-MRA for routine evaluation of PAVMs.

Our study has several limitations. MRA acquisitions were performed on a 1.5 T system. With a 3 T system, higher signal-to-noise ratios can be achieved. This could result in superior image quality based on a higher spatial and temporal resolution. In addition, it enables a broader coverage of the lung reducing the risk of false negative readings. Unfortunately, a 3 T system was not available during the study. Furthermore, there was a difference in experience in reading CE-MRA investigations between both readers. This study showed that image interpretation is reader-dependent, mainly resulting in false positives by the less experienced reader. Reader 1 has both a large experience in chest radiology and PAVM embolotherapy. He represents the level of experience that can be expected in an expert center. Reader 2, although being trained in an expert center, has less experience and could be regarded as representing nonexpert centers. HHT guidelines recommend that PAVM screening, diagnosis and treatment should be performed in expert centers. Furthermore, both readers were aware of the fact that the subjects had a positive TTCE and thus a high chance of having PAVMs with a FAD $\geq$ 2 mm. This could have induced a review bias lowering the threshold for diagnosing PAVMs. Finally, a limitation was the relatively small number of patients in this study. However, it is largest cohort of consecutive patients investigated so far representing a reasonably number of PAVMs with a FAD $\geq$ 2 mm.

5. Conclusions

CE-MRA seems to be a feasible method for the detection of PAVMs with a FAD $\geq$ 2 mm in HHT patients initially screened with TTCE. We are hopeful that future advancements in CE-MRA technology will reduce false positive rates and allow for more broad use of CE-MRA in PAVM diagnosis and management.

Author Contributions: Conceptualization: D.A.F.v.d.H., M.C.P., R.J.S., J.J.M. Methodology: D.A.F.v.d.H., M.C.P., J.J.M. Validation: J.C.K. Formal Analysis: J.C.K. Investigation: D.A.F.v.d.H., W.K. Data Curation: D.A.F.v.d.H., W.K. Writing–Original Draft Preparation: D.A.F.v.d.H. Writing–Review & Editing: M.C.P., H.W.v.E., R.J.S., J.-A.V. Visualization: D.A.F.v.d.H., H.W.v.E. Supervision: J.-A.V., J.J.M. Project Administration: W.K. All authors have read and agreed to the published version of the manuscript.

Funding: This research received no external funding.

Conflicts of Interest: The authors declare no conflict of interest.

References

1. Cottin, V.; Chinet, T.; Lavolé, A.; Corre, R.; Marchand, E.; Reynaud-Gaubert, M.; Plauchu, H.; Cordier, J.-F. Pulmonary Arteriovenous Malformations in Hereditary Hemorrhagic Telangiectasia. *Medicine* **2007**, *86*, 1–17. [CrossRef] [PubMed]

2. Shovlin, C.; Jackson, J.E.; Bamford, K.B.; Jenkins, I.H.; Benjamin, A.R.; Ramadan, H.; Kulinskaya, E. Primary determinants of ischaemic stroke/brain abscess risks are independent of severity of pulmonary arteriovenous malformations in hereditary haemorrhagic telangiectasia. *Thorax* **2008**, *63*, 259–266. [CrossRef] [PubMed]

3. Faughnan, M.E.; Palda, V.A.; Garcia-Tsao, G.; Geisthoff, U.W.; McDonald, J.; Proctor, D.D.; Spears, J.; Brown, D.H.; Buscarini, E.; Chesnutt, M.S.; et al. International guidelines for the diagnosis and management of hereditary haemorrhagic telangiectasia. *J. Med Genet.* **2011**, *48*, 73–87. [CrossRef] [PubMed]

4. Müller-Hülsbeck, S.; Marques, L.; Maleux, G.; Osuga, K.; Pelage, J.-P.; Wohlgemuth, W.A.; Andersen, P.E. CIRSE Standards of Practice on Diagnosis and Treatment of Pulmonary Arteriovenous Malformations. *Cardiovasc. Interv. Radiol.* **2019**, *43*, 353–361. [CrossRef] [PubMed]

5. Bélanger, C.; Chartrand-Lefebvre, C.; Soulez, G.; Faughnan, M.E.; Tahir, M.R.; Giroux, M.-F.; Gilbert, P.; Perreault, P.; Bouchard, L.; Oliva, V.L.; et al. Pulmonary arteriovenous malformation (PAVM) reperfusion after percutaneous embolization: Sensitivity and specificity of non-enhanced CT. *Eur. J. Radiol.* **2016**, *85*, 150–157. [CrossRef] [PubMed]

6. Letourneau-Guillon, L.; Faughnan, M.E.; Soulez, G.; Giroux, M.-F.; Oliva, V.L.; Boucher, L.-M.; Dubois, J.; Prabhudesai, V.; Therasse, E. Embolization of Pulmonary Arteriovenous Malformations with Amplatzer Vascular Plugs: Safety and Midterm Effectiveness. *J. Vasc. Interv. Radiol.* **2010**, *21*, 649–656. [CrossRef] [PubMed]

7. Woodward, C.S.; Pyeritz, R.E.; Chittams, J.L.; Trerotola, S.O. Treated Pulmonary Arteriovenous Malformations: Patterns of Persistence and Associated Retreatment Success. *Radiology* **2013**, *269*, 919–926. [CrossRef] [PubMed]

8. Tau, N.; Atar, E.; Mei-Zahav, M.; Bachar, G.N.; Dagan, T.; Birk, E.; Bruckheimer, E. Amplatzer Vascular Plugs Versus Coils for Embolization of Pulmonary Arteriovenous Malformations in Patients with Hereditary Hemorrhagic Telangiectasia. *Cardiovasc. Interv. Radiol.* **2016**, *39*, 1110–1114. [CrossRef] [PubMed]

9. Stein, E.J.; Chittams, J.L.; Miller, M.; Trerotola, S.O. Persistence in Coil-Embolized Pulmonary Arteriovenous Malformations with Feeding Artery Diameters of 3 mm or Less: A Retrospective Single-Center Observational Study. *J. Vasc. Interv. Radiol.* **2017**, *28*, 442–449. [CrossRef] [PubMed]

10. Brinjikji, W.; Latino, G.A.; Parvinian, A.; Gauthier, A.; Pantalone, R.; Yamaki, V.; Apala, D.R.; Prabhudesai, V.; Cyr, V.; Chartrand-Lefèbvre, C.; et al. Diagnostic Yield of Rescreening Adults for Pulmonary Arteriovenous Malformations. *J. Vasc. Interv. Radiol.* **2019**, *30*, 1982–1987. [CrossRef] [PubMed]

11. Hanneman, K.; Faughnan, M.E.; Prabhudesai, V. Cumulative Radiation dose in Patients with Hereditary Hemorrhagic Telangiectasia and Pulmonary Arteriovenous Malformations. *Can. Assoc. Radiol. J.* **2014**, *65*, 135–140. [CrossRef] [PubMed]

12. Singh, R.; Digumarthy, S.R.; Muse, V.V.; Kambadakone, A.R.; Blake, M.A.; Tabari, A.; Hoi, Y.; Akino, N.; Angel, E.; Madan, R.; et al. Image Quality and Lesion Detection on Deep Learning Reconstruction and Iterative Reconstruction of Submillisievert Chest and Abdominal CT. *Am. J. Roentgenol.* **2020**, *214*, 566–573. [CrossRef] [PubMed]

13. Velthuis, S.; Buscarini, E.; Mager, J.J.; Vorselaars, V.M.; Van Gent, M.W.; Gazzaniga, P.; Manfredi, G.; Danesino, C.; Diederik, A.L.; Vos, J.A.; et al. Predicting the size of pulmonary arteriovenous malformations on chest computed tomography: A role for transthoracic contrast echocardiography. *Eur. Respir. J.* **2014**, *44*, 150–159. [CrossRef] [PubMed]

14. Jackson, C.L.; Huber, J.F. Correlated Applied Anatomy of the Bronchial Tree and Lungs with a System of Nomenclature. *Dis. Chest* **1943**, *9*, 319–326. [CrossRef]

15. R Core Team. *R: A Language and Environment for Statistical Computing*; R Foundation for Statistical Computing: Vienna, Austria, 2014.

16. Schneider, G.; Uder, M.; Koehler, M.; Kirchin, M.A.; Massmann, A.; Buecker, A.; Geisthoff, U. MR Angiography for Detection of Pulmonary Arteriovenous Malformations in Patients with Hereditary Hemorrhagic Telangiectasia. *Am. J. Roentgenol.* **2008**, *190*, 892–901. [CrossRef] [PubMed]

17. Ohno, Y.; Hatabu, H.; Takenaka, D.; Adachi, S.; Hirota, S.; Sugimura, K. Contrast-enhanced MR perfusion imaging and MR angiography: Utility for management of pulmonary arteriovenous malformations for embolotherapy. *Eur. J. Radiol.* **2002**, *41*, 136–146. [CrossRef]

18. Kawai, T.; Shimohira, M.; Kan, H.; Hashizume, T.; Ohta, K.; Kurosaka, K.; Muto, M.; Suzuki, K.; Shibamoto, Y. Feasibility of Time-Resolved MR Angiography for Detecting Recanalization of Pulmonary Arteriovenous Malformations Treated with Embolization with Platinum Coils. *J. Vasc. Interv. Radiol.* **2014**, *25*, 1339–1347. [CrossRef] [PubMed]

19. Himohira, M.; Kawai, T.; Hashizume, T.; Ohta, K.; Nakagawa, M.; Ozawa, Y.; Sakurai, K.; Shibamoto, Y. Reperfusion Rates of Pulmonary Arteriovenous Malformations after Coil Embolization: Evaluation with Time-Resolved MR Angiography or Pulmonary Angiography. *J. Vasc. Interv. Radiol.* **2015**, *26*, 856–864. [CrossRef] [PubMed]

20. Hamamoto, K.; Matsuura, K.; Chiba, E.; Okochi, T.; Tanno, K.; Tanaka, O. Feasibility of Non-contrast-enhanced MR Angiography Using the Time-SLIP Technique for the Assessment of Pulmonary Arteriovenous Malformation. *Magn. Reson. Med. Sci.* **2016**, *15*, 253–265. [CrossRef] [PubMed]

Publisher's Note: MDPI stays neutral with regard to jurisdictional claims in published maps and institutional affiliations.

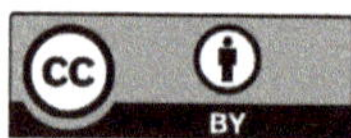

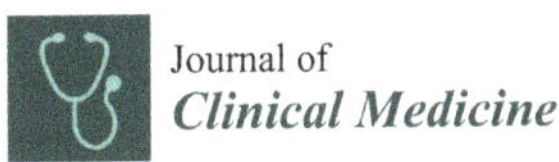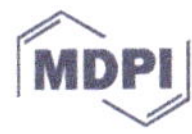

Journal of
Clinical Medicine

Review

The Role of Liver Imaging in Hereditary Hemorrhagic Telangiectasia

Joelle Harwin [1], Mark D. Sugi [1,2], Steven W. Hetts [1,2], Miles B. Conrad [1,2] and Michael A. Ohliger [1,2,*]

1   Department of Radiology and Biomedical Imaging, University of California, San Francisco, CA 94143, USA; Joelle.harwin@ucsf.edu (J.H.); mark.sugi@ucsf.edu (M.D.S.); Steven.hetts@ucsf.edu (S.W.H.); miles.conrad@ucsf.edu (M.B.C.)

2   Department of Radiology, Zuckerberg San Francisco General Hospital, San Francisco, CA 94110, USA

*   Correspondence: michael.ohliger@ucsf.edu

Received: 7 October 2020; Accepted: 4 November 2020; Published: 21 November 2020

Abstract: Hereditary hemorrhagic telangiectasia (HHT) is an autosomal dominant vascular disorder characterized by spontaneous epistaxis, telangiectasia, and visceral vascular malformations. Hepatic vascular malformations are common, though a minority are symptomatic. Symptoms are dependent on the severity and exact type of shunting caused by the hepatic malformation: Arteriosystemic shunting leads to manifestations of high output cardiac failure, and arterioportal shunting leads to portal hypertension. Radiologic imaging, including ultrasound, computed tomography (CT), and magnetic resonance imaging (MRI), is an important tool for assessing liver involvement. Doppler ultrasonography is the first-line screening modality for HHT-related liver disease, and it has a standardized scale. Imaging can determine whether shunting is principally to the hepatic vein or the portal vein, which can be a key determinant of patients' symptoms. Liver-related complications can be detected, including manifestations of portal hypertension, focal liver masses as well as ischemic cholangiopathy. Ultrasound and MRI also have the ability to quantify blood flow through the liver, which in the future may be used to determine prognosis and direct antiangiogenic therapy.

Keywords: HHT; liver; MRI; ultrasound; AVM; bevacizumab; Osler–Weber–Rendu

1. Introduction

Hereditary hemorrhagic telangiectasia (HHT), also called Osler–Weber–Rendu, is an autosomal dominant disorder characterized by arteriovenous malformations (AVMs) throughout the body [1]. The hallmark lesion of HHT is the telangiectasia, a direct connection between the arteriole and venule, bypassing the capillary bed [2]. HHT most commonly involves mutations of two genes: endoglin (*ENG*, on chromosome 9, HHT1) or activin A receptor type II-like 1 (*ACVRL1/ALK1*, on chromosome 12, HHT2). The proteins encoded by *ENG* and *ACVRL1*, endoglin and activin receptor-like kinase 1 (*ALK1*) are endothelial receptors involved in the transforming growth factor beta (TGF-β) signaling pathway [3,4]. The TGF-β signaling pathway, which is involved in angiogenesis and in maintaining vascular integrity, is defective or impaired in patients with HHT [5]. Although mutations in endoglin and *ALK1* are the most common, there are over 600 mutations within at least four different genes which may result in HHT [6–8].

The Curaçao diagnostic criteria are used to clinically diagnose HHT [9] and are based upon the presence of four findings: (1) spontaneous and recurrent epistaxis, (2) multiple mucocutaneous telangiectases at characteristic sites, (3) visceral involvement, and (4) a first-degree relative with HHT. Depending on the number of criteria that are met, the diagnosis is categorized as "definite" (3 or more criteria), "suspected" (2 criteria), or "unlikely" (1 criterion). The diagnosis may be confirmed by genetic analysis; however, because all genetic mutations have not been discovered that cause HHT, genetic testing does not exclude the disease if the diagnosis is suspected clinically. Typical sites of involvement of HHT include mucocutaneous telangiectases causing epistaxis and gastrointestinal bleeding, and AVMs in the lungs, brain, and liver.

Liver involvement with HHT is common but usually asymptomatic. Of individuals with HHT, 44-74% have hepatic vascular malformations (VMs), but only 8% show symptoms [1]. Liver involvement occurs most often in females and in patients with the HHT2 genotype, and these patients average 48 years old [1,10]. The most common complications of severe liver involvement are high-output cardiac failure (HOCF) and portal hypertension [11]. Less common complications include ischemic cholangitis and bile duct necrosis [12]. Variations in the clinical presentation of symptomatic patients with hepatic VMs reflect the unique characteristics of the blood supply to the liver as well as the vessels involved: hepatic arteries, veins, and portal veins [12].

The purpose of this review is to discuss the nature of liver involvement with HHT and discuss ways in which imaging can aid in the diagnosis of HHT, its complications, as well as monitoring of therapy.

2. Blood Flow in the Liver

The physiologic manifestations of HHT in the liver reflect the unique nature of its blood supply. The liver receives blood from the hepatic artery and portal vein, with a majority of blood flow (75–80%) normally coming from the portal vein [13]. Blood flows from the hepatic artery through the liver parenchyma, drains into the hepatic vein and inferior vena cava, and then empties into the right heart. The portal vein drains blood from the intestines and empties nutrient-rich blood into the liver, where it then drains to the hepatic vein and into the heart. Distinct contributions from the hepatic artery and portal vein can be seen by imaging at different times following injection of an intravenous contrast agent. The hepatic artery fills with contrast first, followed by the portal vein and then the hepatic veins (Figure 1). Alterations in this timing can signify the presence of a shunt. Hepatic VMs can result in vascular communications between any two of these three vessels (hepatic artery, portal vein, hepatic vein). The physiologic consequences of VMs are ultimately determined by where these abnormal connections occur.

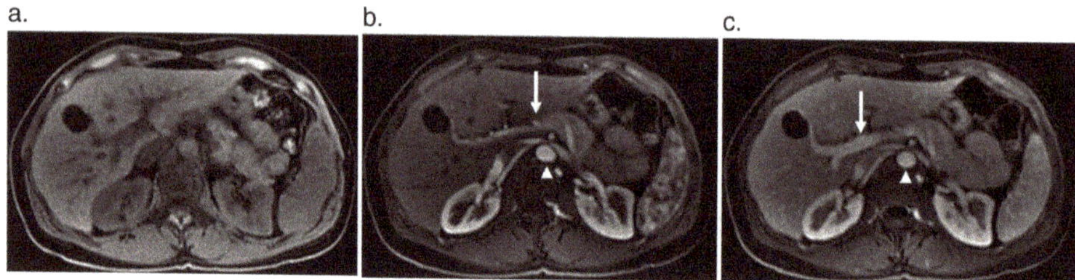

Figure 1. Contrast enhancement phases in a normal liver without vascular shunting on dynamic axial T_1 fat-saturated magnetic resonance imaging. (**a**) Pre-contrast phase. (**b**) Arterial phase shows enhancement of the aorta (arrowhead) and hepatic artery (arrow). (**c**) Portal venous phase shows enhancement of the portal vein (arrow) and slightly diminished enhancement of the aorta (arrowhead) relative to the arterial phase.

3. Hepatic Vascular Malformations

Rather than presenting with single, discrete VMs, liver involvement in HHT is typically diffuse and heterogeneous. Histologically, VMs result in both microscopic changes, such as ectatic sinusoids, and macroscopic vascular anomalies [2]. Diffusely distributed hepatic VMs are relatively characteristic of HHT and unusual in other vascular disorders; therefore, diffuse involvement with VMs should always raise suspicion for underlying HHT [8]. Liver telangiectases are early manifestations of hepatic involvement in HHT [14]. Telangiectases may progress to form more complex vascular malformations and shunts, with up to 21% of patients demonstrating an increase in size and complexity of hepatic VMs after long-term follow-up [4].

Liver vascular shunts are abnormal direct connections where blood bypasses the liver parenchyma. Two major shunt patterns are observed, which lead to different clinical presentations: (1) arteriosystemic (hepatic artery to hepatic vein) and (2) arterioportal (hepatic artery to portal vein) [15]. As mentioned previously, an individual's ensuing clinical symptoms and course is dependent upon on the type and severity of the hepatic VM. These shunt types may coexist, but clinically, one shunt type often dominates [16]. Certain shunts are more commonly associated with specific complications.

3.1. Arteriosystemic Shunt

An arteriosystemic shunt occurs when the hepatic artery is in direct communication with the hepatic vein (Figure 2). This causes arterial blood to bypass the liver parenchyma and capillary bed and drain directly into the systemic venous system and right heart. This results in decreased systemic vascular resistance and increased cardiac preload and stroke volume, the combination of which may cause HOCF [17]. Because HOCF is the most common complication resulting from hepatic VMs, international guidelines recommend obtaining an echocardiogram at the time of hepatic VM diagnosis [10]. These guidelines also recommended further characterization of cardiac and pulmonary pressures with right heart catheterization in individuals with signs or symptoms of HOCF [10]. At cardiac catheterization, patients with HOCF demonstrate increased right atrial, pulmonary wedge, and pulmonary artery pressures [18]. An additional complication evident in HHT patients with HOCF is an increased rate of atrial fibrillation, occurring in approximately 1.6/100 persons [10].

a.   b.   c.

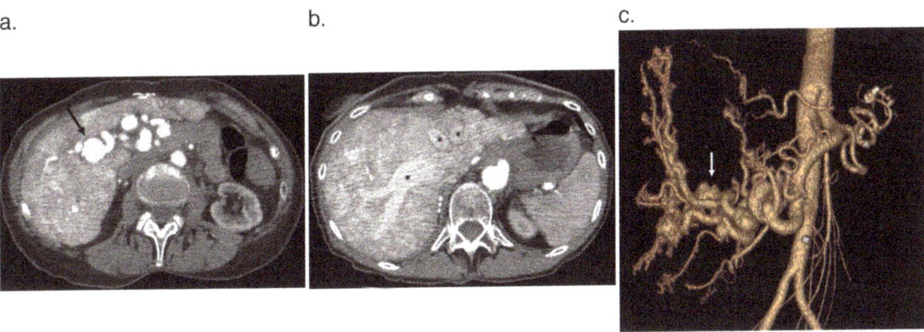

Figure 2. Arteriosystemic shunts on arterial phase CT angiogram of the abdomen in a 73-year-old woman with HHT. (**a**) Marked dilation and tortuosity of the hepatic artery with right hepatic artery aneurysm (arrow). (**b**) Early filling of the hepatic veins (*) on the arterial phase of contrast suggests hepatic arterial to hepatic venous shunting. (**c**) Coronal arterial phase 3D reconstruction demonstrates the marked dilation of the hepatic arteries. The hepatic artery aneurysm is denoted by the arrow.

3.2. Arterioportal Shunt

An arterioportal shunt occurs when the hepatic artery is in direct communication with the portal vein (Figure 3). In this type of shunt, the portal vein is exposed to high arterial pressures and also experiences increased blood flow. This leads to presinusoidal portal hypertension, which may lead to the development of ascites, varices, and splenomegaly [12,19].

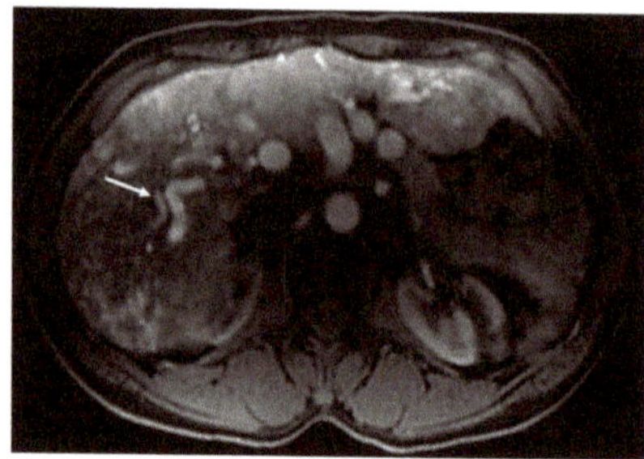

Figure 3. Arterioportal shunt from the hepatic artery to portal vein in a 51-year-old woman with HHT. Axial T_1 MR image with fat saturation acquired during the arterial phase of contrast shows early filling of a right portal vein branch (arrow) adjacent to the dilated hepatic artery, and associated perfusion anomaly in the right hepatic lobe.

4. Imaging in HHT

Ultrasonography (US), computerized tomography (CT), and magnetic resonance imaging (MRI) each has a role in evaluating the liver in patients with HHT [20]. US is the most common initial screening test, given its broad availability and established grading system [4]. CT and MRI are useful for more targeted evaluations, including for evaluation of focal liver lesions. In addition to targeted evaluations of HHT-related lesions, these examinations are often performed to evaluate suspected abnormalities unrelated to HHT (such as abdominal pain), and therefore understanding the expected imaging findings in patients that HHT is extremely important [21].

4.1. Ultrasound

US imaging with grey scale and Doppler evaluation has been a standard screening test for liver AVMs and in the initial work up of patients suspected of having liver involvement due to HHT [10]. US can detect the location of large VMs in the liver, and Doppler imaging permits the evaluation of the direction and magnitude of blood flow [22]. US can also detect focal liver lesions, evaluate the biliary tree, and look for manifestations of portal hypertension such as splenomegaly, ascites, and portal varices.

Dilation of the extrahepatic proper hepatic artery, defined as a diameter greater than 4–5 mm, is one of the earlier manifestations of hepatic VMs [14,15]. This dilated artery can be demonstrated on US. It has been suggested that an additional way to evaluate a dilated proper hepatic artery is by comparing its diameter to that of the splenic artery. Usually, the diameter of the proper hepatic artery is smaller than that of the splenic artery; a reversal of this relationship should raise the suspicion for hepatic VMs [15]. In normal individuals, the diameters of the intrahepatic arteries are usually less than 1.5 mm and can be very challenging to accurately measure on US. With more advanced VMs, dilated intrahepatic arterial branches become more apparent. Another early sign of hepatic VMs is increased velocity within the proper hepatic artery, with some studies suggesting peak flow velocity greater than 100 cm/s as indicative of HHT [15].

On US, arteriosystemic or arterioportal shunts may also be indicated by a low arterial resistive index [14], which is a measure of the end diastolic flow compared to the peak systolic flow. When shunting occurs, the end diastolic flow increases, leading to a diminished resistive index, reflecting a smaller difference between the blood flow in systole and diastole. Another manifestation of arteriosystemic shunts is "arterialization" of the venous waveform, as well as dilation and turbulent flow within the portal and hepatic veins (Figure 4) [14]. In an arterioportal shunt, Doppler US may demonstrate formation of portosystemic collaterals, such as a recanalized paraumbilical vein and even reversal of flow in the portal vein. It is important to note that these findings can also be present in true cirrhosis (e.g., cirrhosis that arises in the setting of viral hepatitis, alcoholic or non-alcoholic fatty liver disease).

a.   b.

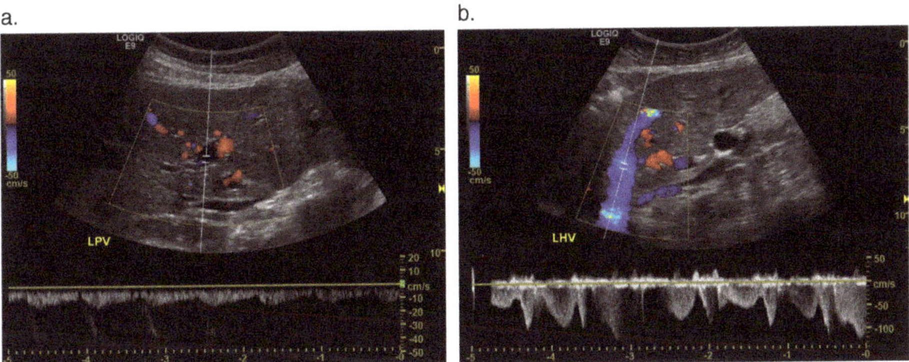

Figure 4. Hepatic vascular malformations on spectral Doppler ultrasound (US) in a 69-year-old woman with HHT. (**a**) Evaluation of the left portal vein shows reversed, pulsatile flow due to arterioportal shunting. (LPV = left portal vein). (**b**) Evaluation of the left hepatic vein shows arterialized waveforms due to artery to hepatic vein (arteriosystemic) shunting. (LHV = left hepatic vein).

Standardized criteria for grading the severity of hepatic VMs based on ultrasound findings has been proposed and demonstrates good interobserver agreement [14,20]. Grading criteria are based upon proper hepatic artery dilation (extrahepatic verses intrahepatic); peak flow velocity; and resistive indices of the proper hepatic artery, degree of hepatic peripheral hypervascularization, and dilation and/or flow abnormalities within the hepatic or portal veins [4]. On Doppler ultrasound, portosystemic shunts may be demonstrated as tubular structures with internal blood flow, communicating between the portal venous branches and hepatic venous branches.

Ultrasound assessment of hepatic VMs can also benefit from injection of intravenous contrast. Contrast-enhanced ultrasound (CEUS) uses microbubbles as intravascular contrast, which are timed to obtain different phases of contrast enhancement such as arterial, parenchymal, and venous [23]. CEUS may offer improved detection of small arteriovenous shunts and can be used to guide real-time intervention [24,25]. CEUS is also becoming increasingly accepted as an effective alternative to multiphase contrast enhanced MR and CT [26]. In HHT, quantitative perfusion imaging with CEUS has been used to identify two distinct subtypes of patients with hepatic VMs [27]. Further research is required to establish the prognostic significance of these groups.

4.2. CT and MRI

Although they are not typically first-line screening modalities, CT and MRI can also be used for the evaluation of hepatic VMs. These modalities permit detailed evaluation of vascular anatomy as well as alterations in perfusion that occur with vascular shunting [28,29]. As discussed previously, CT and MRI examinations are typically obtained in different vascular phases following administration of intravenous contrast. These different phases emphasize either hepatic arterial or portal venous blood flow. In a retrospective review of CT scans from 333 patients with HHT acquired over 15 years, 54.1% had liver involvement [21]. Of patients with liver involvement, 47% had telangiectases alone, while the remainder had telangiectases plus large confluent vascular masses, hepatic shunts, or other perfusion abnormalities. CT and MRI are also sensitive to involvement of other organs such as pancreas and gastrointestinal tract (seen in up to 18% of HHT patients in this series).

As with ultrasound, CT and MRI can also assess for the size of the hepatic artery and other visceral blood vessels [20]. Early contrast filling of the hepatic vein or portal vein on early (arterial) contrast phases can be evidence of arteriosystemic or arterioportal shunting, respectively (Figure 5) [1].

In addition to the evaluation of vascular shunting, MRI and CT are sensitive to abnormalities of the biliary tree (seen in cholangiopathy) or focal hepatic masses, described in more detail below. Finally, anatomic information obtained using MRI can be complemented by quantitative evaluation of blood flow through the hepatic artery or celiac artery [30]. Another strategy used to evaluate vascular malformations in MRI (though not specific to HHT) is to measure the difference in aortic flow before and after the VM [31].

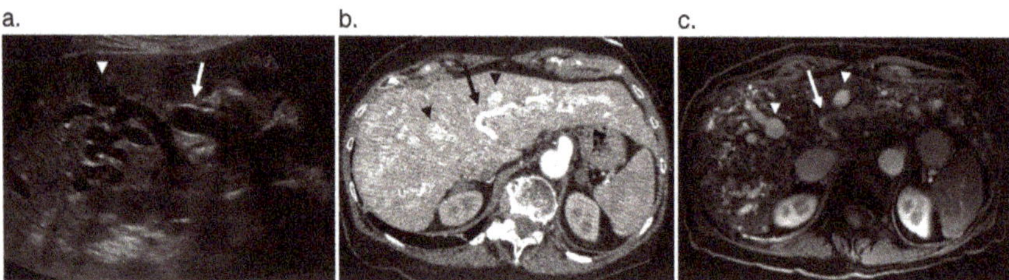

Figure 5. Correlative US, CT, and MR imaging in a 69-year-old woman with HHT. (**a**) Longitudinal grayscale US, (**b**) axial CT angiogram, and (**c**) axial T_1 fat-saturated gadolinium-enhanced arterial phase images show dilation of the hepatic artery (arrow) and hepatic veins (arrowheads) in this patient with multiple arteriosystemic shunts.

4.3. Catheter Angiography

Conventional angiography, with direct arterial visualization, is rarely necessary in evaluating hepatic VMs, given the excellent alternative non-invasive imaging options. However, angiography can be useful in distinguishing between arterioportal, arteriosystemic, and portosystemic shunts (Figure 6). Angiography is often unnecessary because therapeutic embolization of liver AVMs has fallen out of favor due to a high complication rate, described in detail below.

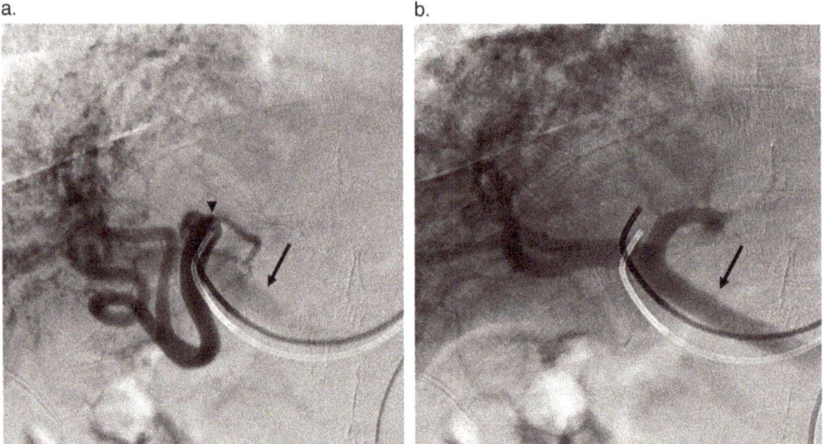

Figure 6. Arterioportal shunt angiography in a 69-year-old woman with HHT. (**a**) Selective catheterization and injection of the hepatic artery (arrowhead) shows dilation of the hepatic arterial system and early contrast opacification of the main portal vein (arrow). (**b**) Portal venous phase shows further opacification of the main portal vein (arrow) and intrahepatic portal veins.

5. Treatment of Hepatic Vascular Malformations

Treatment for symptomatic hepatic VMs is based on targeting the clinical symptoms. For example, in an arteriosystemic shunt resulting in HOCF, management is directed towards HOCF with employment of diuretics, salt restriction, etc. [10]. In an arterioportal shunt resulting in portal hypertension, treatment may involve fluid restriction, beta blockers, etc. Of individuals with symptomatic hepatic VMs, 63% have a complete response to first-line treatment [10].

Currently, treatment is not recommended for asymptomatic individuals with hepatic VMs because the majority do not develop complications [10]. Antiangiogenic therapy is being used with increasing frequency for the therapy of HOCF secondary to hepatic VMs. Bevacizumab is a monoclonal antibody targeting circulating vascular endothelial growth factor (VEGF), which stimulates angiogenesis. Intravenous bevacizumab has been shown to decrease cardiac output in persons with symptomatic hepatic VMs resulting in HOCF [32]. However, there is very limited data on the long-term safety of bevazicumab when used for HHT, particularly because periodic maintenance infusions are required [33]. Despite this, bevacizumab is increasingly used as long-term maintenance therapy for HOCF and as a bridge to orthotopic liver transplant for others [6]. It is thought that tyrosine kinase signaling pathways are also involved in angiogenesis. Pazopanib, an oral tyrosine kinase inhibitor most commonly prescribed for the treatment of renal cell carcinoma, has also been shown to potentially reduce bleeding (epistaxis and anemia) in HHT [34] and has also been used for treatment of liver AVMs refractory to bevacizumab.

In severely symptomatic patients who fail first line therapy, more aggressive treatments have been pursued. The curative treatment is orthotopic liver transplant (OLT), which has 82–92% survival rate [10]. With regard to endovascular therapy, hepatic VMs are often considered "do not touch" lesions due to the high risk of mortality and complication. Hepatic artery embolization is associated with a 10% rate of mortality and 20% rate of complication requiring re-intervention [35]. Therefore, such interventions are only recommended in late stage HOCF only when medical therapies fail and OLT is not an option [10].

6. Imaging of Liver-Specific Complications on HHT

6.1. Pseudocirrhosis

Alterations in liver blood flow caused by VMs in HHT can lead to either diffuse or focal hepatocellular regenerative activity, with fibrosis surrounding the abnormal vasculature [12]. On imaging, hepatic nodules and fibrosis mimic the appearance of cirrhosis. However, in HHT this appearance has been termed "pseudocirrhosis," as the normal hepatocellular architecture is preserved (Figure 7) [12,16,36]. Unlike in true cirrhosis, there is not the same increased risk of hepatocellular carcinoma (HCC) in pseudocirrhosis.

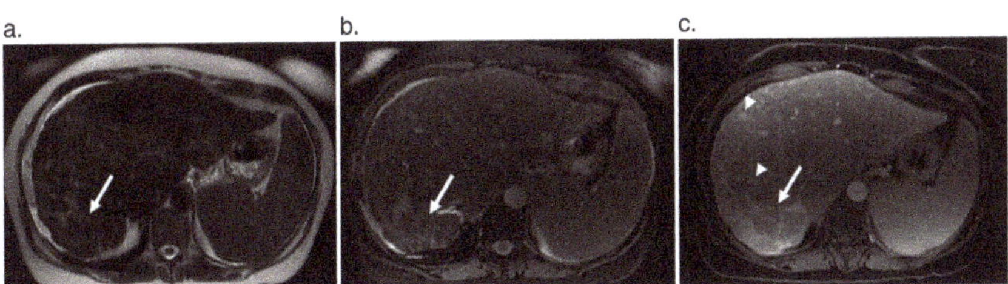

Figure 7. Chronic liver injury with nodular regenerative hyperplasia, pseudocirrhosis, and peripheral fibrosis in a 54-year-old woman with HHT. (**a**) Axial T_1-weighted MR image shows parenchymal nodularity most prominent in the posterior right hepatic lobe (arrow). (**b**) Axial T_2-weighted fat-saturated MR image shows a reticular pattern of increased signal in the posterior right hepatic lobe (arrow). (**c**) Delayed enhancement on the axial T_1 fat-saturated gadolinium-enhanced MR image (arrow), along with multiple telangiectases (arrowheads).

6.2. Focal Nodular Hyperplasia

Focal nodular hyperplasia (FNH) is a common benign liver mass and represents a disorganized proliferation of hepatocytes that can occur in response to VMs. FNH has a 100-fold higher incidence in individuals with HHT [37]. Evaluation with multiphase cross-sectional imaging is usually recommended for evaluation of focal liver lesions. FNH has a highly characteristic imaging appearance on MRI, with early arterial enhancement and a T_2-hyperintense "central scar" (representing disordered mixture of blood vessels and bile ducts) [29]. It is important for radiologists and clinicians to keep in mind the high incidence of FNH in HHT patients in order to avoid unnecessary biopsies.

Although FNH is benign, the imaging characteristics can pose a diagnostic dilemma, especially on a background of "pseudocirrhosis" (Figure 8). For example, lesions in HHT patients may not have the T_2 hyperintense "scar [38]". In such instances, differentiating benign FNH from malignant HCC (or other tumors) is challenging. One solution is to obtain further imaging with gadoxetate-enhanced MRI. Gadoxetate disodium is a gadolinium-based contrast agent that is actively taken up by hepatocytes. Because FNH is composed of proliferating hepatocytes, gadoxetate is readily taken up by these cells. Most hepatic malignant tumors (such as HCC or metastases) lack the transporter for gadoxetate, and therefore, gadoxetate remains extracellular. This results in unique imaging appearances with FNH retaining contrast (hyperintense) on the delayed "hepatobiliary phase" of gadoxetate-enhanced MRI (Figure 9), while HCC or other genuine neoplasms are usually hypointense relative to surrounding parenchyma. It is so essential to radiologically differentiate FNH from potential HCC due to the differences in management. While suspicious lesions require biopsy, a biopsy is not recommended in FNH on a background of hepatic VMs due to the bleeding risk.

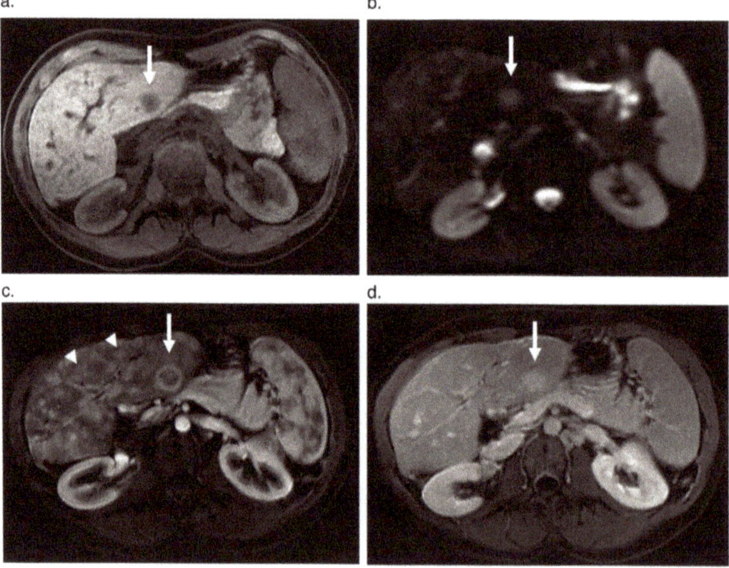

Figure 8. Focal nodular hyperplasia (FNH) mimicking cholangiocarcinoma in a 41-year-old woman with HHT. (**a**) Pre-contrast axial T_1-weighted MR image shows a focal T_1 hypointense lesion in segment III of the left hepatic lobe (arrow). (**b**) The lesion shows restricted diffusion at diffusion-weighted MR imaging (arrow). (**c**) Axial T_1 weighted gadolinium-enhanced MR image with fat saturation shows corresponding peripheral enhancement (arrow) as well as numerous confluent vascular masses (arrowheads). (**d**) The segment III lesion is hyper-enhancing on delayed phase (arrow). The confluent vascular masses are notably isointense to liver parenchyma at this phase. Ultrasound-guided biopsy of the segment III lesion showed features of FNH.

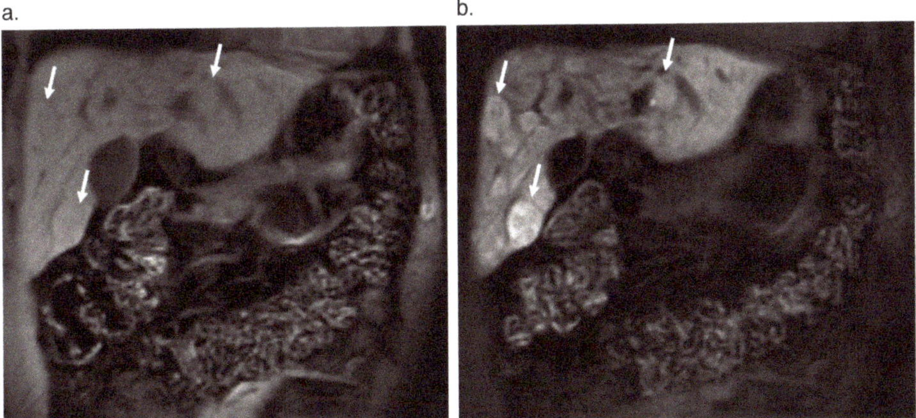

Figure 9. Focal nodular hyperplasia (FNH) in a 61-year-old woman with HHT. (**a**) Numerous hepatic lesions (arrows) are essentially imperceptible given signal characteristics similar to that of background parenchyma on pre-contrast-enhanced coronal T_1-weighted MR image. (**b**) The lesions (arrows) are hyper-enhancing on the hepatobiliary phase of the gadoxetate-enhanced coronal T_1-weighted MR image due to expected retention of contrast, compatible with multifocal FNH.

6.3. Cholangiopathy

An additional and feared complication of arterioportal or arteriosystemic shunts is cholangiopathy. The hepatic artery is the only blood supply to the bile ducts. Therefore, if blood is shunted from the hepatic artery to the portal or systemic veins, the bile ducts have decreased perfusion. In severe cases, this can result in bile duct ischemia/necrosis, biliary strictures, cholangitis, and even liver abscesses (Figure 10) [10,15].

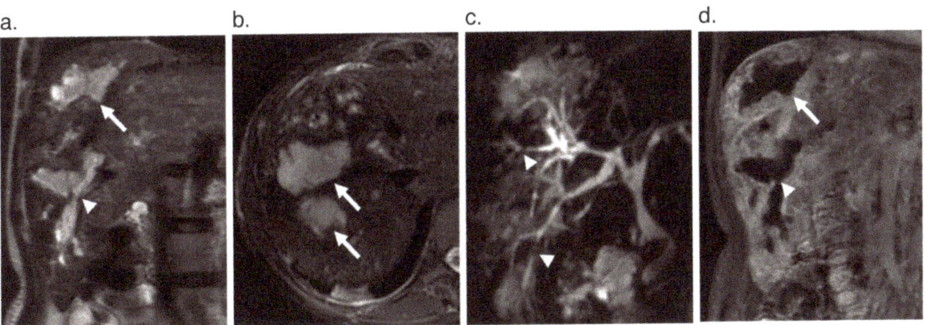

Figure 10. Ischemic cholangiopathy in a 36-year-old woman with HHT. Marked dilation of the intrahepatic bile ducts (arrows) and focal stenoses of the biliary tree (arrowheads) are seen on (**a**) coronal T_2-weighted SSFSE MR images, (**b**) axial T_2-weighted SSFSE MR images, (**c**) coronal MRCP maximum-intensity projection image, and (**d**) coronal T_1-weighted gadolinium-enhanced MR image. (SSFSE = single shot fast spin echo, MRCP = magnetic resonance cholangiopancreatography).

7. Summary and Future Direction

Hepatic VMs are common in patients with HHT, although a majority of them are asymptomatic. Arterial-systemic shunting between the hepatic artery and hepatic vein contributes to HOCF, a major cause of morbidity and mortality for HHT patients. Arterial-portal shunting can lead to portal hypertension. Liver-specific abnormalities include pseudocirrhosis, FNH, and ischemic cholangiopathy.

Non-invasive imaging with US, CT, and MRI plays a valuable role in assessing the hepatic manifestations of HHT. US is the preferred initial screening modality for liver VMs. All three methods can be useful for detecting and distinguishing the type of shunting that is present as well as for the detection of focal lesions as well as the physiologic consequences of portal hypertension.

Because the severity and type of liver shunting is an important determinant of the clinical presentation, particularly the development of HOCF, there is considerable interest in determining whether imaging assessment of hepatic VMs can help predict treatment response in patients undergoing anti-angiogenic therapy. As described above, quantitative assessment of flow and vascular morphology using US or MRI has the potential to help understand the role of the liver in determining the clinical response to these novel therapies.

Author Contributions: All authors contributed significantly to the creation of this manuscript, including drafting of text, preparing figures, and editing of manuscript. All authors have read and agreed to the published version of the manuscript.

Funding: No specific funding was provided for this manuscript.

Conflicts of Interest: Authors declare no relevant conflicts of interest. MAO has received travel support from General Electric, but unrelated to the topic and content of this manuscript.

References

1. Siddiki, H.; Doherty, M.G.; Fletcher, J.G.; Stanson, A.W.; Vrtiska, T.J.; Hough, D.M.; Fidler, J.L.; McCollough, C.; Swanson, K.L. Abdominal Findings in Hereditary Hemorrhagic Telangiectasia: Pictorial Essay on 2D and 3D Findings with Isotropic Multiphase CT. *Radiographics* **2008**, *28*, 171–183. [CrossRef]

2. Choi, H.H.-I.; Manning, M.A.; Mehrotra, A.K.; Wagner, S.; Jha, R.C. Primary Hepatic Neoplasms of Vascular Origin: Key Imaging Features and Differential Diagnoses with Radiology-Pathology Correlation. *Am. J. Roentgenol.* **2017**, *209*, W350–W359. [CrossRef] [PubMed]

3. Fernández-L, A.; Sanz-Rodriguez, F.; Blanco, F.J.; Botella, L.M.; Bernabeu, C. Hereditary Hemorrhagic Telangiectasia, a Vascular Dysplasia Affecting the TGF- Signaling Pathway. *Clin. Med. Res.* **2006**, *4*, 66–78. [CrossRef] [PubMed]

4. Null, N. EASL Clinical Practice Guidelines: Vascular diseases of the liver. *J. Hepatol.* **2016**, *64*, 179–202. [CrossRef]

5. Driesche, S.V.D.; Mummery, C.L.; Westermann, C.J. Hereditary hemorrhagic telangiectasia: An update on transforming growth factor β signaling in vasculogenesis and angiogenesis. *Cardiovasc. Res.* **2003**, *58*, 20–31. [CrossRef]

6. Metze, D.; Cury, V.F.; Gomez, R.S.; Marco, L.; Robinson, D.; Melamed, E.; Leung, A.K.C.; Nam, J.-H.; Matsubara, Y.; Tada, K.; et al. Hereditary Hemorrhagic Telangiectasia. *Encycl. Mol. Mech. Dis.* **2009**, *25*, 830–831.

7. Faughnan, M.E.; Palda, V.A.; Garcia-Tsao, G.; Geisthoff, U.W.; McDonald, J.; Proctor, D.D.; Spears, J.; Brown, D.H.; Buscarini, E.; Chesnutt, M.S.; et al. International guidelines for the diagnosis and management of hereditary haemorrhagic telangiectasia. *J. Med. Genet.* **2009**, *48*, 73–87. [CrossRef]

8. Govani, F.S.; Shovlin, C.L. Hereditary haemorrhagic telangiectasia: A clinical and scientific review. *Eur. J. Hum. Genet.* **2009**, *17*, 860–871. [CrossRef]

9. Shovlin, C.L.; Guttmacher, A.E.; Buscarini, E.; Faughnan, M.E.; Hyland, R.H.; Westermann, C.J.J.; Kjeldsen, A.D.; Plauchu, H. Diagnostic criteria for hereditary hemorrhagic telangiectasia (Rendu-Osler-Weber syndrome). *Am. J. Med. Genet.* **2000**, *91*, 66–67. [CrossRef]

10. Faughnan, M.E.; Mager, J.J.; Hetts, S.W.; Palda, V.A.; Lang-Robertson, K.; Buscarini, E.; Deslandres, E.; Kasthuri, R.S.; Lausman, A.; Poetker, D.; et al. Second International Guidelines for the Diagnosis and Management of Hereditary Hemorrhagic Telangiectasia. *Ann. Intern. Med.* **2020**. [CrossRef]

11. Buscarini, E.; Leandro, G.; Conte, D.; Danesino, C.; Daina, E.; Manfredi, G.; Lupinacci, G.; Brambilla, G.; Menozzi, F.; De Grazia, F.; et al. Natural History and Outcome of Hepatic Vascular Malformations in a Large Cohort of Patients with Hereditary Hemorrhagic Teleangiectasia. *Dig. Dis. Sci.* **2011**, *56*, 2166–2178. [CrossRef] [PubMed]

12. Garcia-Tsao, G. Liver involvement in hereditary hemorrhagic telangiectasia (HHT). *J. Hepatol.* **2007**, *46*, 499–507. [CrossRef] [PubMed]

13. Vernon, H.; Wehrle, C.; Kasai, A. Anatomy, Abdomen and Pelvis, Liver (updated 31 July 2020). In *StatPearls [Internet]*; StatPearls Publishing: Treasure Island, FL, USA, 2020.

14. Buscarini, E.; Danesino, C.; Olivieri, C.; Lupinacci, G.; De Grazia, F.; Reduzzi, L.; Blotta, P.; Gazzaniga, P.; Pagella, F.; Grosso, M.; et al. Doppler Ultrasonographic Grading of Hepatic Vascular Malformations in Hereditary Hemorrhagic Telangiectasia—Results of Extensive Screening. *Ultraschall der Med. Eur. J. Ultrasound* **2004**, *25*, 348–355. [CrossRef] [PubMed]

15. Naganuma, H.; Ishida, H.; Kuroda, H.; Suzuki, Y.; Ogawa, M. Hereditary hemorrhagic telangiectasia: How to efficiently detect hepatic abnormalities using ultrasonography. *J. Med. Ultrason.* **2020**, *47*, 421–433. [CrossRef]

16. Garcia-Tsao, G.; Korzenik, J.R.; Young, L.; Henderson, K.J.; Jain, D.; Byrd, B.; Pollak, J.S.; White, R.I. Liver Disease in Patients with Hereditary Hemorrhagic Telangiectasia. *N. Engl. J. Med.* **2000**, *343*, 931–936. [CrossRef]

17. Alcazar, R.; De La Torre, M.; Peces, R. Symptomatic intrarenal arteriovenous fistula detected 25 years after percutaneous renal biopsy. *Nephrol. Dial. Transplant.* **1996**, *11*, 1346–1348. [CrossRef]

18. Reddy, Y.N.; Melenovsky, V.; Redfield, M.M.; Nishimura, R.A.; Borlaug, B.A. High-Output Heart Failure. *J. Am. Coll. Cardiol.* **2016**, *68*, 473–482. [CrossRef]

19. Xu, B.-G.; Liang, J.; Jia, K.-F.; Han, T. Liver cirrhosis in a patient with hepatic hereditary hemorrhagic telangiectasia and Budd–Chiari syndrome: A case report. *BMC Gastroenterol.* **2020**, *20*, 1–6. [CrossRef]

20. Buscarini, E.; Gandolfi, S.; Alicante, S.; Londoni, C.; Manfredi, G. Liver involvement in hereditary hemorrhagic telangiectasia. *Abdom. Radiol.* **2018**, *43*, 1920–1930. [CrossRef]

21. Welle, C.L.; Welch, B.T.; Brinjikji, W.; Ehman, E.C.; Venkatesh, S.K.; Johnson, M.P.; Iyer, V.N.; Leise, M.D.; Wood, C.P. Abdominal manifestations of hereditary hemorrhagic telangiectasia: A series of 333 patients over 15 years. *Abdom. Radiol.* **2019**, *44*, 2384–2391. [CrossRef]

22. Schelker, R.C.; Barreiros, A.P.; Hart, C.; Herr, W.; Jung, E.-M. Macro- and microcirculation patterns of intrahepatic blood flow changes in patients with hereditary hemorrhagic telangiectasia. *World J. Gastroenterol.* **2017**, *23*, 486–495. [CrossRef] [PubMed]

23. Kearns, K.N.; Sokolowski, J.D.; Chadwell, K.; Chandler, M.; Kiernan, T.; Prada, F.; Kalani, M.Y.S.; Park, M.S. The role of contrast-enhanced ultrasound in neurosurgical disease. *Neurosurg. Focus* **2019**, *47*, E8. [CrossRef] [PubMed]

24. Oe, Y.; Orr, L.; Laifer-Narin, S.; Hyodo, E.; Koczo, A.; Homma, S.; Kandel, J.J.; Meyers, P. Contrast-enhanced sonography as a novel tool for assessment of vascular malformations. *J. Angiogenes. Res.* **2010**, *2*, 25. [CrossRef] [PubMed]

25. Wiesinger, I.; Schreml, S.; Wohlgemuth, W.A.; Stroszczynski, C.; Jung, E. Perfusion quantification of vascular malformations using contrast-enhanced ultrasound (CEUS) with time intensity curve analysis before and after treatment: First results. *Clin. Hemorheol. Microcirc.* **2016**, *62*, 283–290. [CrossRef] [PubMed]

26. Lyshchik, A.; Kono, Y.; Dietrich, C.F.; Jang, H.-J.; Kim, T.K.; Piscaglia, F.; Vezeridis, A.; Willmann, J.K.; Wilson, S.R. Contrast-enhanced ultrasound of the liver: Technical and lexicon recommendations from the ACR CEUS LI-RADS working group. *Abdom. Radiol.* **2018**, *43*, 861–879. [CrossRef] [PubMed]

27. Schelker, R.C.; Andorfer, K.; Putz, F.; Herr, W.; Jung, E.-M. Identification of two distinct hereditary hemorrhagic telangiectasia patient subsets with different hepatic perfusion properties by combination of contrast-enhanced ultrasound (CEUS) with perfusion imaging quantification. *PLoS ONE* **2019**, *14*, e0215178. [CrossRef]

28. Scardapane, A.; Ianora, A.S.; Sabba, C.; Moschetta, M.; Suppressa, P.; Castorani, L.; Angelelli, G. Dynamic 4D MR angiography versus multislice CT angiography in the evaluation of vascular hepatic involvement in hereditary haemorrhagic telangiectasia. *La Radiol. Med.* **2011**, *117*, 29–45. [CrossRef]

29. Wu, J.S.; Saluja, S.; Garcia-Tsao, G.; Chong, A.; Henderson, K.J.; White, R.I. Liver Involvement in Hereditary Hemorrhagic Telangiectasia: CT and Clinical Findings Do Not Correlate in Symptomatic Patients. *Am. J. Roentgenol.* **2006**, *187*, W399–W405. [CrossRef]

30. Kutaiba, N.; Gow, P.J.; French, J.; Lim, R.P. Putting a new spin: MRI monitoring of hepatic artery and portal vein flow for response to bevacizumab in hereditary hemorrhagic telangiectasia. *Clin. Case Rep.* **2014**, *3*, 32–33. [CrossRef]

J. Clin. Med. **2020**, *9*, 3750

31. Edwards, E.A.; Phelps, A.S.; Cooke, D.; Frieden, I.J.; Zapala, M.A.; Fullerton, H.J.; Shimano, K.A. Monitoring Arteriovenous Malformation Response to Genotype-Targeted Therapy. *Pediatrics* **2020**, *146*, e20193206. [CrossRef]
32. Dupuis-Girod, S.; Ginon, I.; Saurin, J.-C.; Marion, D.; Guillot, E.; Decullier, E.; Roux, A.; Carette, M.-F.; Gilbert-Dussardier, B.; Hatron, P.-Y.; et al. Bevacizumab in Patients With Hereditary Hemorrhagic Telangiectasia and Severe Hepatic Vascular Malformations and High Cardiac Output. *JAMA* **2012**, *307*, 948–955. [CrossRef] [PubMed]
33. Buscarini, E.; Vascern-Hht, O.B.O.; Botella, L.M.; Geisthoff, U.; Kjeldsen, A.D.; Mager, H.J.; Pagella, F.; Suppressa, P.; Zarrabeitia, R.; Dupuis-Girod, S.; et al. Safety of thalidomide and bevacizumab in patients with hereditary hemorrhagic telangiectasia. *Orphanet J. Rare Dis.* **2019**, *14*, 1–14. [CrossRef] [PubMed]
34. Faughnan, M.E.; Gossage, J.R.; Chakinala, M.M.; Oh, S.P.; Kasthuri, R.; Hughes, C.C.W.; McWilliams, J.P.; Parambil, J.G.; Vozoris, N.; Donaldson, J.; et al. Pazopanib may reduce bleeding in hereditary hemorrhagic telangiectasia. *Angiogenesis* **2019**, *22*, 145–155. [CrossRef] [PubMed]
35. Chavan, A.; Luthe, L.; Gebel, M.; Barg-Hock, H.; Seifert, H.; Raab, R.; Kirchhoff, T.; Schmuck, B. Complications and clinical outcome of hepatic artery embolisation in patients with hereditary haemorrhagic telangiectasia. *Eur. Radiol.* **2013**, *23*, 951–957. [CrossRef] [PubMed]
36. Cooney, T.; Sweeney, E.C.; Coll, R.; Greally, M. 'Pseudocirrhosis' in hereditary haemorrhagic telangiectasia. *J. Clin. Pathol.* **1977**, *30*, 1134–1141. [CrossRef] [PubMed]
37. Buscarini, E.; Danesino, C.; Plauchu, H.; De Fazio, C.; Olivieri, C.; Brambilla, G.; Menozzi, F.; Reduzzi, L.; Blotta, P.; Gazzaniga, P.; et al. High prevalence of hepatic focal nodular hyperplasia in subjects with hereditary hemorrhagic telangiectasia. *Ultrasound Med. Biol.* **2004**, *30*, 1089–1097. [CrossRef]
38. Scardapane, A.; Ficco, M.; Sabba, C.; Lorusso, F.; Moschetta, M.; Maggialetti, N.; Suppressa, P.; Angelelli, G.; Ianora, A.A.S. Hepatic nodular regenerative lesions in patients with hereditary haemorrhagic telangiectasia: Computed tomography and magnetic resonance findings. *La Radiol. Med.* **2012**, *118*, 1–13. [CrossRef]

Publisher's Note: MDPI stays neutral with regard to jurisdictional claims in published maps and institutional affiliations.

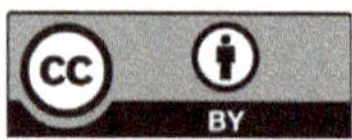

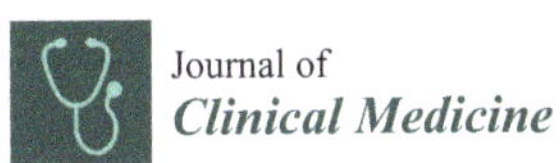

Journal of
Clinical Medicine

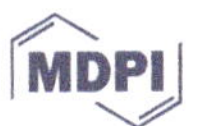

Review

Approach to Pulmonary Arteriovenous Malformations: A Comprehensive Update

Shamaita Majumdar and Justin P. McWilliams *

UCLA Department of Radiological Sciences, Los Angeles, CA 90095, USA; shamaitamajumdar@mednet.ucla.edu
* Correspondence: JuMcWilliams@mednet.ucla.edu; Tel.: +1-310-267-8773

Received: 26 April 2020; Accepted: 15 June 2020; Published: 19 June 2020

Abstract: Pulmonary arteriovenous malformations (PAVMs) are abnormal direct vascular communications between pulmonary arteries and veins which create high-flow right-to-left shunts. They are most frequently congenital, usually in the setting of hereditary hemorrhagic telangiectasia (HHT). PAVMs may be asymptomatic or present with a wide variety of clinical manifestations such as dyspnea, hypoxemia, or chest pain. Even when asymptomatic, presence of PAVMs increases patients' risk of serious, potentially preventable complications including stroke or brain abscess. Transcatheter embolotherapy is considered the gold standard for treatment of PAVMs. Though previous guidelines have been published regarding the management of PAVMs, several aspects of PAVM screening and management remain debated among the experts, suggesting the need for thorough reexamination of the current literature. The authors of this review present an updated approach to the diagnostic workup and management of PAVMs, with an emphasis on areas of controversy, based on the latest literature and our institutional experience.

Keywords: pulmonary arteriovenous malformations; hereditary hemorrhagic telangiectasia; transcatheter embolotherapy; screening; guidelines

---

1. Introduction

Pulmonary arteriovenous malformations (PAVMs) are structurally abnormal, direct vascular communications between pulmonary arteries and veins, which bypass capillary beds to create low-resistance, high-flow continuous intrapulmonary right-to-left shunts [1–3].

The majority of PAVMs (70% or more) are associated with the autosomal dominant disorder hereditary hemorrhagic telangiectasia (HHT), also known as Osler-Weber-Rendu syndrome [2,4–6]. HHT mutations, which most commonly affect the *ENG* gene (HHT Type 1) or *ACVRL1* gene (HHT type 2), disrupt key regulators in angiogenesis, resulting in the development of congenital PAVMs and other vascular anomalies [1,7]. PAVMs affect about 50% of HHT patients overall [8], with a higher incidence and number of PAVMs in patients with *ENG* mutations [9]. Acquired causes of PAVMs account for approximately 20% of cases and include trauma, cardiothoracic surgery, hepatic cirrhosis, metastatic cancer, mitral stenosis, infection, amyloidosis, and chronic thromboembolic disease [2,3]. The wide variety of conditions associated with acquired PAVM suggests a common underlying developmental mechanism which triggers an angiogenic cascade within the pulmonary vasculature [3]. The remaining minority of PAVMs which cannot be classified as congenital or acquired are categorized as idiopathic.

PAVM angioarchitecture is classified as simple or complex based on the segmental pulmonary artery anatomy, which is important for planning endovascular interventions [5,10]. Simple PAVMs are supplied by a single segmental pulmonary artery. The single segmental pulmonary artery will often branch distally into one to three subsegmental branches all supplying the PAVM [5]. Complex PAVMs are supplied by two or more segmental pulmonary arteries. Diffuse PAVM is a rare subtype of complex PAVM characterized by involvement of an entire segment, or sometimes an entire lung, by tangles of malformed vasculature [3]. PAVMs often have a lower lobe predominance [11].

PAVMs are most frequently asymptomatic, but may be associated with a wide spectrum of clinical manifestations, and if left untreated, they can result in serious complications. Physiologic consequences correlate with the size of PAVM and degree of right-to-left shunting, which can limit oxygenation and natural filtration in the lung. Patients may present with varying degrees of dyspnea, cyanosis, clubbing, or chest pain [2,3]. Due to decreased filtration of vasoactive substances into the systemic circulation, migraines are a common neurologic manifestation of PAVM [1]. More serious complications include brain abscess, paradoxical embolism resulting in stroke or transient ischemic attack (TIA), and less frequently, hemoptysis or intrapulmonary hemorrhage [10,12]. HHT patients with PAVMs are several hundred-fold more likely to develop brain abscess compared to the general population [13,14]. The risk of brain abscess is significantly correlated with number of PAVMs, and larger feeding artery size is significantly correlated with risk of ischemic stroke [15]. Current indications for treatment of PAVM include any (solitary or multiple) PAVM with feeding artery diameter ≥2–3 mm, measurable increase in PAVM size, paradoxical emboli, symptomatic hypoxemia, or any of the other aforementioned serious complications [16].

Embolization is the standard of care for treatment of PAVMs, with surgery reserved for refractory cases which have repeatedly failed embolotherapy [17]. This review aims to present updated recommendations for the diagnostic workup and management of PAVMs, with an emphasis on screening protocol and aspects of care within particular subsets of patients, based on the most recent literature and the experiences at our institution, which has been an HHT Center of Excellence since 2010.

2. Methods

A comprehensive narrative review of the last 10 years of literature relevant to pulmonary AVM diagnosis and management was undertaken using PubMed search term (pulmonary arteriovenous malformations) for date range 1 April 2010 to the date of review on 1 April 2020 (Figure 1). The literature search yielded 384 results. After excluding duplicative cohorts, letters, comments, and erratum, the remaining 364 articles were screened by titles, abstracts, and keywords. A total of 201 publications were identified as within the scope of the topic and the full texts were reviewed for eligibility. 73 articles were deemed relevant to PAVM screening and management. Citations of these 73 papers were examined for key articles which may have been published outside of the specified date range. Particular attention was given to articles relevant to areas of controversy, including PAVM screening, size criteria for PAVM treatment, management of PAVMs in pediatric and pregnant patients, treatment of persistent and diffuse PAVMs, management of PAVMs in the setting of pulmonary hypertension, and choice of embolic devices for PAVM embolization. The final literature sample included 110 articles relevant to PAVM screening and aspects of management, with a focus on areas on controversy.

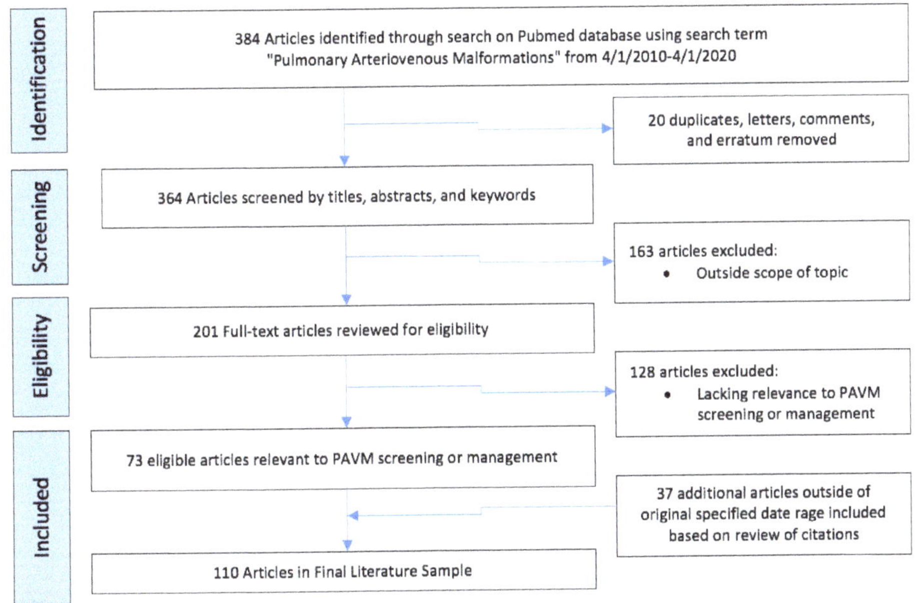

Figure 1. Flowchart for literature selection for narrative review.

3. Screening Protocol in Patient with Suspicion for PAVM

3.1. Transthoracic Contrast Echocardiography

The International Guidelines for Diagnosis and Management of HHT recommend that clinicians screen all patients with possible or confirmed HHT for PAVMs [18]. Transthoracic contrast echocardiography (TTCE) is the screening test of choice for PAVM, with a sensitivity of up to 98.6% and high rates of inter-observer agreement [19,20]. According to the 2011 International Guidelines, TTCE is considered positive if there is any detection of bubbles in the left atrium, and all positive screening tests should subsequently be confirmed with CT and recommended for antibiotic prophylaxis [18]. In patients with negative initial screening, repeat screening should be considered after pregnancy, within 5 years preceding planned pregnancy, and otherwise every 5–10 years. However, recent studies have brought into question whether confirmatory CT and antibiotic prophylaxis are necessary for mildly positive TTCE screening studies.

The TTCE shunt grading system is divided into a 0–3 scale, depending on the degree of left ventricular opacification after administration of a contrast agent. Grade 1 shunts demonstrate minimal opacification with less than 30 bubbles on any single frame. Grade 2 shunts correspond to moderate opacification with 30–100 bubbles. Grade 3 shunts have extensive opacification with >100 bubbles. A 2016 survey assessing current practices among 33 practitioners at HHT Centers of Excellence worldwide showed that for patients with Grade 1 screening echocardiograms, 41% recommend follow up with contrast enhanced CT, 22% recommend noncontrast CT, and 25% recommend repeat TTCE in 5–10 years, suggesting inconsistency among practices [21].

Velthuis et al. demonstrated a relationship between the grade of right-to-left shunt on TTCE and the prevalence of cerebral complications (ischemic stroke, TIA, brain abscess) in patients screened for HHT [22]. Out of 1038 patients, 530 had shunts detected on TTCE. Grade 1 shunts were not associated with an increased prevalence of cerebral manifestations, whereas grade 2 and 3 shunts were both independent predictors for prevalence of cerebral complication. 58 patients had shunting only with Valsalva maneuver, suggesting a diagnosis of patent foramen ovale (PFO) rather than pulmonary shunt, and none of these patients had any subsequent complication. Another study by Velthuis et al. prospectively investigated whether TTCE shunt grade could predict size of PAVMs on chest CT in 510 patients [23]. The positive predicted value for presence of PAVM on chest CT was 13.4% for grade 1 shunts, compared to 45.3% and 92.5% for grade 2 and 3 shunts, respectively. Moreover, none of the grade 1 shunts subsequently needed embolization, whereas 25.3% of grade 2 shunts and 77.4% of grade 3 shunts required endovascular closure of PAVM. Other studies have reported similar observations, for example that increased shunt grade predicts presence of PAVM on chest CT [24–26], and that patients with grade 1 shunts do not receive intervention, whereas those with grade 2 and 3 shunts often do [27–30].

These studies strongly suggest that grade 1 shunts are not associated with cerebral complications and do not predict presence of treatable PAVMs. As a result, we suggest that in patients with grade 1 shunts on screening TTCE, a conservative strategy withholding chest CT and antibiotic prophylaxis is justified and appropriate [31]. Repeat TTCE screening should be performed every 5 years to monitor for increased shunting. In patients with grade 2 shunts or higher on screening TTCE, diagnostic chest CT should be performed. Lastly, patients who demonstrate TTCE shunting only with Valsalva most likely have a diagnosis of PFO rather than PAVM, so the maneuver should be avoided during PAVM screening, and subsequent chest CT is not necessary.

3.2. Contrast Versus Noncontrast Thoracic CT

As mentioned previously, for patients undergoing confirmatory chest CT after screening TTCE, there is inconsistency among providers on whether to perform this study with or without contrast [21]. Currently, unenhanced multidetector chest CT with thin-cut 1–2 mm reconstructions is considered the gold standard for confirming PAVM [2,3,18]. Noncontrast CT is sufficient for identifying the highly characteristic feeding artery and draining vein, with a saccular or fistulous connection in between [10]. However, some institutions choose to perform CT with a modified pulmonary angiography protocol (CTPA) to better define the PAVM angioarchitecture and aid in treatment planning [2,3]. Furthermore, contrast can be a useful, though not absolutely necessary, tool for follow-up of embolized PAVMs, by assessing the presence or absence of contrast enhancement in the PAVM sac and/or draining vein. If contrast is used, care must be taken to avoid injection of air bubbles which could risk neurologic complication.

Overall, we maintain that CT can be performed either with or without contrast for screening and diagnosis of PAVMs. The use of contrast can help screen for extrapulmonary vascular anomalies, better define PAVM angioarchitecture, and provide additional variables to assess treatment success on follow-up CT, but has the disadvantage of increased cost and possibility of air embolism, allergy or nephrotoxicity.

4. Management of PAVM by Sub-Populations

4.1. Small PAVMs

The 2011 HHT consensus guidelines recommended embolization of PAVMs with a feeding artery diameter 3 mm or greater, with the caveat that targeting PAVMs with a feeding artery as low as 2 mm may be appropriate in some cases [18]. Older literature commonly referenced the notion that cerebral ischemic events did not occur in patients having PAVMs with feeding artery diameter below 3 mm [32]. However, subsequent studies suggest that even small PAVMs can sometimes result in complications. One case in 2004 described embolization of a PAVM with feeding artery diameter of 1.8 mm in a patient with recurrent embolic strokes, with no further strokes post-treatment [33]. In 2004, Mager et al. reported long-term outcomes after embolization of 349 PAVMs in a cohort of 112 patients [34]. PAVMs targeted in this study had feeding artery diameter ≥3 mm or had caused bleeding or systemic complications. In 38 patients, smaller visualized PAVMs were initially left untreated; 16 of these 38 patients (42%) later required reintervention due to increasing shunt or complication. In 74 patients, all of the visible PAVMs including small lesions were treated at the initial procedure, and only 4% of patients in this group required reintervention. These data suggest that patients are much more likely to require reintervention when all visible PAVMs are not embolized at the time of initial procedure. Three of the five complications reported in the study were definitive sequelae of small untreated PAVMs, including one brain abscess and two TIAs. A 2006 study by Pollak et al. reported that nearly 20% of small PAVMs will grow over time, and that up to half of these may result in symptomatic events or complications [35]. A study in 2008 examining risk factors for stroke and brain abscess in HHT patients with PAVMs found that all patients who experienced stroke or abscess in spite of previous embolization had small untreated PAVMs with feeding artery diameter ≤2–3 mm, and embolization of all angiographically visible PAVMs was associated with significantly reduced ischemic stroke rate [36].

Overall, current evidence suggests that serious complications including stroke and brain abscess may occur in PAVMs with feeding artery diameter <3 mm. Given this risk, we feel it is reasonable to perform embolization for any PAVM with feeding artery diameter 2 mm or larger, and any symptomatic PAVM. Furthermore, several studies suggest that embolization of all angiographically visible PAVMs at the time of initial procedure will significantly reduce the likelihood of needing reintervention and risk of complication. Thus, if an embolization procedure is being performed, we recommend that all visible PAVMs (including those smaller than 2 mm) be occluded at the same session, if technically feasible.

4.2. Pediatric Patients

The 2011 International Guidelines recommend that PAVM screening be performed at the time of the initial clinical evaluation for HHT for both adults and children, with TTCE as the initial screening test and confirmatory CT performed for positive TTCE [18,37]. However, these guidelines pose some drawbacks for the pediatric population. As previously discussed, many studies have shown that TTCE is often positive in the absence of treatable PAVM, particularly for low grade shunts [23–25]. Since any positive TTCE study mandated subsequent CT, this potentially exposes the child to unnecessary or avoidable radiation. Furthermore, the placement of intravenous lines, which is necessary for TTCE, may be stressful for pediatric patients.

Mowers et al. completed a retrospective 14-year longitudinal study of PAVMs in 129 children with HHT [38]. The study utilized standard screening methods, with initial TTCE screening, followed by confirmatory CT for any positive TTCE shunt graded 2 or above. Negative patients were rescreened every 5 years, and all PAVMs with a supplying artery greater than 3 mm were embolized. 59% (76/129) of children screened positive on TTCE and were diagnosed with PAVM. Of those, 38 (50%) had small (<3 mm) PAVMs which were left untreated, and 38 (50%) had large PAVMs ≥ 3 mm which were embolized. 15 children had symptomatic PAVMs, all of which were large. All patients in the untreated cohort remained asymptomatic. Nine of the 38 treated patients had initial negative screening, but had PAVMs which grew larger at follow-up and were subsequently embolized. 21% (8/38) of the embolization group required repeat intervention, primarily due to persistence of the treated PAVM. No children in the study suffered treatment complications or adverse events in follow-up.

Hosman et al. completed an 18-year prospective study using a more conservative method of screening in 175 children with HHT [39]. In the conservative approach, screening was performed every 5 years using history and physical to detect dyspnea, cyanosis, and clubbing, pulse oximetry to detect hypoxemia, and chest radiography to screen for visible PAVM. Positive abnormalities were found in 50/175 (28%) children with HHT, and these 50 patients subsequently received diagnostic CT. 39 out of 50 patients who underwent CT were found to have PAVMs, suggesting highly efficient detection rate using this screening method. 33/39 (85%) children with PAVMs underwent embolization, 29 of them before the age of 18. 19/29 (66%) treated patients required multiple interventions due to persistence. 57 HHT patients who did not have PAVM detected through childhood screening received TTCE screening after age 18. In 6/57 (11%) of these patients, a PAVM was detected in adult screening and 2/57 (3.5%) were ultimately embolized. No children in the cohort suffered brain abscess, stroke, hemoptysis or hemothorax due to PAVM.

Based on these studies, we can conclude that both standard and conservative approaches are acceptable screening methods for PAVM in children. Standard screening with TTCE every 5 years, followed by noncontrast low-dose CT for grade 2 or higher shunts is safe and effective at detecting PAVM, but risks exposing a larger percentage of pediatric patients to radiation. Conservative screening with physical exam, pulse oximetry, and chest radiograph every 5 years is also safe and effective, with the added benefit of decreased likelihood of exposure to CT radiation. However, with the conservative algorithm, there is a small chance of missing a treatable AVM which might not be detected until adulthood.

Regarding frequency of screening, the existing recommendations state that for patients with initial negative TTCE screen, screening should be repeated after puberty, and otherwise every 5–10 years. However, recent longitudinal studies suggest that PAVMs can grow during puberty and that a more frequent screening interval during childhood may be appropriate. Mowers et al. reported that, out of 31 children with HHT with negative initial screening who were followed for more than a year, nine of them (29%) went on to develop new PAVMS on subsequent TTCE screen, with a mean time to detection of 5.6 years [38]. Another study showed that, among 37 children with known PAVMs followed with interval CT scans, PAVM size seemed to grow approximately 10% per year and double in size every 5–6 years [40]. Since evidence suggests that PAVMs are expected to grow during childhood, increasing the risk of worsening symptoms or complications, we maintain that pediatric patients should be rescreened for PAVMs at 5-year intervals.

In the pediatric population, there remains significant controversy regarding treatment approach. Current guidelines state that symptomatic children should always be treated, whereas treatment of asymptomatic children should be considered on a case-by-case basis. The prevalence and symptomatology of PAVMs in children is similar in frequency and distribution to adults, and serious complications from PAVMs do occur, particularly in PAVMs $\geq$ 3 mm [38,41]. One series followed 42 children with PAVMs treated with embolization (diameter $\geq$ 3 mm) for an average of 7 years [41]. Prior to clinical assessment or embolic treatment, several children within the study group had suffered serious complications related to PAVMs: 60% (25/42) of patients presented with cyanosis; hemoptysis had occurred in 7% (3/42) and neurologic complications had occurred in 19% (8/42). This study demonstrated significant improvement in oxygenation after embolization, particularly in patients with focal PAVMs, and only one post-treatment neurologic event, which occurred in a patient with diffuse PAVMs. Persistence at follow-up occurred in 15% of PAVMs, emphasizing the need for long-term follow-up post-treatment. Several other studies also suggest that PAVM-related complications in children tend to occur only with large PAVMs, and that small untreated PAVMs may not pose as significant of a threat as in adults [39,42,43].

Our own institutional practice is to screen infants and young children clinically using history, physical, and pulse oximetry, and to start TTCE screening at age 10–12, with repeat TTCE every 5 years thereafter. We prefer to treat symptomatic PAVMs and any PAVM $\geq$ 3 mm in pediatric patients, and to monitor smaller asymptomatic PAVMs until age 18 to reduce childhood radiation exposure. When embolization is required, we perform dense distal embolization of the PAVM to mitigate the high rates of persistence at follow-up.

4.3. PAVMs in Pregnancy

PAVMs have been observed to cause increased morbidity during pregnancy [44]. Physiologic changes of pregnancy result in increased blood volume and cardiac output, particularly in the second and third trimester, which may raise pressure within the PAVM. Moreover, high progesterone levels are thought to increase venous distensibility. These physiologic factors can promote enlargement and rupture of PAVMs during pregnancy. Numerous cases of PAVM-related complications during pregnancy have been reported in the literature, most frequently hemothorax [45–51]. However, despite acknowledgement of this greater risk during pregnancy, international consensus guidelines do not provide specific recommendations about treatment of PAVMs during pregnancy [18]. The British Thoracic Society guidelines advise clinicians to consider pregnancy a relative contraindication to elective embolization due to radiation and preterm labor risk, with the caveat that benefits may outweigh risks in setting of life-threatening hemoptysis [1]. They further contend that most PAVM pregnancies do well even in the setting of significant hypoxemia, but recommend management as a "high-risk" pregnancy, quoting a 1% risk of maternal death. However, our review of existing literature suggests this may be an underestimation, and that treatment of PAVM during pregnancy is both safe and warranted given the morbidity and mortality risk.

The risk of death with PAVM pregnancy quoted by the British Thoracic Society was determined from a 2008 review by Shovlin et al. [52]. This study reported 5 deaths out of 484 pregnancies in women with HHT, approximately 1%. However, out of 484 pregnancies, 23 cases (in 16 patients) were prospectively followed during the pregnancy, and 15 of the 16 patients in this prospective group had had their PAVMs embolized prior to pregnancy. Although no deaths occurred in the prospective group, inclusion of these pretreated cases is not a valid assessment of mortality risk for untreated PAVM. 239 of the 484 cases were previous pregnancies in women currently attending HHT clinic, constituting the retrospective study group. All patients in this subgroup had to be alive given they were present in clinic post-pregnancy, so their inclusion again is not valid to assess mortality. 222 pregnancies in the study were assessed in first-degree relatives with known HHT. In this group, 5 deaths occurred out of 222 cases, a rate of approximately 2.3%. The number of patients with PAVMs in this third study group was not known. Several may not have had PAVMs at all, and others may have had their PAVMs treated prior to pregnancy. Thus, estimates drawn from this study may underestimate the true mortality risk of untreated PAVM in pregnancy.

Earlier data does support the notion that untreated PAVMs are dangerous during pregnancy. A 1995 study by the same group reviewed maternal complications of 161 pregnancies in HHT women with and without PAVMs [53]. In 138 pregnancies without PAVM, no deaths occurred, and there was one ischemic stroke of unknown cause (0.7%). Of the 23 pregnancies with untreated PAVM, 8 (23%) resulted in nonfatal complications comprised of 6 pulmonary shunt increases and 2 ischemic strokes. 2 of the 23 PAVM cases resulted in fatal pulmonary hemorrhages, an 8.7% maternal death rate.

A 2014 study surveyed women with HHT regarding complications during pregnancy, including 38 women with known PAVMs [54]. Eight women with PAVMs had been screened and treated prior to pregnancy, and no complications were noted in a total of 17 pregnancies in this group. Thirty women with PAVMs had not been treated pre-pregnancy; out of 64 pregnancies in this group, 11 complications were deemed to be PAVM-related, including 2 cases of hemoptysis, 5 hemothoraces (1 post-partum), 2 TIAs, and 1 post-partum myocardial infarction. While this survey-based study cannot be used to estimate mortality rate, the findings do suggest that untreated PAVM poses a high morbidity risk during pregnancy.

The data from these three studies can be roughly combined to make conservative risk estimates for untreated pulmonary AVMs in pregnancy (Figure 2) [52–54]. A mortality estimate can be calculated based on the data from first-degree relatives in the 2008 survey (222 pregnancies) combined with the retrospective data from the 1995 study (23 pregnancies), which yields 7 deaths in 245 patients (2.9%). For non-fatal complications, a morbidity estimate can be calculated based on the retrospective data and the data from first-degree relatives in the 2008 survey (461 pregnancies), retrospective data from the 1995 study (23 pregnancies), and retrospective data from the 2014 survey (64 pregnancies), which yields 30 nonfatal complications in 548 pregnancies (5.5%). These risk estimates, although imperfect, do underscore the danger of untreated PAVMs in pregnancy. A recent review examining pregnancy in HHT concluded similarly that the current maternal mortality and morbidity risks quoted in the literature are likely underestimations, and that these cases should be considered high risk [51].

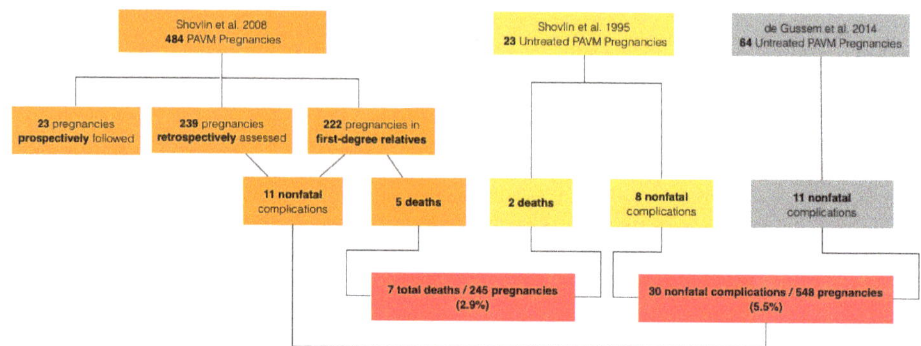

Figure 2. Flowchart representation of mortality and morbidity risk estimates for untreated pulmonary arteriovenous malformations in pregnancy.

The British Thoracic Society describes pregnancy as a relative contraindication to elective embolization due to radiation exposure and risk of preterm labor [1]. However, studies have shown that complications from PAVM embolization are rare. One study examining outcomes of 205 PAVM embolization procedures in non-pregnant patients reported a ≤1% procedural complication rate, that being a single TIA [35]. Gershon et al. published a case series describing the embolization of 13 PAVMs in 7 pregnant patients, gestational age 16–36 weeks, reporting no complications [44]. Furthermore, there are no reports in the literature of PAVM embolization procedures causing preterm labor, adverse maternal outcome, or adverse fetal outcome. From the existing literature, the morbidity risk of PAVM embolization appears to be very low, and the mortality risk is essentially nonexistent.

A second topic of frequent concern is radiation risk, but deterministic effects of radiation exposure in fetuses are only seen with high radiation doses [55]. The risks of radiation exposure decrease with gestational age. For example, at 8–15 weeks gestation, decreased intelligence quotient (IQ) is seen at 100 mGy and growth retardation at >250 mGy [55]. However, from 16 weeks gestation through term, decreased IQ is typically observed above 100 mGy and growth retardation is only observed at >1500 mGy [55]. The fetal radiation dose from PAVM embolization is estimated to be less than 1–2 mGy, well below all deterministic thresholds. Cancer risk is thought to increase by 0.01% for every 1 mGy of fetal radiation dose, meaning approximately 0.02% risk of cancer [55]. In other words, PAVM embolization has an estimated 1 in 5000 risk of cancer induction, and no deterministic effects, compared to a greater than 1 in 50 risk of maternal, and possibly fetal, death from untreated PAVM during pregnancy. From the existing evidence, we believe that the benefit of PAVM embolization during pregnancy greatly outweighs the risk. Regarding optimal timing of therapy, a review of 26 case reports of untreated PAVM complications in pregnancy found that 8% of complications occurred in the first trimester, 85% percent in the second or third trimester, and the remainder were unknown [44]. We feel that early in the second trimester may be the ideal time to treat pregnant mothers with PAVM, as this stage of fetal development has the least susceptibility to radiation and is generally a stable period with low risk of preterm labor.

A third area of concern in the context of pregnancy and angiography is the safety of contrast agents. In general, iodinated contrast media are considered safe for pregnant and lactating mothers, with the same risk factors for adverse reactions as the general population [56]. Although transplacental transfer of iodinated contrast has been observed, there is no evidence to suggest teratogenic effects in humans [56]. Nonionic iodinated contrast agents are preferred when contrast is needed in pregnant women, as they do not affect neonatal thyroid function [56].

Finally, it should be noted that PAVMs which were treated prior to pregnancy can have complications during pregnancy. In the aforementioned 2008 trial by Shovlin et al. 23 pregnancies in

16 patients with PAVMs were prospectively followed, and 15 of these patients had been embolized before pregnancy. Two nonfatal PAVM hemorrhages were observed in this group [52]. The previously discussed 2014 survey study reported no deaths and no complications in 17 pregnancies among 8 women treated prior to pregnancy. These numbers are too small to provide definitive risk estimates, but they should raise awareness that previously treated AVMs, especially those treated in the distant past and demonstrating systemic arterial reperfusion, can bleed during pregnancy. Any hemoptysis in a patient with treated pulmonary AVM should immediately raise suspicion for bronchial reperfusion with hemorrhage, and should prompt emergency room visit and definitive management.

In conclusion, evidence demonstrates that the risk of untreated PAVM in pregnancy is high, while the risk of PAVM embolization is vanishingly low. We believe that patients with untreated PAVMs should be treated prior to pregnancy whenever possible. Pregnant patients who have not been screened for PAVM should undergo screening with TTCE or low-dose noncontrast chest CT. If PAVMs are discovered during pregnancy, they should be treated. We have provided a case example of successful PAVM embolization during pregnancy from our institution (Figure 3). Patients who are symptomatic from their PAVMs should be treated immediately, regardless of gestational age. There is insufficient data to determine what PAVM size should be treated during pregnancy in an asymptomatic patient; our institution uses the same 3 mm feeding artery cut-off that we use for pediatric patients with asymptomatic PAVM, while patients with smaller PAVM are monitored closely and treated in the post-partum period. In patients with PAVMs treated during pregnancy, we recommend follow-up evaluation within 6 months postpartum, followed by a repeat screen every 3–5 years or prior to the next pregnancy. Patients with negative PAVM screening before or during pregnancy should continue to have standard repeat screening after pregnancy.

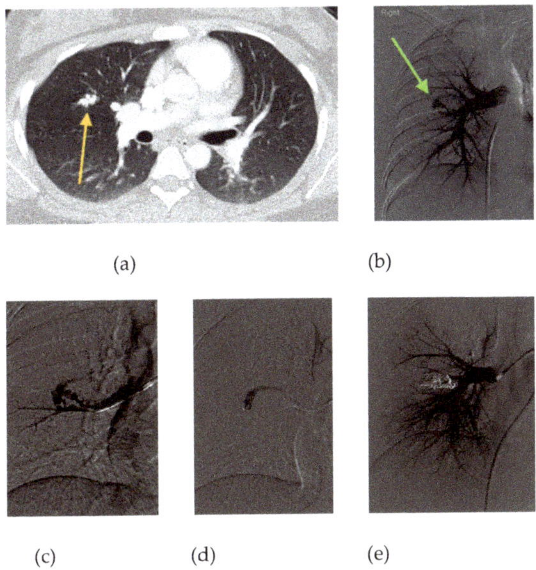

(a)   (b)

(c)   (d)   (e)

Figure 3. 20-year-old female, who is 6 months pregnant presents with mild dyspnea. (**a**) Chest CT performed to rule out pulmonary embolism reveals complex PAVM with 3 mm feeding artery (orange arrow). (**b**) Initial pulmonary angiogram confirms PAVM in the right middle lobe (green arrow). (**c**) Angiogram shows selection of the supplying artery with a catheter. (**d**) Microcatheter placement into PAVM nidus. (**e**) Final angiogram shows complete occlusion of PAVM following embolization with 11 microcoils and 1 microvascular plug. Estimated fetal radiation dose was <5 mGy, scatter only with no direct irradiation. Remainder of pregnancy was uneventful and the patient delivered a healthy baby girl at 39 weeks gestational age.

4.4. Persistent PAVMs

While embolization is the standard of care for PAVM treatment, up to 25% of initially successful cases experience persistence, meaning return of flow to the PAVM in follow-up [34,57,58]. Some providers believe that the presence of embolic material in persistent PAVMs can effectively filter clinically significant paradoxical emboli, rendering them less dangerous, while others theorize that persistent PAVMs may pose a higher risk owing to the potential for in-situ thrombus formation resulting from diminished flow [59,60]. The relative risk compared to native PAVMs is uncertain, but significant complications have been ascribed to persistent PAVMs, and re-treatment should be performed whenever feasible [57]. One commonly-used criterion for persistence is the failure of the draining vein or sac to regress by >70% on follow-up CT [57,61,62]. Persistence usually occurs in one of two patterns, recanalization or reperfusion. In recanalization, there is return of flow through previously placed embolic material supplying the PAVM. This is the most common pattern of persistence, seen in 88–91% of cases [57,63]. In reperfusion, flow reaches the PAVM by means of accessory arteries passing around the embolic material. Persistent PAVMs of either type have been shown to be difficult to treat, with variable success rates after repeat embolization ranging from 40% to 80% [35,57,63,64]. Studies report higher likelihood of retreatment success with recanalization compared to reperfusion [57].

A third, less common pattern of persistence is systemic-to-pulmonary reperfusion, usually arising from bronchial, internal mammary, or subclavian artery collaterals [57]. Although systemic-to-pulmonary reperfusion represents a left-to-left shunt and carries no risk of paradoxical embolization, the systemic pressure and fragile collateral arteries can lead to hemoptysis [35,58,63]. Asymptomatic patients can be counseled and monitored, while symptomatic patients should undergo systemic artery embolization or resection of the involved segment. Caution should be exercised during embolization of systemic-to-pulmonary collaterals, as multifocal strokes have been encountered from the use of particulate embolization [35].

The characteristics and treatment outcomes of persistent PAVMs described in the literature reveal several patterns which can be used to guide interventional management. Most complex PAVMs persist in a reperfusion rather than recanalization pattern, suggesting that at the time of initial embolization, thorough investigation of collateral branches and accessory feeder vessels to complex PAVMs should be performed, to reduce the risk of later reperfusion [65]. The most recent data reaffirms that persistent PAVMs are difficult to treat, but indicates that distal embolization beyond the existing embolic results in more durable occlusion [65]. This is consistent with similar findings from previous reports [57,63]. It is hypothesized that distal embolization may be more successful by allowing placement of embolic material directly into the PAVM sac or nidus, resulting in more durable occlusion regardless of angioarchitecture [65–68]. However, it should be noted that the distal embolization technique is not always technically feasible, since the previously deposited embolic material may prevent distal access [57,63,65]. One study reports a high success rate treating recanalized PAVMs using coils in conjunction with Amplatzer vascular plugs [61]. In either case, dense packing and complete stasis in the targeted AVM should be the desired endpoint [16].

Lastly, a recent study by Haddad et al. described a relationship between smoking and PAVM persistence at follow-up [69]. In 102 HHT patients with 373 treated PAVMs, five-year persistence-free survival rates in nonsmokers, smokers of 1–20 pack-years, and smokers of more than 20 pack-years were 12%, 22%, and 38% respectively [69]. The study demonstrated a dose-response and temporal relationship between smoking and PAVM persistence, likely related to effects on the vascular endothelium. While the total number of smokers in the study was relatively low and further studies are needed to confirm the findings, we recommend advising patients of these possible risks as further reason for smoking cessation.

4.5. Diffuse PAVMs

Diffuse PAVMs are a rare subtype of complex PAVM, with a slight female predilection, in which one or more segments of the lung is diffusely involved by PAVMs [70,71]. Patients with this pattern of involvement can experience severe hypoxemia and are at far higher risk of serious complications including adverse neurologic events compared to those with focal PAVMs [70]. Due to the vast complexity of the malformation angioarchitecture, embolization in these patients is more technically challenging compared to standard embolization in focal or even multifocal PAVM cases.

Pierucci et al. has described the natural history and outcomes of 36 patients who underwent embolization for diffuse PAVMs [71]. Among the 10 patients with unilateral diffuse PAVM, 30% had experienced complications such as brain abscess or hemoptysis. Comparatively, of 26 patients with bilateral diffuse PAVM, 70% had had complications including abscess and stroke, suggesting a higher rate of adverse events with increasing lung involvement. Regarding procedural technique, the authors of study embolized all visible focal PAVMs with diameter >3 mm. In areas of diffuse PAVM, they utilized an approach called peripheral blood flow redistribution, treating only the most severely involved regions, using dense coil packing to perform peripheral-to-central occlusion of the target artery, thereby redistributing pulmonary blood flow to less involved portions of lung [71]. At a mean 8.5 year follow-up, oxygenation had significantly improved in both the unilateral cohort (from 87% to 95%) and bilateral cohort (79% to 85%). All nine deaths which occurred during the study period were in the bilateral cohort, 3 of which were PAVM-related complications (11%).

A second series reviewed 39 patients with diffuse or multifocal PAVM, including a subset of 22 patients with true diffuse PAVM, around 60% of whom had suffered neurologic complications [72]. This study used similar techniques, combining embolization of all large focal PAVMs and peripheral blood flow redistribution in areas of diffuse PAVM involvement. At mean 3.5 year follow-up, 80% of patients endorsed improvement in dyspnea symptoms. 10% of treated patients experienced ischemic or infectious complications due to reperfusion of embolized PAVMs or enlargement of untreated PAVMs.

Given the anatomic complexity and technical challenge of treating diffuse PAVM endovascularly, lung transplantation for diffuse PAVM has been described, typically in settings where PAVMs were not amenable to embolization or surgical resection [73–75]. The Registry of the International Society for Heart and Lung Transplantation reports a median survival around 8 years for lung transplant overall [76]. Most case studies on lung transplant for diffuse PAVM have only reported outcomes at short term follow-up, on the order of 1–3 years. A prospective study by Shovlin et al. reported long term outcomes of a small cohort of 6 patients with diffuse PAVM who were considered for lung transplantation [77]. The cohort was young (≤47 years), hypoxemic with baseline oxygen saturation less than 86%, and had all undergone maximal transcatheter embolization. One patient in the cohort received single lung transplant, but died within 4 weeks of surgery. The remaining 5 non-transplanted patients had a median 21 year survival, ranging from 16–27 years, considerably longer than the overall median survival reported for lung transplant. The marked longevity demonstrated by the non-transplanted cohort compared to the reported median survival with lung transplant is an important factor which patients and providers must consider; the option to pursue lung transplant for diffuse PAVM is a multifactorial decision which should give weight to survival outcomes, symptomatology, and quality of life in a case-by-case basis.

In patients with diffuse PAVMs, we believe that transcatheter embolotherapy should be first-line treatment. Embolization of all focal PAVMs ≥ 3 mm should be performed to reduce risk of stroke and brain abscess. Additionally, peripheral-to-central occlusion targeting areas of diffuse involvement can be considered, to achieve peripheral blood flow redistribution to less involved lung segments. This second approach can achieve modest improvements in dyspnea and hypoxemia in patients who have few lung segments involved. However, in patients with truly diffuse bilateral PAVM affecting all lung segments, transcatheter embolotherapy may not achieve meaningful improvements in hypoxemia, as there are no normal lung segments for redistribution (Figure 4). In these patients, embolization of only focal PAVMs ≥ 3 mm may be preferable, followed by expectant management. In all patients with diffuse PAVM, even after embolotherapy, adverse PAVM-related outcomes still occur with relatively high frequency; treated patients should be advised to seek prompt medical attention for symptoms suggestive of stroke, bleeding or brain abscess.

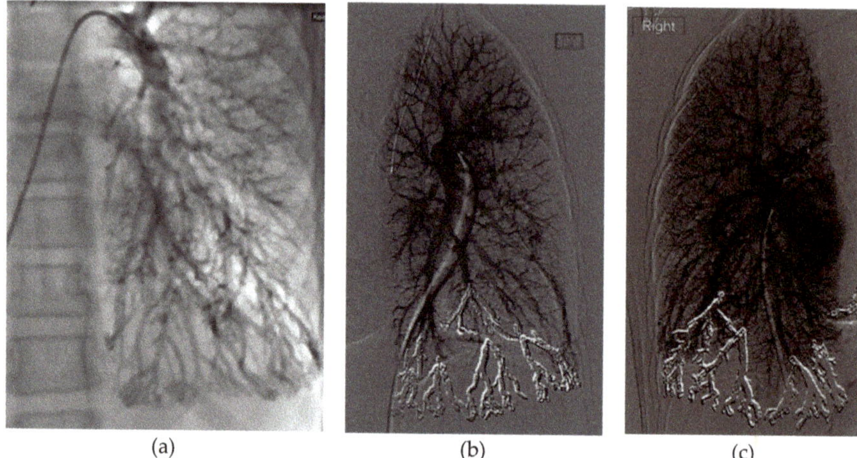

(a)   (b)   (c)

Figure 4. 9-year-old female with genetically confirmed HHT, mild growth and developmental delay, presenting with dyspnea on exertion and chronic hypoxemia (baseline oxygen saturation of 60–80%) requiring supplemental oxygen. CT chest (not shown) showed diffuse PAVMs affecting all segments of both lungs. (**a**) Initial pulmonary angiogram of the left lung demonstrates diffuse PAVMs, most pronounced in the basal left lower lobe and lingula. (**b**) Final pulmonary angiogram of the left lung following peripheral-to-central embolization of the left lower lobe and lingula with implantation of 20 coils. (**c**) Final pulmonary angiogram of the contralateral right lung, performed 1 month after the left-sided embolization. Similar to the left lung, embolization was performed of the dominant PAVMs of the right lower lobe basilar segments. Despite the extensive embolization, the patient had no improvement in baseline oxygen saturation or functional status.

4.6. Pulmonary Hypertension

Pulmonary hypertension (PH), defined as mean pulmonary arterial pressure (mPAP) ≥25 mmHg [78], is relatively common among HHT patients, with reported rates between 1.5–13% [10,79–81]. Screening for PH can be performed at the time of routine TTCE [79]. Many of these HHT patients have secondary PH, often as a result of high-output cardiac failure secondary to hepatic arteriovenous malformations (AVMs) [8,10,80,82]. A smaller proportion of patients, about 1%, have heritable or primary PH; this is usually seen with the *ACVRL1* mutation (HHT type 2) [83–86]. The coexistence of PAVMs and PH poses a clinical dilemma, as there is a paucity of data examining the evolution of PH following PAVM embolization. The presence of PAVMs may have a protective effect in the setting of severe PH, by providing a low resistance "pop-off valve" which could help decrease right ventricular afterload [10]. Treatment of PAVMs in these patients could hypothetically increase the pulmonary vascular resistance, worsening PH. Alternatively, the improved oxygenation and decrease in cardiac output following PAVM embolization could outweigh the potential increase in pulmonary vascular resistance, thereby mitigating an increase in pulmonary pressures [87–89].

There are several conflicting reports in the existing literature. Cases have described fatal increases in pulmonary arterial pressure following PAVM embolization in the setting of severe baseline PH, defined by some as mPAP ≥ 40 mmHg [78,90]. Others report adverse outcomes of not treating, wherein worsening PH led to continued growth and eventual fatal rupture of untreated PAVM [91]. In a series of 43 patients, embolization of PAVMs did not generally lead to a significant increase in pulmonary artery pressure, in the setting of baseline mild-to-moderate PH [88]; notably, patients with baseline severe PH were excluded from the study. Within our own institution, we have experienced one case in which PH worsened following PAVM closure (Figure 5).

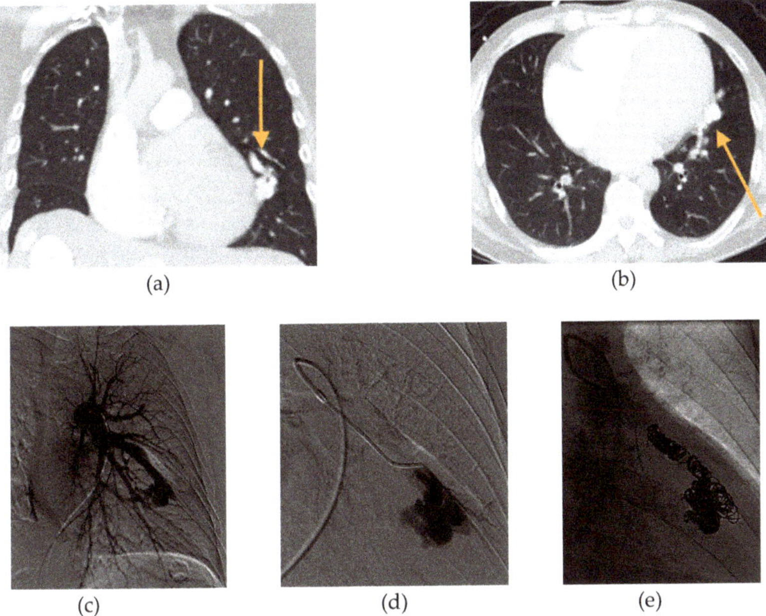

Figure 5. 49-year-old male with history of nonischemic cardiomyopathy, severe mitral and triscuspid regurgitation, PAVM, and PH presented with acute hypoxemic respiratory failure. (**a**) Axial and (**b**) coronal CT angiogram images revealing a large PAVM in the lingula (orange arrows). (**c**) Initial pulmonary angiogram of the left lung demonstrates that a large proportion of pulmonary arterial flow passes through the PAVM, acting as a "pop-off" valve. (**d**) Selective angiogram shows selection of the feeding artery with filling of the complex PAVM sac. Prior to embolization, patient's oxygen saturation on 4 L nasal cannula was 89%. Pre-embolization main pulmonary artery pressure (PAP) was 53/21 mmHg (mPAP 33 mmHg). (**e**) Final pulmonary angiogram shows occlusion of PAVM with combined coiling and deployment of an 8 mm Amplatzer plug in the arterial feeder. Following embolization, PAP increased 72/37 mmHg (mPAP 50 mmHg). Oxygen saturation on 4 L nasal cannula improved to 99%. The patient was weaned to room air and discharged in good condition. Two years later, he was admitted on multiple occasions for acute decompensated heart failure. At 3.5 years after embolization, he died from acute renal failure secondary to cardiorenal syndrome.

Before treating HHT patients with PH, one should seek to determine the etiology, and whether there is significant hepatic vascular involvement. Some reports suggest that occlusion of low-resistance PAVMs in the setting of high cardiac output could lead to worsening PH [58,90]. During PAVM embolization procedures in patients with PH, pre-embolization and post-embolization pressures can be obtained and compared. In cases where the effect of embolization is uncertain, temporary occlusion of the feeding artery can be performed with a balloon occlusion catheter while monitoring the cardiovascular response, to predict the risk of pulmonary hemodynamic changes prior to embolization [58]. There may also be a role for endothelin-receptor antagonists to mitigate worsening of PH following PAVM embolization in at-risk patients, though further study is needed [86].

We recommend that patients with coexisting PH and PAVM be considered for therapy on a case-by-case basis. Existing evidence suggests that embolotherapy of PAVMs is indicated in patients with mild-to-moderate PH. Though the data remains inconclusive, severe baseline PH (mPAP $\geq$ 40 mmHg) and larger PAVM size may result in increased likelihood of worsening PH after closure, and embolization in such cases should be carefully weighed.

5. Embolic Devices

Coils are a well-established option for PAVM embolization, promoting luminal thrombosis through both reduction of vascular flow and intrinsic prothrombotic properties of the coil design. They are relatively easy to use and adapt exceptionally well to the shape of the vascular lumen. Regarding coil size, the diameter of the initial coil should not be smaller than the feeding artery diameter, as this increases the risk of paradoxical embolization [92]. Conversely, coils with too large of a diameter may lead to inadequate packing, or rarely complications such as vessel rupture [92]. For pushable coils, 20–30% coil oversizing relative to feeding vessel diameter is recommended [16,92]. With newer, longer detachable coil designs, coil size can be closely matched to the vessel diameter, as the longer coils provide more vessel wall contact to prevent migration. In general, long and soft coils can provide maximal packing density with low migration risk. However, currently published data do not demonstrate differences in safety, technical feasibility, or reperfusion rates at 1-year follow up based on type of coil utilized [93,94]. Some studies have reported high persistence rates for PAVMs treated with coils, up to 49% at 2-year follow-up [64]. A 2017 study by Stein et al. reported high persistence rates around 21% in small PAVMs ≤ 3 mm treated with coils alone [95]. Recent data suggests that all patients with embolization coils placed after 1984 can safely undergo 1.5 T magnetic resonance imaging (MRI) [96].

Amplatzer vascular plugs (AVPs) are dense expandable nitinol mesh vascular occlusion devices that reduce blood flow in a target vascular lumen to promote thrombosis [92]. It is recommended to oversize vascular plugs by 30–50% relative to the target vessel diameter at the occlusion site [92]. The vascular occlusion induced by AVPs is not instantaneous, and may take several minutes, particularly in high-flow settings [92]. Sometimes, the large amount of flow in the AVM can prevent occlusion or lead to later recanalization of the AVP; the addition of one or more coils proximal to the plug can help prevent this occurrence [61]. Compared to coils, AVPs appear to have a lower risk of device migration [3,97]. Vascular plugs may also have less metallic artifact compared to coils, which can be advantageous when evaluating treated PAVMs on follow-up imaging [3]. On the other hand, vascular plugs require rigid deployment systems with larger caliber sheaths and catheters, which can lead to technical difficulties, particularly limiting the ability to perform distal embolization [3]. One study evaluating efficacy of AVPs in PAVM treatment reported an 84% treatment success rate, defined as >70% sac size regression on follow-up CT [98]. A more recent study of 88 embolized simple PAVMs reported treatment success rates between 83.3–100% using various types of AVPs [99]. Other studies report low recanalization rates ranging between 5–7% [100,101]. One study found AVPs to be very effective in treatment of 24 large PAVMs with feeding artery diameter ≥8 mm, reporting no persistence, migration, or complications in follow-up [102]. Studies show that vascular plugs are less likely to recanalize compared to coils, and that vascular plug alone or in combination with coils might be a better primary option for PAVM embolization when technically feasible [16,103,104]. A 2012 study achieved high rates of technical success treating complex PAVMs by first performing venous sac embolization with detachable coils, followed by occlusion of the large feeding arteries using AVPs [105]. As with coils, AVPs placed after 1984 can be safely imaged using 1.5 T MRI [96].

Another device option for PAVM treatment is the Microvascular Plug (MVP) (Medtronic, Minneapolis, USA), a detachable plug consisting of a nitinol skeleton partially coated with polytetrafluoroethylene (PTFE) (Table 1). Advantages of MVPs in embolization of PAVMs include microcatheter-based deployment, resheathability, immediate occlusion even in the setting of intraprocedural anticoagulation, and less metal artifact compared to coils [106,107]. Furthermore, it is thought that the PTFE coating may help prevent delayed recanalization. Studies have shown the use of MVPs to be safe and technically successful in the treatment of PAVMs [106,108]. A 2015 series describing the use of MVPs to embolize 20 PAVMs in 7 patients demonstrated immediate cessation of flow through the feeding artery in 91% (21/23) of cases, with no device migration [106]. More recent studies have described similar findings using MVPs to treat PAVMs with feeding artery diameters >2 mm; they report technical success rates of 98–100% with immediate stasis of feeding vessels, and low persistence rates of 0–6%, considerably lower than rates seen with traditional coils [108–110]. A summary of the data presented in this section is provided in Table 1.

Table 1. Summary of literature on PAVM embolization outcomes of various embolic devices published in the last 10 years.

Study	Total # PAVMs Embolized	# Persistent PAVMs Embolized	Mean PAVM Feeding Artery Diameter (mm, ±SD) *	Embolic Devices	Technical Success **	Mean Follow-Up, Years	Persistence Rate at Follow-Up	Complications [†]
Letourneau-Guillon 2010 [101]	35	0	5.0 (3.0–10.0)	AVP	97%	1.1	7%	Major: None Minor: Chest pain (4)
Trerotola 2010 [61]	37	0	Not reported (all ≥ 5 mm)	AVP + coils	100%	1.1	0%	Major: None Minor: Chest pain (7)
Tapping 2011 [100]	19	2	Not reported (3.0–12.0 mm)	AVP type I (8) AVP type II (11)	100%	2.3 (Type I) 1.5 (Type II)	5% (Type I) 0% (Type II)	Major: None Minor: Chest pain (1)
Hundt 2012 [105]	11	0	4.4 ± 1.4	AVP + coils	91%	Not specified	12.5%	Major: None Minor: Chest pain (4) Hemoptysis (1)
Kucukay 2014 [102]	24	0	11.5 ± 2.2	AVP	100%	3.0	0%	Major: None Minor: Chest pain (5)
Shimohira 2015 [64]	24	12	3.8 (1.4–5.2)	Coils	100%	2 (median)	49% (primary embolization) 100% (repeat embolization)	Not reported
Conrad 2015 [106]	20	0	3.5 (1.9–5.0)	MVP (19) MVP + coils (1)	100%	0.3	10%	Major: None Minor: Microemboli to toe (1)
Tau 2016 [104]	63	0	Not reported	Coils (37) AVP (21) AVP + coils (5)	100%	7.7	18.9% (coils) 0% (AVP) 0% (AVP + coils)	Major: None Minor: None
Stein 2017 [95]	141	0	2.4 ± 1.1	Coils	100%	1.6	21%	Major: None Minor: Chest pain (21) Groin infection (1) Hematoma (Not specified) Effusion (Not specified) Flushing (Not specified)
Mahdjoub 2018 [108]	39	6	2.3 ± 0.7	MVP	98%	1.0	6%	Not reported

117

Table 1. *Cont.*

Study	Total # PAVMs Embolized	# Persistent PAVMs Embolized	Mean PAVM Feeding Artery Diameter (mm, ±SD) *	Embolic Devices	Technical Success **	Mean Follow-Up, Years	Persistence Rate at Follow-Up	Complications [†]
Andersen 2019 [103]	322	30	Not reported (all ≥ 2 mm)	Coils (213) AVP (89) Detachable balloon (13) AVP + coils (7)	100%	4.8	11.7% (Coils) 4.5% (AVP) 0% (Balloon) 14.3% (AVP + coils)	Not reported
Bailey 2019 [110]	119	0	3.3 ± 1.2	MVP	100%	0.9	0%	Major: None Minor: Chest pain (1)
Ratnani 2019 [109]	157	0	2.3 (1.0–5.9, MVP) 2.8 (1.0–7.6, Other)	MVP (92) Coils (24) AVP (35) AVP + coils (6)	100% (MVP) 100% (Coils) 97% (AVP) 100% (AVP + coils)	1.4 (MVP) 3.3 (Other)	2% (MVPs) 46.7% (Coils) 15% (AVP) 20% (AVP + coils)	Major: None Minor: Asymptomatic Pulmonary Infarcts (1)
Lee 2019 [98]	19	0	3.1 ± 0.7	AVP	100%	1.2	16%	Major: None Minor: Tachycardia (1) Chest pain (1)
Kennedy 2020 [94]	46	0	4.3 ± 1.5 (Nester) 4.4 ± 1.4 (Interlock)	Nester coils (26) Interlock coils (20)	100%	1.2	0% (Nester) 5.6% (Interlock)	Major: None Minor: Chest pain (5) Migraine (3) Minor hemoptysis (1)
Adachi 2020 [99]	88	0	4.1 ± 2.1	Coils (50) AVP (20) AVP + coils (18)	100%	3.2	22% (Coils) 10% (AVP) 39% (AVP + coils)	Major: None Minor: Not reported

* Range is provided when standard deviation was not specified. ** Technical success defined as complete angiographic occlusion of PAVM at end of procedure. [†] Value in parenthesis indicates the number of cases of a given complication. [#] Symbol defined as "Number of".

6. Follow-Up

Follow-up is important for patients with HHT to monitor for reperfusion of treated PAVM and growth of existing or previously microscopic PAVMs. As previously mentioned in the screening protocol discussion, patients with negative initial screening or suspected microscopic PAVMs (grade 1 shunts on initial screening TTCE) should have repeat TTCE screening every 5 years.

In patients with initial negative screening CT, or a CT showing a very small PAVM not indicated for treatment, there is conflicting evidence on what constitutes an appropriate surveillance interval. Previous guidelines recommended 3–5 year CT follow-up. However, a 2019 study by Curnes et al. has reported a lack of growth over time for small untreated PAVMs in adults [111]. For each patient in the study, they compared 2 CT exams with the longest interval between them (mean 8.4 years, range 3.1–14.1 years) to assess growth, analyzing a total of 88 PAVMs in 21 patients. They found that untreated PAVMs grew slowly, if at all, and that any demonstrated growth was minimal and clinically inconsequential [111]. Similar findings were reported by Ryan et al. in a 2017 study investigating the natural history of small and microscopic untreated PAVMs in adults [112]. The findings from Curnes et al. and Ryan et al. challenge the guideline of 3–5 year CT follow-up for small untreated PAVMs, suggesting that this interval could be safety extended up to 5–10 years [111,112].

Another study assessed the diagnostic yield of rescreening adult HHT patients with initial negative screening CT [113]. They found that in 172 HHT patients, there is a low rate of newly detected PAVMs, approximately 0.7%/patient-year, most of which are small and not amenable to treatment. No treatable PAVMs were identified at the 5-year mark, and only 1 treatable PAVM was identified after 6 years, further supporting the notion that a longer screening interval of 5–10 years may be warranted [113]. In addition, a survey of providers at HHT Centers of Excellence worldwide has shown that around one fifth of providers already choose to obtain follow-up imaging in 10 years for patients who demonstrate PAVM stability on 2 CT scans in a 5-year period [21]. This is the regimen we follow at our institution.

The existing guidelines state that for patients who have undergone recent embolization of their PAVMs, follow-up CT should be performed within 6–12 months of treatment, then repeated every 3 years [18]. We feel that this interval can be increased in many patients, thereby reducing radiation exposure and reducing costs. At our institution, we recommend initial follow-up with CT within 6 months of embolization, followed by a repeat CT in 3–5 years based on likelihood of persistence, favoring shorter follow-up times for larger and more complex PAVMs. We use the common definition of successful PAVM treatment, that being more than 70% shrinkage of the draining vein or sac [57,61,62]. Either non-contrast or contrast-enhanced CT can be used.

One study has investigated whether graded TTCE can be used post-embolotherapy as a follow-up tool to predict the need for repeat treatment [114]. In 32 patients with prior PAVM embolization, graded TTCE was performed and the results were compared to their most recent chest CT. Two patients had PAVMs requiring repeat embolotherapy (feeding artery diameter ≥3 mm) due to untreated PAVM growth or treated PAVM persistence. All patients with negative TTCE had no visible PAVMs on CT. Both patients who did require repeat embolotherapy had grade 3 shunts on TTCE. The study suggests that post-embolotherapy TTCE can be used to predict the need for repeat embolotherapy and presence of treatable PAVM on CT. These results are promising and may provide an avenue for post-embolotherapy patients to avoid repeated radiation exposure.

Lastly, some authors suggest the use of time-resolved magnetic resonance imaging (MRI) for follow-up, particularly in patients treated with coils as there may be less induced metallic artifact with this modality [3,16,115,116]. A recent pilot study compared the use of ferumoxytol-enhanced MR angiography (MRA) to CT angiography (CTA) for PAVM detection [81]. The two modalities were comparable in detection rate for PAVMs > 2 mm, and ferumoxytol-enhanced MRA was able to detect several persistent PAVMs which were missed by CTA due to beam-hardening artifact from embolization coils. The data are preliminary, but both time-resolved MR and ferumoxytol-enhanced MR may prove to be feasible alternatives to CT for PAVM imaging, especially in the post-embolization setting, while avoiding the use of radiation and nephrotoxic contrast [117].

7. Conclusions

PAVMs are important to detect and challenging to treat. As the vast majority of PAVMs occur in the setting of HHT, particular attention should be given to screening and surveillance of PAVMs in this patient population. Detailed review of the current literature suggests that contemporary practices often deviate from previously published guidelines on PAVM management.

Grade 1 shunts on initial screening TTCE are not associated with cerebral complications and do not predict presence of treatable PAVMs, and therefore chest CT can be withheld. The same is true of shunts which are seen only with Valsalva maneuver. In these patients, TTCE screening can be repeated every 5 years.

Chest CT should be performed in patients with grade 2 shunts or higher on screening TTCE. CT can be performed sufficiently with or without contrast.

Serious complications including stroke and brain abscess often occur in PAVMs with feeding artery diameter ≥3 mm. These complications can also occur with smaller feeding artery diameters, though it is less common. It is recommended to treat any PAVM with feeding artery 2 mm or greater, and any symptomatic PAVM. Furthermore, embolization of all angiographically visible PAVMs at the time of initial procedure appears to significantly reduce the likelihood of reintervention and risk of ischemic stroke.

Both standard and conservative approaches are acceptable screening methods for PAVM in pediatric patients. Standard screening with TTCE, followed by CT for grade 2 or higher shunts, is safe and effective at detecting PAVM, but risks exposing a larger percentage of pediatric patients to radiation. Conservative screening with physical exam, pulse oximetry, and chest radiograph every 5 years is also safe, effective, and may reduce radiation exposure. However, with the conservative algorithm, there is a slightly higher risk of occasionally missing a treatable AVM which is not detected until adulthood.

PAVMs are expected to grow during childhood, potentially increasing associated risks and symptoms. Pediatric patients should be rescreened for PAVMs at 5-year intervals.

We recommend treatment of symptomatic AVMs and asymptomatic PAVMs ≥ 3 mm in pediatric patients, and monitoring of smaller asymptomatic PAVMs until age 18 to reduce childhood radiation exposure.

For untreated PAVM in pregnancy, both the morbidity and mortality exceed 1%, while the risk of PAVM embolization is much lower. Thus, pregnant patients with untreated PAVMs should be treated, prior to pregnancy if possible. If PAVMs are discovered during pregnancy, they should be treated. Symptomatic patients should be treated as needed, regardless of gestational age. Otherwise, early in the second trimester may be the ideal time to treat pregnant mothers with PAVM, as this stage of fetal development has the least susceptibility to radiation and is generally a stable period with low risk of preterm labor. Unscreened pregnant patients with HHT should undergo screening.

Persistent PAVMs are difficult to treat, with high rates of reperfusion or recanalization following repeat embolization. Embolization distal to the existing embolic results in a better rate of durable occlusion, especially when treating the recanalization pattern of persistence.

Patients with diffuse PAVMs are very high risk for adverse events. In patients with diffuse PAVM affecting only one segment or a few segments, the optimal treatment strategy combines embolization of focal PAVMs ≥ 3 mm and peripheral-to-central occlusion of the most severely affected segment(s) to achieve peripheral blood flow redistribution and improve hypoxemia. In patients with truly diffuse bilateral PAVM affecting all lung segments, attempts at blood flow redistribution are unlikely to achieve meaningful improvements in hypoxemia, though embolization of focal PAVMs ≥ 3 mm should be pursued to reduce risk of paradoxical embolization. Even after treatment, patients with diffuse PAVM remain high risk for complications.

Patients with coexisting PH and PAVM should be considered for therapy on a case-by-case basis. Treatment is typically indicated in patients with mild-to-moderate PH. Severe baseline PH should prompt careful consideration of risks versus benefits, due to the possibility of worsening PH after closure.

For patients with initial negative screening CT or small untreatable PAVM on CT, there is conflicting evidence regarding what constitutes an appropriate screening interval. The most recent studies demonstrate slow growth of small untreated PAVMs, challenging the recommendation to obtain follow-up CTs every 3–5 years, and suggesting that a longer screening interval of 5–10 years may be warranted for these patients.

For follow-up of treated PAVMs, we recommend initial follow-up with CT within 6 months of embolization. This should be followed by a repeat CT every 3–5 years based on perceived likelihood of persistence, favoring the 3 year follow-up interval for more complex PAVMs, and 5 years for all others.

Emerging data suggests that MR may have similar diagnostic accuracy as CT for follow-up of treated PAVMs, in particular for PAVMs with feeding artery diameter >2 mm. Preliminary data also suggests that serial graded TTCE has potential to be used as a post-embolotherapy follow-up tool, with high predictive accuracy for presence of treatable PAVMs on CT. These methods provide avenues to avoid repeated radiation exposure and nephrotoxic contrast.

Author Contributions: Conceptualization, S.M. and J.P.M.; writing—original draft preparation, S.M.; writing—review and editing, S.M. and J.P.M. All authors have read and agreed to the published version of the manuscript.

Funding: This research received no external funding.

Conflicts of Interest: S.M. declares no conflict of interest. J.P.M. has received a speaker honorarium from Penumbra, Inc.

References

1. Shovlin, C.L.; Condliffe, R.; Donaldson, J.W.; Kiely, D.G.; Wort, S.J. British Thoracic Society clinical statement on pulmonary arteriovenous malformations. *Thorax* **2017**, *72*, 1154–1163. [CrossRef] [PubMed]
2. Saboo, S.S.; Chamarthy, M.; Bhalla, S.; Park, H.; Sutphin, P.; Kay, F.; Battaile, J.; Kalva, S.P. Pulmonary arteriovenous malformations: Diagnosis. *Cardiovasc. Diagn. Ther.* **2018**, *8*, 325. [CrossRef]
3. Contegiacomo, A.; del Ciello, A.; Rella, R.; Attempati, N.; Coppolino, D.; Larici, A.R.; Di Stasi, C.; Marano, G.; Manfredi, R. Pulmonary arteriovenous malformations: What the interventional radiologist needs to know. *Radiol. Med.* **2019**, *124*, 973–988. [CrossRef]
4. Tellapuri, S.; Park, H.S.; Kalva, S.P. Pulmonary arteriovenous malformations. *Int. J. Cardiovasc. Imaging* **2019**, *64*, 1–8. [CrossRef] [PubMed]
5. White, J.R.; Pollak, J.S.; Wirth, J.A. Pulmonary arteriovenous malformations: Diagnosis and transcatheter embolotherapy. *J. Vasc. Interv. Radiol.* **1996**, *7*, 787–804. [CrossRef]
6. Wong, H.; Chan, R.; Klatt, R.; Faughnan, M. Idiopathic pulmonary arteriovenous malformations: Clinical and imaging characteristics. *Eur. Respir. J.* **2011**, *38*, 368–375. [CrossRef] [PubMed]
7. Ruiz-Llorente, L.; Gallardo-Vara, E.; Rossi, E.; Smadja, D.M.; Botella, L.M.; Bernabeu, C. Endoglin and alk1 as therapeutic targets for hereditary hemorrhagic telangiectasia. *Expert Opin. Ther. Targets* **2017**, *21*, 933–947. [CrossRef] [PubMed]
8. Dupuis-Girod, S.; Cottin, V.; Shovlin, C.L. The lung in hereditary hemorrhagic telangiectasia. *Respiration* **2017**, *94*, 315–330. [CrossRef]
9. Mu, W.; Cordner, Z.A.; Yuqi Wang, K.; Reed, K.; Robinson, G.; Mitchell, S.; Lin, D. Characterization of pulmonary arteriovenous malformations in ACVRL1 versus ENG mutation carriers in hereditary hemorrhagic telangiectasia. *Genet. Med.* **2018**, *20*, 639–644. [CrossRef] [PubMed]
10. Circo, S.; Gossage, J.R. Pulmonary vascular complications of hereditary haemorrhagic telangiectasia. *Curr. Opin. Pulm. Med.* **2014**, *20*, 421–428. [CrossRef]
11. Salibe-Filho, W.; Piloto, B.M.; Oliveira, E.P.; Castro, M.A.; Affonso, B.B.; Motta-Leal-Filho, J.M.D.; Bortolini, E.; Terra-Filho, M. Pulmonary arteriovenous malformations: Diagnostic and treatment characteristics. *J. Bras. Pneumol.* **2019**, *45*, e20180137. [CrossRef]

12. Alicea-Guevara, R.; Cruz Caliz, M.; Adorno, J.; Fernandez, R.; Rivera, K.; Gonzalez, G.; Hernandez-Castillo, R.A.; Fernandez, R.; Castillo Latorre, C. Life-threatening hemoptysis: Case of Osler–Weber–Rendu Syndrome. *Oxf. Med. Case Rep.* **2018**, *2018*, omx108. [CrossRef] [PubMed]

13. Meier, N.M.; Foster, M.L.; Battaile, J.T. Hereditary hemorrhagic telangiectasia and pulmonary arteriovenous malformations: Clinical aspects. *Cardiovasc. Diagn. Ther.* **2018**, *8*, 316–324. [CrossRef] [PubMed]

14. Kjeldsen, A.D.; Tørring, P.M.; Nissen, H.; Andersen, P.E. Cerebral abscesses among Danish patients with hereditary haemorrhagic telangiectasia. *Acta Neurol. Scand.* **2014**, *129*, 192–197. [CrossRef]

15. Etievant, J.; Si-Mohamed, S.; Vinurel, N.; Dupuis-Girod, S.; Decullier, E.; Gamondes, D.; Khouatra, C.; Cottin, V.; Revel, D. Pulmonary arteriovenous malformations in hereditary haemorrhagic telangiectasia: Correlations between computed tomography findings and cerebral complications. *Eur. Radiol.* **2018**, *28*, 1338–1344. [CrossRef]

16. Muller-Hulsbeck, S.; Marques, L.; Maleux, G.; Osuga, K.; Pelage, J.P.; Wohlgemuth, W.A.; Andersen, P.E. CIRSE standards of practice on diagnosis and treatment of pulmonary arteriovenous malformations. *Cardiovasc. Interv. Radiol.* **2020**, *43*, 353–361. [CrossRef]

17. Gossage, J.R.; Kanj, G. Pulmonary arteriovenous malformations: A state of the art review. *Am. J. Respir. Crit. Care Med.* **1998**, *158*, 643–661. [CrossRef]

18. Faughnan, M.; Palda, V.; Garcia-Tsao, G.; Geisthoff, U.; McDonald, J.; Proctor, D.; Spears, J.; Brown, D.; Buscarini, E.; Chesnutt, M. International guidelines for the diagnosis and management of hereditary haemorrhagic telangiectasia. *J. Med. Genet.* **2011**, *48*, 73–87. [CrossRef] [PubMed]

19. Gossage, J.R. Role of contrast echocardiography in screening for pulmonary arteriovenous malformation in patients with hereditary hemorrhagic telangiectasia. *Chest* **2010**, *138*, 769–771. [CrossRef]

20. Vorselaars, V.M.M.; Velthuis, S.; Huitema, M.P.; Hosman, A.E.; Westermann, C.J.J.; Snijder, R.J.; Mager, J.J.; Post, M.C. Reproducibility of right-to-left shunt quantification using transthoracic contrast echocardiography in hereditary haemorrhagic telangiectasia. *Neth. Heart J.* **2018**, *26*, 203–209. [CrossRef] [PubMed]

21. Chick, J.F.B.; Reddy, S.N.; Pyeritz, R.E.; Trerotola, S.O. A survey of pulmonary arteriovenous malformation screening, management, and follow-up in hereditary hemorrhagic telangiectasia centers of excellence. *Cardiovasc. Interv. Radiol.* **2017**, *40*, 1003–1009. [CrossRef] [PubMed]

22. Velthuis, S.; Buscarini, E.; Van Gent, M.W.; Gazzaniga, P.; Manfredi, G.; Danesino, C.; Schonewille, W.J.; Westermann, C.J.; Snijder, R.J.; Mager, J.J. Grade of pulmonary right-to-left shunt on contrast echocardiography and cerebral complications: A striking association. *Chest* **2013**, *144*, 542–548. [CrossRef] [PubMed]

23. Velthuis, S.; Buscarini, E.; Mager, J.J.; Vorselaars, V.M.; Van Gent, M.W.; Gazzaniga, P.; Manfredi, G.; Danesino, C.; Diederik, A.L.; Vos, J.A. Predicting the size of pulmonary arteriovenous malformations on chest computed tomography: A role for transthoracic contrast echocardiography. *Eur. Respir. J.* **2014**, *44*, 150–159. [CrossRef]

24. Zukotynski, K.; Chan, R.P.; Chow, C.-M.; Cohen, J.H.; Faughnan, M.E. Contrast echocardiography grading predicts pulmonary arteriovenous malformations on CT. *Chest* **2007**, *132*, 18–23. [CrossRef]

25. Parra, J.A.; Bueno, J.; Zarauza, J.; Fariñas-Alvarez, C.; Cuesta, J.M.; Ortiz, P.; Zarrabeitia, R.; del Molino, A.P.; Bustamante, M.; Botella, L.M. Graded contrast echocardiography in pulmonary arteriovenous malformations. *Eur. Respir. J.* **2010**, *35*, 1279–1285. [CrossRef]

26. Van Gent, M.W.F.; Post, M.C.; Snijder, R.J.; Westermann, C.J.J.; Plokker, H.W.M.; Mager, J.J. Real prevalence of pulmonary right-to-left shunt according to genotype in patients with hereditary hemorrhagic telangiectasia: A transthoracic contrast echocardiography study. *Chest* **2010**, *138*, 833–839. [CrossRef]

27. Fernandopulle, N.; Mertens, L.; Klingel, M.; Manson, D.; Ratjen, F. Echocardiography grading for pulmonary arteriovenous malformation screening in children with hereditary hemorrhagic telangiectasia. *J. Pediatr.* **2018**, *195*, 288–291. [CrossRef] [PubMed]

28. Parra, J.A.; Cuesta, J.M.; Zarrabeitia, R.; Fariñas-Álvarez, C.; Bueno, J.; Marqués, S.; Parra-Fariñas, C.; Botella, M.L.; Bernabéu, C.; Zarauza, J. Screening pulmonary arteriovenous malformations in a large cohort of Spanish patients with hemorrhagic hereditary telangiectasia. *Int. J. Cardiol.* **2016**, *218*, 240–245. [CrossRef]

29. Van Gent, M.W.; Post, M.C.; Snijder, R.J.; Swaans, M.J.; Plokker, H.W.; Westermann, C.J.; Overtoom, T.T.; Mager, J.J. Grading of pulmonary right-to-left shunt with transthoracic contrast echocardiography: Does it predict the indication for embolotherapy? *Chest* **2009**, *135*, 1288–1292. [CrossRef]

30. Karam, C.; Sellier, J.; Mansencal, N.; Fagnou, C.; Blivet, S.; Chinet, T.; Lacombe, P.; Dubourg, O. Reliability of contrast echocardiography to rule out pulmonary arteriovenous malformations and avoid CT irradiation in pediatric patients with hereditary hemorrhagic telangiectasia. *Echocardiography* **2015**, *32*, 42–48. [CrossRef] [PubMed]

31. Velthuis, S.; Buscarini, E.; Gossage, J.R.; Snijder, R.J.; Mager, J.J.; Post, M.C. Clinical implications of pulmonary shunting on saline contrast echocardiography. *J. Am. Soc. Echocardiogr.* **2015**, *28*, 255–263. [CrossRef]

32. Moussouttas, M.; Fayad, P.; Rosenblatt, M.; Hashimoto, M.; Pollak, J.; Henderson, K.; Ma, T.-Z.; White, R. Pulmonary arteriovenous malformations: Cerebral ischemia and neurologic manifestations. *Neurology* **2000**, *55*, 959–964. [CrossRef]

33. Todo, K.; Moriwaki, H.; Higashi, M.; Kimura, K.; Naritomi, H. A small pulmonary arteriovenous malformation as a cause of recurrent brain embolism. *Am. J. Neuroradiol.* **2004**, *25*, 428–430. [PubMed]

34. Mager, J.J.; Overtoom, T.T.; Blauw, H.; Lammers, J.W.; Westermann, C.J. Embolotherapy of pulmonary arteriovenous malformations: Long-term results in 112 patients. *J. Vasc. Interv. Radiol.* **2004**, *15*, 451–456. [CrossRef] [PubMed]

35. Pollak, J.S.; Saluja, S.; Thabet, A.; Henderson, K.J.; Denbow, N.; White, R.I., Jr. Clinical and anatomic outcomes after embolotherapy of pulmonary arteriovenous malformations. *J. Vasc. Interv. Radiol.* **2006**, *17*, 35–45. [CrossRef]

36. Shovlin, C.L.; Jackson, J.E.; Bamford, K.B.; Jenkins, I.H.; Benjamin, A.R.; Ramadan, H.; Kulinskaya, E. Primary determinants of ischaemic stroke/brain abscess risks are independent of severity of pulmonary arteriovenous malformations in hereditary haemorrhagic telangiectasia. *Thorax* **2008**, *63*, 259–266. [CrossRef] [PubMed]

37. Al-Saleh, S.; Dragulescu, A.; Manson, D.; Golding, F.; Traubici, J.; Mei-Zahav, M.; MacLusky, I.B.; Faughnan, M.E.; Carpenter, S.; Ratjen, F. Utility of contrast echocardiography for pulmonary arteriovenous malformation screening in pediatric hereditary hemorrhagic telangiectasia. *J. Pediatr.* **2012**, *160*, 1039–1043. [CrossRef] [PubMed]

38. Mowers, K.L.; Sekarski, L.; White, A.J.; Grady, R.M. Pulmonary arteriovenous malformations in children with hereditary hemorrhagic telangiectasia: A longitudinal study. *Pulm. Circ.* **2018**, *8*. [CrossRef]

39. Hosman, A.E.; de Gussem, E.M.; Balemans, W.A.; Gauthier, A.; Westermann, C.J.; Snijder, R.J.; Post, M.C.; Mager, J.J. Screening children for pulmonary arteriovenous malformations: Evaluation of 18 years of experience. *Pediatr. Pulmonol.* **2017**, *52*, 1206–1211. [CrossRef]

40. Ratjen, A.; Au, J.; Bscn, S.C.; John, P.; Ratjen, F. Growth of pulmonary arteriovenous malformations in pediatric patients with hereditary hemorrhagic telangiectasia. *J. Pediatr.* **2019**. [CrossRef]

41. Faughnan, M.E.; Thabet, A.; Mei-Zahav, M.; Colombo, M.; MacLusky, I.; Hyland, R.H.; Pugash, R.A.; Chait, P.; Henderson, K.J.; White, R.I., Jr. Pulmonary arteriovenous malformations in children: Outcomes of transcatheter embolotherapy. *J. Pediatr.* **2004**, *145*, 826–831. [CrossRef] [PubMed]

42. Giordano, P.; Lenato, G.M.; Suppressa, P.; Lastella, P.; Dicuonzo, F.; Chiumarulo, L.; Sangerardi, M.; Piccarreta, P.; Valerio, R.; Scardapane, A. Hereditary hemorrhagic telangiectasia: Arteriovenous malformations in children. *J. Pediatr.* **2013**, *163*, 179–186. [CrossRef]

43. Ibrahim, S.M.; Henderson, K.J.; Rashid, S.; Hussein, S.M.; White, R.I., Jr.; Pollak, J.S. Correlation of oxygen saturation and serious adverse events in pediatric patients with documented or suspected pulmonary arteriovenous malformation. *Angiogenesis* **2015**, *18*, 537–538.

44. Gershon, A.S.; Faughnan, M.E.; Chon, K.S.; Pugash, R.A.; Clark, J.A.; Bohan, M.J.; Henderson, K.J.; Hyland, R.H.; White, R.I., Jr. Transcatheter embolotherapy of maternal pulmonary arteriovenous malformations during pregnancy. *Chest* **2001**, *119*, 470–477. [CrossRef] [PubMed]

45. Moore, B. Pulmonary arterio-venous fistula. *Thorax* **1969**, *24*, 381. [CrossRef] [PubMed]

46. Ference, B.A.; Shannon, T.M.; White, R.I., Jr.; Zawin, M.; Burdge, C.M. Life-threatening pulmonary hemorrhage with pulmonary arteriovenous malformations and hereditary hemorrhagic telangiectasia. *Chest* **1994**, *106*, 1387–1390. [CrossRef]

47. Swinburne, A.; Fedullo, A.; Gangemi, R.; Mijangos, J. Hereditary telangiectasia and multiple pulmonary arteriovenous fistulas: Clinical deterioration during pregnancy. *Chest* **1986**, *89*, 459–460. [CrossRef]

48. Gammon, R.B.; Miksa, A.K.; Keller, F.S. Osler-Weber-Rendu disease and pulmonary arteriovenous fistulas: Deterioration and embolotherapy during pregnancy. *Chest* **1990**, *98*, 1522–1524. [CrossRef]

49. Laroche, C.M.; Wells, F.; Shneerson, J. Massive hemothorax due to enlarging arteriovenous fistula in pregnancy. *Chest* **1992**, *101*, 1452–1454. [CrossRef]

50. Chanatry, B.J. Acute hemothorax owing to pulmonary arteriovenous malformation in pregnancy. *Anesth. Analg.* **1992**, *74*, 613–615. [CrossRef]

51. Dupuis, O.; Delagrange, L.; Dupuis-Girod, S. Hereditary haemorrhagic telangiectasia and pregnancy: A review of the literature. *Orphanet J. Rare Dis.* **2020**, *15*, 5. [CrossRef] [PubMed]

52. Shovlin, C.; Sodhi, V.; McCarthy, A.; Lasjaunias, P.; Jackson, J.; Sheppard, M. Estimates of maternal risks of pregnancy for women with hereditary haemorrhagic telangiectasia (Osler–Weber–Rendu syndrome): Suggested approach for obstetric services. *BJOG Int. J. Obstet. Gynaecol.* **2008**, *115*, 1108–1115. [CrossRef] [PubMed]

53. Shovlin, C.; Winstock, A.; Peters, A.; Jackson, J.; Hughes, J. Medical complications of pregnancy in hereditary haemorrhagic telangiectasia. *Qjm Int. J. Med.* **1995**, *88*, 879–887.

54. De Gussem, E.M.; Lausman, A.Y.; Beder, A.J.; Edwards, C.P.; Blanker, M.H.; Terbrugge, K.G.; Mager, J.J.; Faughnan, M.E. Outcomes of pregnancy in women with hereditary hemorrhagic telangiectasia. *Obstet. Gynecol.* **2014**, *123*, 514–520. [CrossRef] [PubMed]

55. Dauer, L.T.; Thornton, R.H.; Miller, D.L.; Damilakis, J.; Dixon, R.G.; Marx, M.V.; Schueler, B.A.; Vañó, E.; Venkatesan, A.M.; Bartal, G. Radiation management for interventions using fluoroscopic or computed tomographic guidance during pregnancy: A joint guideline of the Society of Interventional Radiology and the Cardiovascular and Interventional Radiological Society of Europe with Endorsement by the Canadian Interventional Radiology Association. *J. Vasc. Interv. Radiol.* **2012**, *23*, 19–32. [CrossRef] [PubMed]

56. Puac, P.; Rodríguez, A.; Vallejo, C.; Zamora, C.A.; Castillo, M. Safety of contrast material use during pregnancy and lactation. *Magn. Reson. Imaging Clin. N. Am.* **2017**, *25*, 787–797. [CrossRef] [PubMed]

57. Woodward, C.S.; Pyeritz, R.E.; Chittams, J.L.; Trerotola, S.O. Treated pulmonary arteriovenous malformations: Patterns of persistence and associated retreatment success. *Radiology* **2013**, *269*, 919–926. [CrossRef] [PubMed]

58. Remy-Jardin, M.; Dumont, P.; Brillet, P.-Y.; Dupuis, P.; Duhamel, A.; Remy, J. Pulmonary arteriovenous malformations treated with embolotherapy: Helical CT evaluation of long-term effectiveness after 2–21-year follow-up. *Radiology* **2006**, *239*, 576–585. [CrossRef] [PubMed]

59. Chan, R.P.; Faughnan, M.; White, R. Pulmonary arteriovenous malformations treated with embolotherapy. *Radiology* **2007**, *244*, 932. [CrossRef]

60. Shimohira, M.; Kawai, T.; Hashizume, T.; Ohta, K.; Suzuki, K.; Shibamoto, Y. Pulmonary arteriovenous malformations: Current technique of transcatheter embolization and subsequent management. *Interv. Radiol.* **2017**, *2*, 116–121. [CrossRef]

61. Trerotola, S.O.; Pyeritz, R.E. Does use of coils in addition to amplatzer vascular plugs prevent recanalization? *Am. J. Roentgenol.* **2010**, *195*, 766–771. [CrossRef] [PubMed]

62. Lee, D.W.; White, R.I.; Egglin, T.K.; Pollak, J.S.; Fayad, P.B.; Wirth, J.A.; Rosenblatt, M.M.; Dickey, K.W.; Burdge, C.M. Embolotherapy of large pulmonary arteriovenous malformations: Long-term results. *Ann. Thorac. Surg.* **1997**, *64*, 930–940. [CrossRef]

63. Milic, A.; Chan, R.P.; Cohen, J.H.; Faughnan, M.E. Reperfusion of pulmonary arteriovenous malformations after embolotherapy. *J. Vasc. Interv. Radiol.* **2005**, *16*, 1675–1683. [CrossRef] [PubMed]

64. Shimohira, M.; Kawai, T.; Hashizume, T.; Ohta, K.; Nakagawa, M.; Ozawa, Y.; Sakurai, K.; Shibamoto, Y. Reperfusion rates of pulmonary arteriovenous malformations after coil embolization: Evaluation with time-resolved MR angiography or pulmonary angiography. *J. Vasc. Interv. Radiol.* **2015**, *26*, 856–864. [CrossRef]

65. Cusumano, L.R.; Duckwiler, G.R.; Roberts, D.G.; McWilliams, J.P. Treatment of recurrent pulmonary arteriovenous malformations: Comparison of proximal versus distal embolization technique. *Cardiovasc. Interv. Radiol.* **2020**, *43*, 29–36. [CrossRef]

66. Hayashi, S.; Baba, Y.; Senokuchi, T.; Nakajo, M. Efficacy of venous sac embolization for pulmonary arteriovenous malformations: Comparison with feeding artery embolization. *J. Vasc. Interv. Radiol.* **2012**, *23*, 1566–1577. [CrossRef] [PubMed]

67. Kajiwara, K.; Urashima, M.; Yamagami, T.; Kakizawa, H.; Matsuura, N.; Matsuura, A.; Ohnari, T.; Ishikawa, M.; Awai, K. Venous sac embolization of pulmonary arteriovenous malformation: Safety and effectiveness at mid-term follow-up. *Acta Radiol.* **2014**, *55*, 1093–1098. [CrossRef]

68. Dinkel, H.P.; Triller, J. Pulmonary arteriovenous malformations: Embolotherapy with superselective coaxial catheter placement and filling of venous sac with Guglielmi detachable coils. *Radiology* **2002**, *223*, 709–714. [CrossRef] [PubMed]

69. Haddad, M.M.; Bendel, E.C.; Harmsen, W.S.; Iyer, V.N.; Misra, S. Smoking significantly impacts persistence rates in embolized pulmonary arteriovenous malformations in patients with hereditary hemorrhagic telangiectasia. *Radiology* **2019**, *292*, 762–770. [CrossRef]

70. Faughnan, M.E.; Lui, Y.W.; Wirth, J.A.; Pugash, R.A.; Redelmeier, D.A.; Hyland, R.H.; White, R.I., Jr. Diffuse pulmonary arteriovenous malformations: Characteristics and prognosis. *Chest* **2000**, *117*, 31–38. [CrossRef]

71. Pierucci, P.; Murphy, J.; Henderson, K.J.; Chyun, D.A.; White, R.I., Jr. New definition and natural history of patients with diffuse pulmonary arteriovenous malformations: Twenty-seven–year experience. *Chest* **2008**, *133*, 653–661. [CrossRef] [PubMed]

72. Lacombe, P.; Lagrange, C.; Beauchet, A.; El Hajjam, M.; Chinet, T.; Pelage, J.-P. Diffuse pulmonary arteriovenous malformations in hereditary hemorrhagic telangiectasia: Long-term results of embolization according to the extent of lung involvement. *Chest* **2009**, *135*, 1031–1037. [CrossRef] [PubMed]

73. Fukushima, H.; Mitsuhashi, T.; Oto, T.; Sano, Y.; Kusano, K.F.; Goto, K.; Okazaki, M.; Date, H.; Kojima, Y.; Yamagishi, H.; et al. Successful lung transplantation in a case with diffuse pulmonary arteriovenous malformations and hereditary hemorrhagic telangiectasia. *Am. J. Transpl.* **2013**, *13*, 3278–3281. [CrossRef] [PubMed]

74. Svetliza, G.; De la Canal, A.; Beveraggi, E.; Giacoia, A.; Ruiz, C.; Caruso, E.; Rodríguez Giménez, J.; Vassallo, B. Lung transplantation in a patient with arteriovenous malformations. *J. Heart Lung Transplant.* **2002**, *21*, 506–508. [CrossRef]

75. Reynaud-Gaubert, M.; Thomas, P.; Gaubert, J.; Pietri, P.; Garbe, L.; Giudicelli, R.; Orehek, J.; Fuentes, P. Pulmonary arteriovenous malformations: Lung transplantation as a therapeutic option. *Eur. Respir. J.* **1999**, *14*, 1425–1428. [CrossRef]

76. Chambers, D.C.; Yusen, R.D.; Cherikh, W.S.; Goldfarb, S.B.; Kucheryavaya, A.Y.; Khusch, K.; Levvey, B.J.; Lund, L.H.; Meiser, B.; Rossano, J.W.; et al. The registry of the international society for heart and lung transplantation: Thirty-fourth adult lung and heart-lung transplantation report—2017; focus theme: Allograft ischemic time. *J. Heart Lung Transplant.* **2017**, *36*, 1047–1059. [CrossRef] [PubMed]

77. Shovlin, C.L.; Buscarini, E.; Hughes, J.M.B.; Allison, D.J.; Jackson, J.E. Long-term outcomes of patients with pulmonary arteriovenous malformations considered for lung transplantation, compared with similarly hypoxaemic cohorts. *BMJ Open Respir. Res.* **2017**, *4*, e000198. [CrossRef]

78. Simonneau, G.; Montani, D.; Celermajer, D.S.; Denton, C.P.; Gatzoulis, M.A.; Krowka, M.; Williams, P.G.; Souza, R. Haemodynamic definitions and updated clinical classification of pulmonary hypertension. *Eur. Respir. J.* **2019**, *53*, 1801913. [CrossRef]

79. Olivieri, C.; Lanzarini, L.; Pagella, F.; Semino, L.; Corno, S.; Valacca, C.; Plauchu, H.; Lesca, G.; Barthelet, M.; Buscarini, E. Echocardiographic screening discloses increased values of pulmonary artery systolic pressure in 9 of 68 unselected patients affected with hereditary hemorrhagic telangiectasia. *Genet. Med.* **2006**, *8*, 183–190. [CrossRef]

80. Revuz, S.; Decullier, E.; Ginon, I.; Lamblin, N.; Hatron, P.Y.; Kaminsky, P.; Carette, M.F.; Lacombe, P.; Simon, A.C.; Rivière, S.; et al. Pulmonary hypertension subtypes associated with hereditary haemorrhagic telangiectasia: Haemodynamic profiles and survival probability. *PLoS ONE* **2017**, *12*, e0184227. [CrossRef]

81. Chizinga, M.; Rudkovskaia, A.A.; Henderson, K.; Pollak, J.; Garcia-Tsao, G.; Young, L.H.; Fares, W.H. Pulmonary hypertension prevalence and prognosis in a cohort of patients with hereditary hemorrhagic telangiectasia undergoing embolization of pulmonary arteriovenous malformations. *Am. J. Respir. Crit. Care Med.* **2017**, *196*, 1353–1356. [CrossRef]

82. De Picciotto, C.; El Hajjam, M.; Karam, C.; Chinet, T.; Bonay, M. Pulmonary gas exchange in hereditary hemorrhagic telangiectasia patients with liver arteriovenous malformations. *Respir. Res.* **2019**, *20*, 137. [CrossRef] [PubMed]

83. Trembath, R.C.; Thomson, J.R.; Machado, R.D.; Morgan, N.V.; Atkinson, C.; Winship, I.; Simonneau, G.; Galie, N.; Loyd, J.E.; Humbert, M. Clinical and molecular genetic features of pulmonary hypertension in patients with hereditary hemorrhagic telangiectasia. *N. Engl. J. Med.* **2001**, *345*, 325–334. [CrossRef]

84. Cottin, V.; Dupuis-Girod, S.; Lesca, G.; Cordier, J.F. Pulmonary vascular manifestations of hereditary hemorrhagic telangiectasia (rendu-osler disease). *Respiration* **2007**, *74*, 361–378. [CrossRef] [PubMed]

85. Sopeña, B.; Pérez-Rodríguez, M.T.; Portela, D.; Rivera, A.; Freire, M.; Martínez-Vázquez, C. High prevalence of pulmonary hypertension in patients with hereditary hemorrhagic telangiectasia. *Eur. J. Intern. Med.* **2013**, *24*, e30–e34. [CrossRef] [PubMed]

86. Yokokawa, T.; Sugimoto, K.; Kimishima, Y.; Misaka, T.; Yoshihisa, A.; Morisaki, H.; Yamada, O.; Nakazato, K.; Ishida, T.; Takeishi, Y. A case of pulmonary hypertension and hereditary hemorrhagic telangiectasia related to an ACVRL1 mutation. *Intern. Med.* **2020**. [CrossRef] [PubMed]

87. Andrivet, P.; Lofaso, F.; Carette, M.; Allegrini, J.; Adnot, S. Haemodynamics and gas exchange before and after coil embolization of pulmonary arteriovenous malformations. *Eur. Respir. J.* **1995**, *8*, 1228–1230. [CrossRef]

88. Shovlin, C.; Tighe, H.; Davies, R.; Gibbs, J.; Jackson, J. Embolisation of pulmonary arteriovenous malformations: No consistent effect on pulmonary artery pressure. *Eur. Respir. J.* **2008**, *32*, 162–169. [CrossRef]

89. Vorselaars, V.M.M.; Velthuis, S.; Mager, J.J.; Snijder, R.J.; Bos, W.J.; Vos, J.A.; van Strijen, M.J.L.; Post, M.C. Direct haemodynamic effects of pulmonary arteriovenous malformation embolisation. *Neth. Heart J.* **2014**, *22*, 328–333. [CrossRef]

90. Haitjerm, T.; Jurrien, M.; Overtoom, T.T.C.; Ernst, J.M.; Westermann, C.J. Unusual complications after embolization of a pulmonary arteriovenous malformation. *Chest* **1996**, *109*, 1401–1404. [CrossRef]

91. Montani, D.; Price, L.; Girerd, B.; Chinet, T.; Lacombe, P.; Simonneau, G.; Humbert, M. Fatal rupture of pulmonary arteriovenous malformation in hereditary haemorrhagic telangiectasis and severe PAH. *Eur. Respir. Rev.* **2009**, *18*, 42–46. [CrossRef] [PubMed]

92. Vaidya, S.; Tozer, K.R.; Chen, J. An overview of embolic agents. *Semin. Interv. Radiol.* **2008**, *25*, 204–215. [CrossRef] [PubMed]

93. Prasad, V.; Chan, R.P.; Faughnan, M.E. Embolotherapy of pulmonary arteriovenous malformations: Efficacy of platinum versus stainless steel coils. *J. Vasc. Interv. Radiol.* **2004**, *15*, 153–160. [CrossRef] [PubMed]

94. Kennedy, S.A.; Faughnan, M.E.; Vozoris, N.T.; Prabhudesai, V. Reperfusion of pulmonary arteriovenous malformations following embolotherapy: A randomized controlled trial of detachable versus pushable coils. *Cardiovasc. Interv. Radiol.* **2020**. [CrossRef]

95. Stein, E.J.; Chittams, J.L.; Miller, M.; Trerotola, S.O. Persistence in coil-embolized pulmonary arteriovenous malformations with feeding artery diameters of 3 mm or less: A retrospective single-center observational study. *J. Vasc. Interv. Radiol.* **2017**, *28*, 442–449. [CrossRef]

96. Alsafi, A.; Jackson, J.E.; Fatania, G.; Patel, M.C.; Glover, A.; Shovlin, C.L. Patients with in-situ metallic coils and Amplatzer vascular plugs used to treat pulmonary arteriovenous malformations since 1984 can safely undergo magnetic resonance imaging. *Br. J. Radiol.* **2019**, *92*, 20180752. [CrossRef]

97. Corvino, F.; Silvestre, M.; Cervo, A.; Giurazza, F.; Corvino, A.; Maglione, F. Endovascular occlusion of pulmonary arteriovenous malformations with the ArtVentive Endoluminal Occlusion System™. *Diagn. Interv. Radiol.* **2016**, *22*, 463. [CrossRef]

98. Lee, S.Y.; Lee, J.; Kim, Y.H.; Kang, U.R.; Cha, J.G.; Lee, J.; Cha, S.I.; Kim, C.H. Efficacy and safety of AMPLATZER vascular plug type IV for embolization of pulmonary arteriovenous malformations. *J. Vasc. Interv. Radiol.* **2019**, *30*, 1082–1088. [CrossRef]

99. Adachi, A.; Ohta, K.; Jahangiri, Y.; Matsui, Y.; Horikawa, M.; Geeratikun, Y.; Chansanti, O.; Yata, S.; Fujii, S.; Steinberger, J.; et al. Treatment of pulmonary arteriovenous malformations: Clinical experience using different embolization strategies. *Jpn. J. Radiol.* **2020**, *38*, 382–386. [CrossRef]

100. Tapping, C.R.; Ettles, D.F.; Robinson, G.J. Long-term follow-up of treatment of pulmonary arteriovenous malformations with AMPLATZER Vascular Plug and AMPLATZER Vascular Plug II devices. *J. Vasc. Interv. Radiol.* **2011**, *22*, 1740–1746. [CrossRef] [PubMed]

101. Letourneau-Guillon, L.; Faughnan, M.E.; Soulez, G.; Giroux, M.F.; Oliva, V.L.; Boucher, L.M.; Dubois, J.; Prabhudesai, V.; Therasse, E. Embolization of pulmonary arteriovenous malformations with amplatzer vascular plugs: Safety and midterm effectiveness. *J. Vasc. Interv. Radiol.* **2010**, *21*, 649–656. [CrossRef] [PubMed]

102. Kucukay, F.; Özdemir, M.; Şenol, E.; Okten, S.; Ereren, M.; Karan, A. Large pulmonary arteriovenous malformations: Long-term results of embolization with AMPLATZER vascular plugs. *J. Vasc. Interv. Radiol.* **2014**, *25*, 1327–1332. [CrossRef]

103. Andersen, P.E.; Duvnjak, S.; Gerke, O.; Kjeldsen, A.D. Long-term single-center retrospective follow-up after embolization of pulmonary arteriovenous malformations treated over a 20-year period: Frequency of re-canalization with various embolization materials and clinical outcome. *Cardiovasc. Interv. Radiol.* **2019**, *42*, 1102–1109. [CrossRef] [PubMed]

104. Tau, N.; Atar, E.; Mei-Zahav, M.; Bachar, G.N.; Dagan, T.; Birk, E.; Bruckheimer, E. Amplatzer vascular plugs versus coils for embolization of pulmonary arteriovenous malformations in patients with hereditary hemorrhagic telangiectasia. *Cardiovasc. Interv. Radiol.* **2016**, *39*, 1110–1114. [CrossRef]

105. Hundt, W.; Kalinowski, M.; Kiessling, A.; Heverhagen, J.T.; Eivazi, B.; Werner, J.; Steinbach, S.; Klose, K.J.; Burbelko, M. Novel approach to complex pulmonary arteriovenous malformation embolization using detachable coils and Amplatzer vascular plugs. *Eur. J. Radiol.* **2012**, *81*, e732–e738. [CrossRef] [PubMed]

106. Conrad, M.B.; Ishaque, B.M.; Surman, A.M.; Kerlan, R.K., Jr.; Hope, M.D.; Dickey, M.A.; Hetts, S.W.; Wilson, M.W. Intraprocedural safety and technical success of the MVP micro vascular plug for embolization of pulmonary arteriovenous malformations. *J. Vasc. Interv. Radiol.* **2015**, *26*, 1735–1739. [CrossRef] [PubMed]

107. Chamarthy, M.R.; Park, H.; Sutphin, P.; Kumar, G.; Lamus, D.; Saboo, S.; Anderson, M.; Kalva, S.P. Pulmonary arteriovenous malformations: Endovascular therapy. *Cardiovasc. Diagn. Ther.* **2018**, *8*, 338–349. [CrossRef]

108. Mahdjoub, E.; Tavolaro, S.; Parrot, A.; Cornelis, F.; Khalil, A.; Carette, M.F. Pulmonary arteriovenous malformations: Safety and efficacy of microvascular plugs. *Am. J. Roentgenol.* **2018**, *211*, 1135–1143. [CrossRef]

109. Ratnani, R.; Sutphin, P.D.; Koshti, V.; Park, H.; Chamarthy, M.; Battaile, J.; Kalva, S.P. Retrospective comparison of pulmonary arteriovenous malformation embolization with the polytetrafluoroethylene-covered nitinol microvascular plug, AMPLATZER plug, and coils in patients with hereditary hemorrhagic telangiectasia. *J. Vasc. Interv. Radiol.* **2019**, *30*, 1089–1097. [CrossRef]

110. Bailey, C.R.; Arun, A.; Towsley, M.; Choi, W.K.; Betz, J.F.; MacKenzie, S.; Areda, M.A.; Duvvuri, M.; Mitchell, S.; Weiss, C.R. MVP micro vascular plug systems for the treatment of pulmonary arteriovenous malformations. *Cardiovasc. Interv. Radiol.* **2019**, *42*, 389–395. [CrossRef]

111. Curnes, N.R.; Desjardins, B.; Pyeritz, R.; Chittams, J.; Sienko, D.; Trerotola, S.O. Lack of growth of small (≤2 mm feeding artery) untreated pulmonary arteriovenous malformations in patients with hereditary hemorrhagic telangiectasia. *J. Vasc. Interv. Radiol.* **2019**, *30*, 1259–1264. [CrossRef]

112. Ryan, D.J.; O'Connor, T.M.; Murphy, M.M.; Brady, A.P. Follow-up interval for small untreated pulmonary arteriovenous malformations in hereditary haemorrhagic telangiectasia. *Clin. Radiol.* **2017**, *72*, 236–241. [CrossRef]

113. Brinjikji, W.; Latino, G.A.; Parvinian, A.; Gauthier, A.; Pantalone, R.; Yamaki, V.; Apala, D.R.; Prabhudesai, V.; Cyr, V.; Chartrand-Lefebvre, C.; et al. Diagnostic yield of rescreening adults for pulmonary arteriovenous malformations. *J. Vasc. Interv. Radiol.* **2019**, *30*, 1982–1987. [CrossRef] [PubMed]

114. DePietro, D.M.; Curnes, N.R.; Chittams, J.; Ferrari, V.A.; Pyeritz, R.E.; Trerotola, S.O. Postembolotherapy pulmonary arteriovenous malformation follow-up: A role for graded transthoracic contrast echocardiography prior to high-resolution chest CT scan. *Chest* **2019**. [CrossRef]

115. Hamamoto, K.; Matsuura, K.; Chiba, E.; Okochi, T.; Tanno, K.; Tanaka, O. Feasibility of non-contrast-enhanced MR angiography using the time-SLIP technique for the assessment of pulmonary arteriovenous malformation. *Magn. Reson. Med. Sci.* **2016**. [CrossRef] [PubMed]

116. Kawai, T.; Shimohira, M.; Kan, H.; Hashizume, T.; Ohta, K.; Kurosaka, K.; Muto, M.; Suzuki, K.; Shibamoto, Y. Feasibility of time-resolved MR angiography for detecting recanalization of pulmonary arteriovenous malformations treated with embolization with platinum coils. *J. Vasc. Interv. Radiol.* **2014**, *25*, 1339–1347. [CrossRef] [PubMed]

117. Khan, S.N.; Finn, J.P.; Bista, B.; Kee, S.; McWilliams, J.P. Comparison of ferumoxytol MR angiography and CT angiography for the detection of pulmonary arterial venous malformations (AVMs) in hereditary hemorrhagic telangiectasia: Initial results. *Radiol. Cardiothorac. Imaging* **2020**, *2*. [CrossRef]

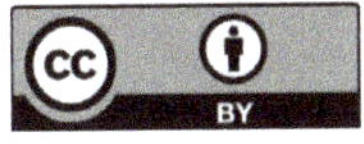

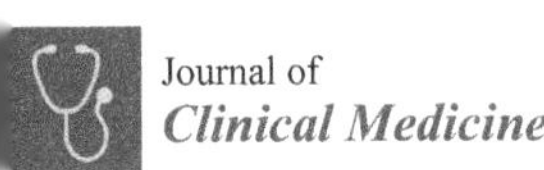

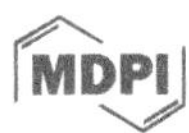

Article

Safety of Catheter Embolization of Pulmonary Arteriovenous Malformations—Evaluation of Possible Cerebrovascular Embolism after Catheter Embolization of Pulmonary Arteriovenous Malformations in Patients with Hereditary Hemorrhagic Telangiectasia/Osler Disease by Pre- and Post-Interventional DWI

Guenther Schneider *, Alexander Massmann, Peter Fries, Felix Frenzel, Arno Buecker and Paul Raczeck

Clinic of Diagnostic and Interventional Radiology, Saarland University Medical Center, Kirrberger Str. 1, 66421 Homburg, Germany; Alexander.Massmann@uks.eu (A.M.); peter.fries@uks.eu (P.F.); felix.frenzel@uks.eu (F.F.); arno.buecker@uks.eu (A.B.); paul.raczeck@uks.eu (P.R.)
* Correspondence: dr.guenther.schneider@uks.eu; Tel.: +49-6481-1624600; Fax: +49-6481-1624606

Citation: Schneider, G.; Massmann, A.; Fries, P.; Frenzel, F.; Buecker, A.; Raczeck, P. Safety of Catheter Embolization of Pulmonary Arteriovenous Malformations— Evaluation of Possible Cerebrovascular Embolism after Catheter Embolization of Pulmonary Arteriovenous Malformations in Patients with Hereditary Hemorrhagic Telangiectasia/Osler Disease by Pre- and Post-Interventional DWI. *J. Clin. Med.* **2021**, *10*, 887. https://doi.org/10.3390/jcm10040887

Academic Editors: Hans-Jurgen Mager, Carmelo Bernabeu and Marco Post

Received: 18 January 2021
Accepted: 17 February 2021
Published: 22 February 2021

Publisher's Note: MDPI stays neutral with regard to jurisdictional claims in published maps and institutional affiliations.

Abstract: Background. This paper aimed to prospectively evaluate the safety of embolization therapy of pulmonary arteriovenous malformations (PAVMs) for the detection of cerebral infarctions by pre- and post-interventional MRI. Method One hundred and five patients (male/female = 44/61; mean age 48.6+/−15.8; range 5–86) with pre-diagnosed PAVMs on contrast-enhanced MRA underwent embolization therapy. The number of PAVMs treated in each patient ranged from 1–8 PAVMs. Depending on the size and localization of the feeding arteries, either Nester-Coils or Amplatzer vascular plugs were used for embolization therapy. cMRI was performed immediately before, and at the 4 h and 3-month post-embolization therapy. Detection of peri-interventional cerebral emboli was performed via T2w and DWI sequences using three different b-values, with calculation of ADC maps. Results Embolization did not show any post-/peri-interventional, newly developed ischemic lesions in the brain. Only one patient who underwent re-embolization and was previously treated with tungsten coils that corroded over time showed newly developed, small, diffuse emboli in the post-interventional DWI sequence. This patient already had several episodes of brain emboli before re-treatment due to the corroded coils, and during treatment, when passing the corroded coils, experienced additional small, clinically inconspicuous brain emboli. However, this complication was anticipated but accepted, since the vessel had to be occluded distally. Conclusion Catheter-based embolization of PAVMs is a safe method for treatment and does not result in clinically inconspicuous cerebral ischemia, which was not demonstrated previously.

Keywords: hereditary hemorrhagic telangiectasia/HHT/osler's disease; cerebral ischemic lesions; catheter based embolization therapy; pulmonary arteriovenous malformations

1. Introduction

Arteriovenous malformations (AVMs) in patients with Hereditary Hemorrhagic Telangiectasia (HHT; Osler's disease) are malformations in which arteries and veins are directly connected, due to the absence of intervening capillaries [1]. The most common clinical symptoms are spontaneous and recurrent epistaxis, as well as Telangiectasias (small AVMs) on the lips, tongue, buccal mucosa, face, chest, and fingers [2]. Larger AVMs become symptomatic in the lungs, liver, gastrointestinal tract, or brain; thus, complications from severe bleeding or shunting with possible consecutive cerebrovascular incidents may occur. Pulmonary arteriovenous malformations (PAVMs) are defined as pathologic communications between pulmonary arteries and pulmonary veins, resulting in a right-to-left

J. Clin. Med. **2021**, *10*, 887. https://doi.org/10.3390/jcm10040887

https://www.mdpi.com/journal/jcm

shunt [3,4]. Larger shunts may result in hypoxemia manifesting with dyspnea, poten-tially increasing the risk of paradoxical cerebral embolization [5], and, in consequence, the risk of increased morbidity and mortality. Of the approaches to treating patients with PAVMs, catheter embolization, either with coils or vascular plugs [6], is considered the treatment of choice because of its high success rate and reduced invasiveness compared to lung surgery [7,8], and because embolization more favorably respects the unaffected lung parenchyma compared to surgical resection [9].

Reperfusion or recanalization of initially successfully treated PAVMs is the most common cause of recurrence after coil embolization [10–12]. However, interventionalists can minimize the risk of reperfusion by using dense "packing" techniques that result in the complete cross-sectional occlusion of feeding arteries [13]. Thus, PAVM embolization with Amplatzer vascular plugs (AVP) has been shown to achieve relatively high mid-term success rates in terms of recurrence or recanalization, even in bilateral treatment [14–17]. In general, a low reperfusion rate is noted in the long-term due to late re-opening [6,18].

The incidence of stroke in patients with HHT ranges between 9 and 18% [19,20]. Although the occurrence of clinically conspicuous stroke seems to be lower in patients with PAVMs treated with embolization therapy than in patients with untreated, persistent PAVMs [19–22], little is yet known about the rate of clinically inconspicuous ischemic brain lesions associated with PAVMs. In contrast, procedure-associated, clinically inconspicu-ous ischemic brain lesions are common in up to 40% of patients undergoing supra-aortal endovascular procedures or neurovascular interventions, such as carotid stenting or en-darterectomy [23,24].

To our knowledge, no data are yet available on the incidence of peri-interventional cerebral ischemia occurring during catheter-based embolization of PAVMs. Therefore, the aim of our investigational study was to prospectively evaluate the incidence of peri-interventional cerebrovascular incidents in patients with HHT referred for catheter-based embolization of PAVMs.

2. Materials and Methods

2.1. Patients

This single-center, prospective study observational was approved by the institutional review board. Written informed consent for both catheter-based embolization and the use of imaging data was obtained from all patients or legal guardians.

All patients included in the study suffered from HHT, confirmed either by genetic testing or, in most cases, based on Curaçao criteria [1,25]. Independently of clinical presen-tation and symptoms, each included patient had at least one PAVM with a feeding artery diameter of at least 2 mm diagnosed by contrast-enhanced MR angiography (CE-MRA), and in a few cases, CT imaging.

Patients were ineligible for inclusion if they had a severe allergy to iodine contrast agents, significantly impaired renal function (GFR < 15 mL/min), and/or severely im-paired blood coagulation (INR > 2) or platelet count (<50.000/dL). Likewise, patients were ineligible for inclusion if they were contraindicated for MRI (e.g., for implanted cardiac pacemakers).

2.2. Embolization Technique

Access through the right common femoral vein was obtained after local anesthesia of the groin region. A 7F sheath was inserted and the common pulmonary artery was probed with the help of a 5F pigtail catheter and a bentson guidewire. Diagnostic pulmonary angiograms were performed to locate and visualize the PAVMs. Afterwards, using a Rosen guidewire, a Cook White Lumax guiding catheter (Cook Medical) or a coaxial system consisting of a Neuron 6F Long Sheath and a Neuron 6F Select Catheter (Penumbra) was inserted, and selective catheterization of the segmental and subsegmental pulmonary artery feeding the PAVM was performed, using the coaxial system. Guidewires which might perforate the aneurysm sac were avoided. The number and diameters of the feeding arteries of the evaluated PAVMs were identified after contrast medium injection. The PAVMs were classified as simple or complex based on the number of feeding arteries, as described elsewhere [26,27].

Depending on the size of the main feeding artery and the anatomical situation, either Nester-Coils (Cook, USA) or Amplatzer vascular plugs II/IV (St. Jude Medical) were used for embolization. These were introduced through a guiding catheter of appropriate size under a water seal. The diameter of the device was chosen to be approximately 30% larger than the size of the main feeding artery. The plug or coil was then placed as distally as possible in the feeding artery with sparing of the PAVM itself.

The choice of embolization device was made according to the length of the available landing zone, which is the distance between the PAVM and the first proximal pulmonary subsegmental artery. In the case of amplatzer vascular plugs, the position of the device was checked by Digital Subtraction Angiography (DSA) immediately after device placement. If the position of the device was deemed adequate and satisfactory, the device was released; otherwise, the device was retrieved and repositioned as necessary.

Post-embolization angiography was performed after satisfactory device placement to confirm the total occlusion of the PAVM.

Immediately before the procedure, each patient received IV injection of 2500 IE Heparin.

The number of PAVMs treated in each patient ranged from one to eight, either treated in one intervention or across multiple interventions, depending on the duration and complexity of the procedure as well as the patient's general condition of compliance during angiography.

2.3. Pre- and Post-Interventional Pulmonary MRI

Pulmonary CE-MRA to evaluate PAVMs before and after intervention was performed on a 1.5 Tesla (T) magnet (Magnetom Aera, Siemens Medical Systems, Erlangen, Germany) with a 16-channel phased-array coil. The imaging protocol consisted of dynamic, time-resolved, contrast-enhanced MRA, and high-resolution, pulmonary arterial- and early venous-phase, contrast-enhanced MRA sequences.

Time-resolved MRA was performed after injection of a small contrast bolus (0.025 mmol/kg of gadobenate dimeglumine [MultiHance™, Bracco] or 0.05 mmol/kg of gadoteridol [ProHance™, Bracco]). The sequence parameters were as follows: repetition time/echo time (TR/TE) = 2.7/1.0 ms, average field of view = 40 × 29 cm, slice thickness = 1.5 mm, 140–160 slices, BW = ±113 kHz. The temporal resolution of the sequence was 3 sec/dataset with a total of 72 slices. k-space sampling was performed via key-hole imaging (TWIST). The true spatial resolution was $1.2 \times 1.2 \times 1.5$ mm^3, which was interpolated to $0.7 \times 0.7 \times 1.0$ mm^3 by zero-filling.

High-resolution, contrast-enhanced Angio 3D MRA was then performed using the timings established in the time-resolved study. Initially, breath-hold, non-contrast enhanced, T1-weighted, spoiled gradient recalled echo (FLASH 3D) images were acquired. The sequence parameters were as follows: TR/TE = 2.81/1.07 ms, average field of view = 40 × 29 cm, slice thickness = 1.3 mm, 140–160 slices, BW 540 kHz. The temporal resolution of the sequence was 2.2 s/dataset with a total number of up to 160 slices. The true spatial resolution was $1.3 \times 1.3 \times 1.5$ mm^3, which was interpolated to $1.1 \times 1.1 \times 1.3$ mm^3 by zero-filling. Thereafter, the identical FLASH 3D sequence was repeated after injection of 0.075 mmol/kg of gadobenate dimeglumine or 0.15 mmol/kg of gadoteridol at a flow rate of 2 mL/s at end-inspiration, followed by a flush of 30 mL normal saline [28]. The scan time varied depending on patient size and the number of slices required. Likewise, the acquisition time varied with the size of the patient and the number of phase-encoded steps needed to maintain resolution. Iterative reconstruction was applied to provide an effective acceleration factor of approximately 4.0, which also varied slightly depending on the number of slices.

The first acquisition was the arterial phase of the pulmonary circulation, and possible shunts between the bronchial arteries and pulmonary veins were also visualized during this phase. Subsequently, a second full acquisition was performed in which normal pulmonary veins were visible. For all acquisitions, patients were instructed to hold their breath at end-inspiration. The total acquisition time for the entire MRA protocol ranged between 5 and 6 min. All examinations were performed as part of the daily clinical routine. Follow-up of all interventional procedures by means of CE-MRA was performed routinely, first at 3 months post-intervention and then at yearly intervals.

2.4. Cerebral MRI

Cerebral MRI was performed immediately before the embolization, as well as at the 4 h and 3-month post-embolization therapy. For detection of peri-interventional cerebral ischemic lesions, T2w imaging (T2-Turbo Spin Echo [TSE], slice thickness 3 mm, TR = 5000 ms, TE = 92 ms, BW 191 kHz) and Diffusion Weighted Imaging (DWI; echo planar imaging sequence, slice thickness 5 mm, TR = 6300 ms, TE= 89 ms, BW: 1132 kHz) using three different b-values (b = 0, 400, 800) with calculation of ADC maps were performed. Any new lesion occurring between the pre- and post-interventional cerebral MRI scans on either sequence was considered a new cerebrovascular incident associated with the intervention. Additional pre- and post-contrast T1-weighted TSE, FLAIR, and susceptibility weighted sequences were acquired as part of the initial screening to rule out cerebral AVMs, including micro-AVMs.

2.5. Statistical Analysis

The characteristics of all participants were transcribed into software (Excel, version2011; Microsoft, Redmond, Wash) for subsequent analysis. Central tendency was measured by the mean, while range and standard deviation were used to measure the dispersion of data.

3. Results

Between 2008 and 2019, a total of 105 patients (male/female = 44/61; mean age 48.6 +/− 15.8 (range 5–86)) met the inclusion criteria and were included in the study. Overall, 289 PAVMs were embolized across these 105 patients. This total included 47 (16.3%) re-perfused PAVMs in 35 (33.3%) patients. A total of 871 embolization coils and 119 vascular plugs were used. No technical difficulties occurred during placement or deployment of the embolization device.

No cerebrovascular incidents directly ascribable to the embolization procedure occurred. Small, diffuse, but clinically inconspicuous acute cerebral lesions were detected in one patient (1/105; 0.95%) on DWI-MRI at 4 h after the interventional procedure, but this patient had previously undergone embolization of a vessel with tungsten coils that had corroded over time. Since re-embolization into the previously placed tungsten coils was considered necessary and unavoidable, the possibility of new cerebral emboli resulting from small particles of corroded tungsten coil released during the re-embolization was anticipated prior to the treatment. The re-embolization of this patient was successful, and no further brain lesion and no clinical symptoms of stroke were encountered over a follow-up period of 8 years.

No other patient, whether undergoing primary embolization or re-embolization, showed any signs or symptoms of cerebrovascular incidents, and no newly developed clinically inconspicuous ischemic brain lesions were observed on MRI.

Clinical examples of diagnosis and treatment are depicted in Figures 1–4.

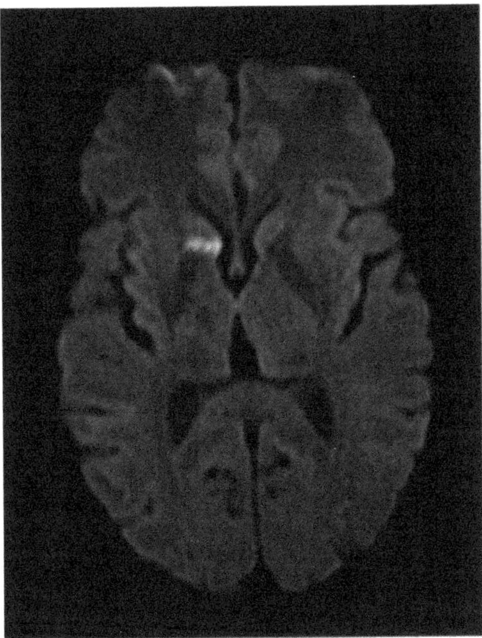

Figure 1. Cerebral DWI (b = 800) demonstrating subacute cerebral ischemia, in this case prior to embolization of multiple PAVMs. The newly developed lesion arose between screening for PAVM and the day of interventional therapy, but the patient did not exhibit any clinical signs or symptoms. This example highlights the importance of DWI for the detection of pre-existing cerebral ischemia, as well as peri-interventional cerebral insult.

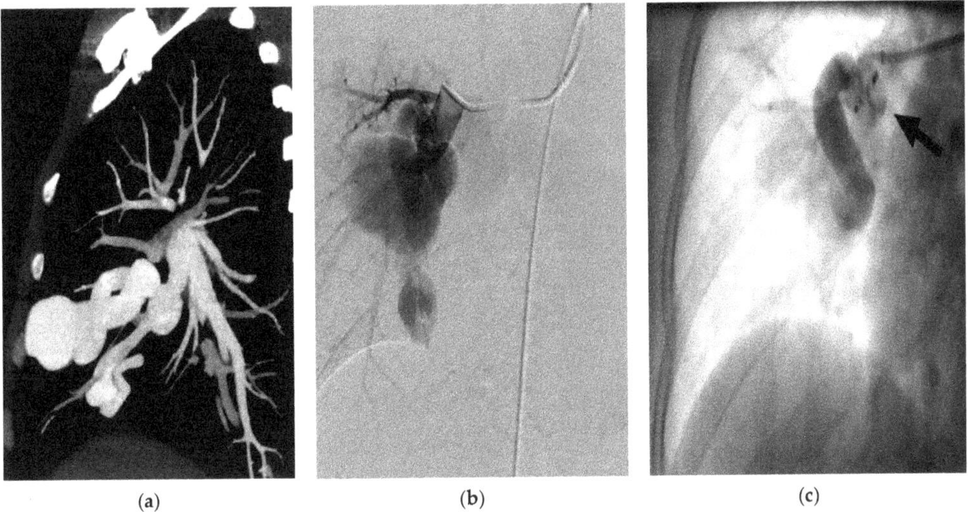

(**a**)   (**b**)   (**c**)

Figure 2. (**a–c**) CT of a patient, demonstrating a giant complex PAVM of the right lung (**a**). The PAVM is depicted after selective catheterization of the feeding artery on DSA after manual contrast medium injection (**b**). DSA of the PAVM directly after positioning of an amplatzer vascular plug II (arrow) with already reduced flow in the PAVM (**c**).

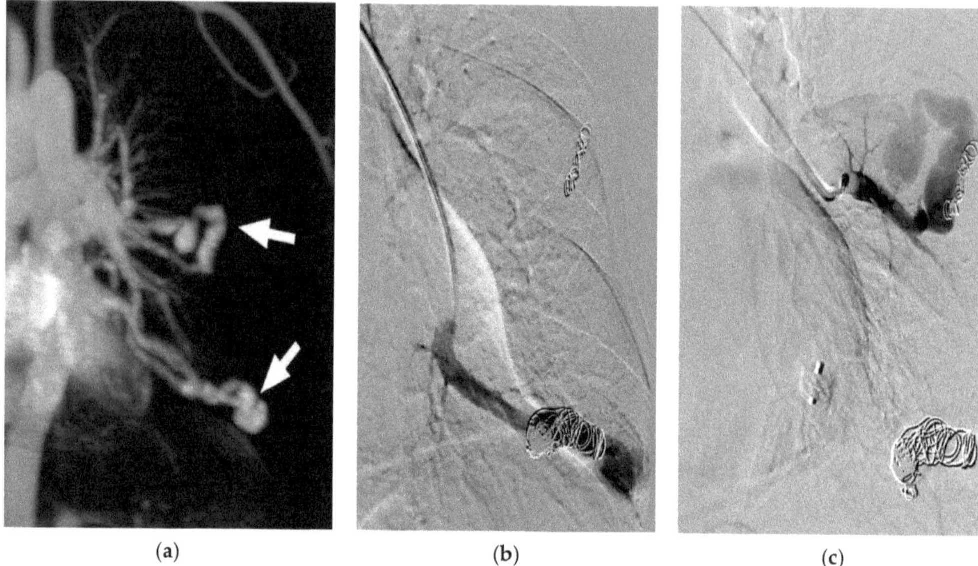

Figure 3. (**a–c**) Re-perfused PAVM after previous treatment elsewhere. Contrast-enhanced MRA (**a**) shows two large, re-perfused PAVMs (arrows) with early enhancement of the draining vein. In (**b**) the DSA of one re-perfused PAVM is shown, depicting insufficient dense packing of coils resulting in reperfusion of the vessel. No guide wire should be used, since small thrombi from the coils might be mobilized and lead to systemic emboli. In (**c**) the second re-perfused PAVM is demonstrated, showing only small coils at the wall of the vessel. Embolization was performed proximal to the treated vessel segment to avoid possible migration of the coils.

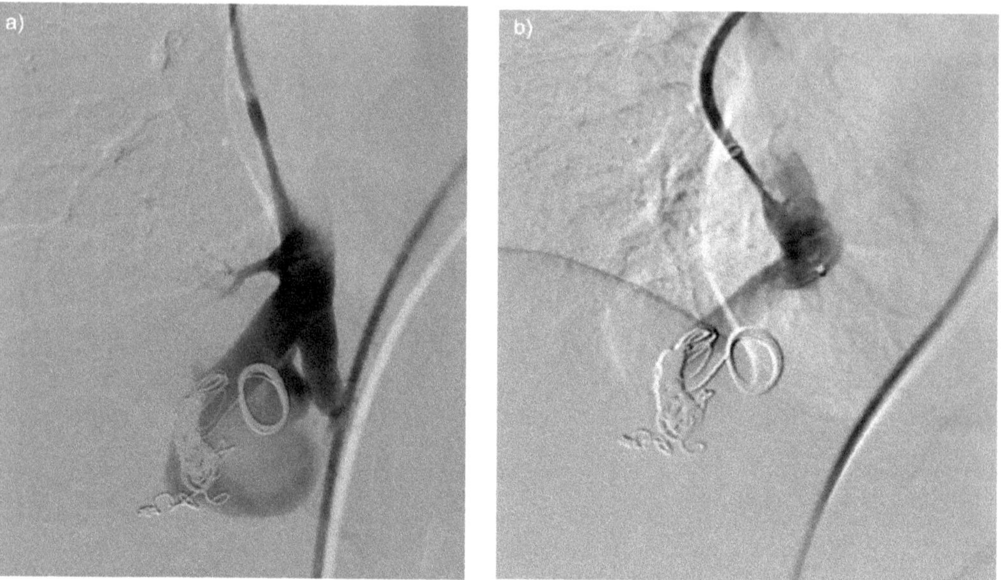

Figure 4. *Cont.*

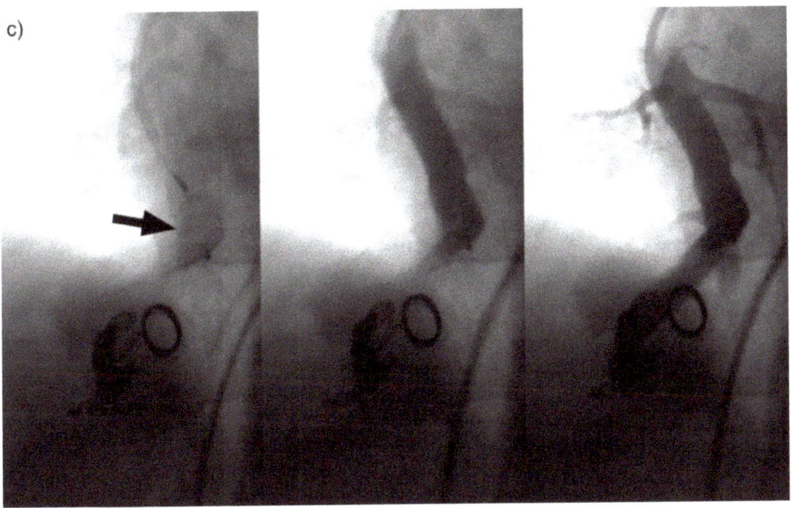

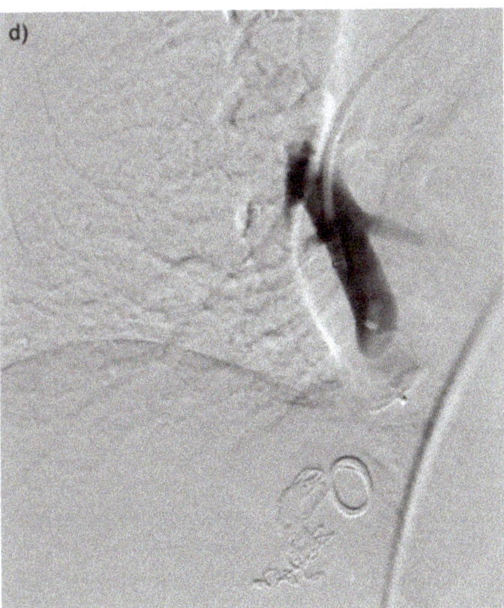

Figure 4. (**a–d**) A giant re-perfused PAVM in the lower right lobe. In this case, pre-interventional DSA (**a**) shows two large feeding vessels originating from a common trunk, resulting in embolization being performed at the level of the bifurcation. With DSA performed just after implantation, (**b**) shows the amplatzer plug II still connected to the wire. Optimal positioning is depicted. The dynamic series in (**c**) shows the vascular plug (arrow) still penetrable to contrast medium, however, flow is already reduced. At 5 min post-implantation of the vascular plug (**d**), the feeding artery of the re-perfused PAVM is completely occluded.

4. Discussion

In general, all vascular interventions involving the thoracic or the supra-aortal regions bear the risk of clinically (in)conspicuous cerebral ischemic lesions, as reported for transcatheter aortic valve implantation or in carotid angioplasty [29,30]. Thus, all patients undergoing thoracic or supra-aortal interventions are prone to dementia and cognitive dysfunction [31,32]. Our prospective study on the occurrence of procedure-associated brain lesions following catheter-based embolization of PAVMs in patients with HHT suggests that this procedure carries a very low risk of cerebrovascular incidents in this patient population. Although our study can only be considered preliminarily, only one individual exhibited newly formed, clinically inconspicuous, small and diffuse cerebral emboli at 4 h after the interventional procedure, and this patient was unique amongst the patients in our cohort due to the presence of corroded tungsten coils from previous interventions. Embolization of the vessel had to be performed proximally and distally to the corroded coils and thus, when forwarding the catheter through the corroded coils, the risk of additional small displaced fragments was unavoidable.

To our knowledge, this is the first study to report on the incidence of peri-procedural cerebrovascular incidents following catheter-based embolization of PAVMs. Although the incidence of ischemic stroke ranges between 9 and 18% in patients with HHT and patent PAVMs [19,20,33–35], our findings suggest that embolization therapy does not significantly impact the rate of further cerebrovascular incidents. Indeed, the one event noted in our series can be ascribed to the embolization material used previously (tungsten coils) rather than to the embolization procedure itself. Given the relatively high number of participants and the high number of complex PAVMs warranting re-embolization therapy due to reperfusion, our results confirm that embolization therapy is safe and highly effective for the treatment of PAVMs in patients with HHT [36–38].

Available data regarding the occurrence of peri-interventional cerebrovascular incidents measured with DWI sequences in cMRI suggest that new ischemic brain lesions occur in up to 34% of patients treated for carotid stenting [23]. However, neurovascular interventions are more prone to acute cerebral embolism. Moreover, studies investigating the implementation of protection devices during carotid stenting have not shown statistically significant reductions in the incidence of acute peri-interventional embolism [30,39,40].

There were some limitations to this study. First, as in all interventional studies, evaluation of peri-procedural complications requires expertise and experience. This was a single-center study with procedures performed and assessed by only a few, very experienced interventional radiologists. It is possible that a greater number of cerebrovascular incidents might have occurred in this same patient cohort, had the interventions been performed by less experienced physicians. However, it should be noted that PAVMs are a complex pathology that warrant a certain degree of interventional experience by the treating physician, and that intervention would usually be undertaken at dedicated institutions by experienced personnel. Second, we only evaluated safety in terms of cerebrovascular incidents. Further studies are needed to evaluate the incidence of other potential complications, such as chest pain, hemoptysis, and hemothorax. Moreover, cMRI readings could not be blinded, since examiners were instructed to carefully look for new, small ischemic lesions in the brain, therefore being aware of the embolization therapy and patient's disease.

In conclusion, to our knowledge, this is the first study to investigate the safety of catheter embolization of PAVMs in patients with HHT in terms of cerebrovascular incidents. Although further multi-center studies in larger patient populations are required to confirm our preliminary results, our observational study reveals a very low rate of clinically inconspicuous cerebral ischemia in patients with HHT undergoing interventional treatment for PAVMs.

Author Contributions: All referenced authors approved to the submitted version of this manuscript and all authors agree to be personally responsible for each respective contribution and ensure the accuracy and integrity of the submitted work. All authors confirm the submitted article is appropriately investigated, resolved and documented. Conceptualization: G.S., P.R.; Methodology: P.R., G.S.; Software: P.R.; Validation: P.R., G.S.; Formal Analysis: A.B., G.S., P.R., F.F., A.M., P.F.; Investigation: G.S., P.R.; Resources: G.S., A.B.; Data Curation: P.R., A.M., F.F., P.F.; Writing—Original Draft Preparation: P.R., G.S.; Writing—Review & Editing: G.S., A.B., F.F., A.M., P.F.; Visualization: P.R., G.S., P.F., A.M., F.F.; Supervision: G.S.; Project Administration: G.S.; Funding Acquisition: not applicable. All authors have read and agreed to the published version of the manuscript.

Funding: This research did not receive any specific funding.

Institutional Review Board Statement: Institutional Review Board approval of the corresponding ethics committee was obtained.

Informed Consent Statement: Informed consent was obtained from all subjects involved in the study.

Data Availability Statement: The data presented in this study are available on request from the corresponding author. The data are not publicly available due to privacy and ethical reasons.

Conflicts of Interest: The authors declare no conflict of interest. There are no sponsors to declare in the choice of this research project, neither in the design of the study, the collection, analyses or interpretation of data, nor in the writing of the manuscript, nor in the decision to publish the results.

Abbreviations

HHT	Hereditary Hemorrhagic Telangiectasia
(P)AVM	(Pulmonary) Arteriovenous Malformation
AVP	Amplatzer Vascular Plug
cMRI	cerebral Magnetic Resonance Imaging
CE-MRA	Contrast Enhanced Magnetic Resonance Angiography
DWI	Diffusion Weighted Imaging
ADC	Apparent Diffusion Coefficient
MR(I)	Magnetic Resonance (Imaging)
GFR	Glomerular Filtration Rate
INR	International Normalized Ratio
DSA	Digital Subtraction Angiography
BW	Body Weight
TSE	Turbo Spin Echo

References

1. McDonald, J.; Pyeritz, R.E. Hereditary Hemorrhagic Telangiectasia. In *Gene Reviews*; University of Washington: Seattle, WA, USA, 1993.
2. McDonald, J.; Bayrak-Toydemir, P.; E Pyeritz, R. Hereditary hemorrhagic telangiectasia: An overview of diagnosis, management, and pathogenesis. *Genet. Med.* **2011**, *13*, 607–616. [CrossRef]
3. Schneider, G.; Uder, M.; Koehler, M.; Kirchin, M.A.; Massmann, A.; Buecker, A.; Geisthoff, U. MR angiography for detection of pulmonary arteriovenous malformations in patients with hereditary hemorrhagic telangiectasia. *Am. J. Roentgenol.* **2008**, *190*, 892–901. [CrossRef]
4. Mager, J.J.; Overtoom, T.T.; Blauw, H.; Lammers, J.W.; Westermann, C.J. Embolotherapy of pulmonary arteriovenous malformations: Long-term results in 112 patients. *J. Vasc. Interv. Radiol.* **2004**, *15*, 451–456. [CrossRef]
5. Abdel Aal, A.K.; Hamed, M.F.; Biosca, R.F.; Saddekni, S.; Raghuram, K. Occlusion time for Amplatzer vascular plug in the management of pulmonary arteriovenous malformations. *Am. J. Roentgenol.* **2009**, *192*, 793–799.
6. Letourneau-Guillon, L.; Faughnan, M.E.; Soulez, G.; Giroux, M.-F.; Oliva, V.L.; Boucher, L.-M.; Dubois, J.; Prabhudesai, V.; Therasse, E. Embolization of pulmonary arteriovenous malformations with amplatzer vascular plugs: Safety and midterm effectiveness. *J. Vasc. Interv. Radiol.* **2010**, *21*, 649–656. [CrossRef]
7. Porstmann, W. *Therapeutic Embolization of Arteriovenous Pulmonary Fistula by Catheter Technique*; Springer: Berlin/Heidelberg, Germany, 1977.
8. Apostolopoulou, S.C.; Kelekis, N.L.; Papagiannis, J.; Hausdorf, G.; Rammos, S. Transcatheter occlusion of a large pulmonary arteriovenous malformation with use of a Cardioseal device. *J. Vasc. Interv. Radiol.* **2001**, *12*, 767–769. [CrossRef]
9. Govani, F.S.; Shovlin, C.L. Hereditary haemorrhagic telangiectasia: A clinical and scientific review. *Eur. J. Hum. Genet.* **2009**, *17*, 860–871. [CrossRef] [PubMed]
10. Woodward, C.S.; Pyeritz, R.E.; Chittams, J.L.; Trerotola, S.O. Treated pulmonary arteriovenous malformations: Patterns of persistence and associated retreatment success. *Radiology* **2013**, *269*, 919–926. [CrossRef] [PubMed]
11. Sagara, K.; Miyazono, N.; Inoue, H.; Ueno, K.; Nishida, H.; Nakajo, M. Recanalization after coil embolotherapy of pulmonary arteriovenous malformations: Study of long-term outcome and mechanism for recanalization. *Am. J. Roentgenol.* **1998**, *170*, 727–730. [CrossRef]
12. Milic, A.; Chan, R.P.; Cohen, J.H.; E Faughnan, M. Reperfusion of Pulmonary Arteriovenous Malformations after Embolotherapy. *J. Vasc. Interv. Radiol.* **2005**, *16*, 1675–1683. [CrossRef] [PubMed]
13. White, R.I. Pulmonary Arteriovenous Malformations: How Do I Embolize? *Tech. Vasc. Interv. Radiol.* **2007**, *10*, 283–290. [CrossRef]

14. Hart, J.L.; Aldin, Z.; Braude, P.; Shovlin, C.L.; Jackson, J. Embolization of pulmonary arteriovenous malformations using the Amplatzer vascular plug: Successful treatment of 69 consecutive patients. *Eur. Radiol.* **2010**, *20*, 2663–2670. [CrossRef] [PubMed]

15. Beck, A.; Dagan, T.; Matitiau, A.; Bruckheimer, E. Transcatheter closure of pulmonary arteriovenous malformations with amplatzer devices. *Catheter. Cardiovasc. Interv.* **2006**, *67*, 932–937. [CrossRef] [PubMed]

16. Rossi, M.; Rebonato, A.; Greco, L.; Stefanini, G.; Citone, M.; Speranza, A.; David, V. A new device for vascular embolization Report on case of two pulmonary arteriovenous fistulas embolization using the amplatzer vascular plug. *Cardiovasc. Interv. Radiol.* **2006**, *29*, 902–906. [CrossRef] [PubMed]

17. Cil, B.; Canyigit, M.; Ozkan, O.S.; Pamuk, G.A.; Dogan, R. Bilateral multiple pulmonary arteriovenous malformations: Endovascular treatment with the Amplatzer Vascular Plug. *J. Vasc. Interv. Radiol.* **2006**, *17*, 141–145. [CrossRef] [PubMed]

18. Tapping, C.R.; Ettles, D.F.; Robinson, G.J. Long-Term Follow-Up of Treatment of Pulmonary Arteriovenous Malformations with AMPLATZER Vascular Plug and AMPLATZER Vascular Plug II Devices. *J. Vasc. Interv. Radiol.* **2011**, *22*, 1740–1746. [CrossRef]

19. Shovlin, C.L.; Letarte, M. Rare diseases bullet 4: Hereditary haemorrhagic telangiectasia and pulmonary arteriovenous malformations: Issues in clinical management and review of pathogenic mechanisms. *Thorax* **1999**, *54*, 714–729. [CrossRef]

20. Shovlin, C.L.; Jackson, J.E.; Bamford, K.B.; Jenkins, I.H.; Benjamin, A.R.; Ramadan, H.; Kulinskaya, E. Primary determinants of ischaemic stroke/brain abscess risks are independent of severity of pulmonary arteriovenous malformations in hereditary haemorrhagic telangiectasia. *Thorax* **2008**, *63*, 259–266. [CrossRef]

21. Lacombe, P.; Lagrange, C.; Beauchet, A.; El, H.M.; Chinet, T.; Pelage, J.P. Diffuse pulmonary arteriovenous malformations in hereditary hemorrhagic telangiectasia: Long-term results of embolization according to the extent of lung involvement. *Chest* **2009**, *135*, 1031–1037. [CrossRef] [PubMed]

22. Lacombe, P.; Lacout, A.; Marcy, P.-Y.; Binsse, S.; Sellier, J.; Bensalah, M.; Chinet, T.; Bourgault-Villada, I.; Blivet, S.; Roume, J.; et al. Diagnosis and treatment of pulmonary arteriovenous malformations in hereditary hemorrhagic telangiectasia: An overview. *Diagn. Interv. Imaging* **2013**, *94*, 835–848. [CrossRef]

23. Grunwald, I.Q.; Papanagiotou, P.; Roth, C.; Fassbender, K.; Karp, K.; Krick, C.; Schieber, H.; Muller, M.; Haass, A.; Reith, W. Lesion load in unprotected carotid artery stenting. *Neuroradiology* **2009**, *51*, 313–317. [CrossRef] [PubMed]

24. Flach, H.Z.; Ouhlous, M.; Hendriks, J.M.; Van Sambeek, M.R.H.M.; Veenland, J.F.; Koudstaal, P.J.; Van Dijk, L.C.; Van Der Lugt, A. Cerebral Ischemia After Carotid Intervention. *J. Endovasc. Ther.* **2004**, *11*, 251–257. [CrossRef] [PubMed]

25. McDonald, J.; Wooderchak-Donahue, W.; VanSant, W.C.; Whitehead, K.; Stevenson, D.A.; Bayrak-Toydemir, P. Hereditary hemorrhagic telangiectasia: Genetics and molecular diagnostics in a new era. *Front. Genet.* **2015**, *6*, 1. [CrossRef]

26. White, R.I., Jr. Pulmonary arteriovenous malformations and hereditary hemorrhagic telangiectasia: Embolotherapy using balloons and coils. *Arch. Intern. Med.* **1996**, *156*, 2627–2628. [CrossRef] [PubMed]

27. White, R.I.; Pollak, J.S.; Wirth, J.A. Pulmonary Arteriovenous Malformations: Diagnosis and Transcatheter Embolotherapy. *J. Vasc. Interv. Radiol.* **1996**, *7*, 787–804. [CrossRef]

28. Schiebler, M.L.; Nagle, S.K.; François, C.J.; Repplinger, M.D.; Hamedani, A.G.; Vigen, K.K.; Yarlagadda, R.; Grist, T.M. Effectiveness of MR angiography for the primary diagnosis of acute pulmonary embolism: Clinical outcomes at 3 months and 1 year. *J. Magn. Reson. Imaging* **2013**, *38*, 914–925. [CrossRef]

29. Lansky, A.J.; Brown, D.; Pena, C.; Pietras, C.G.; Parise, H.; Ng, V.G.; Meller, S.; Abrams, K.J.; Cleman, M.; Margolis, P.; et al. Neurologic Complications of Unprotected Transcatheter Aortic Valve Implantation (from the Neuro-TAVI Trial). *Am. J. Cardiol.* **2016**, *118*, 1519–1526. [CrossRef] [PubMed]

30. Grunwald, I.Q.; Reith, W.; Kühn, A.L.; Balami, J.S.; Karp, K.; Fassbender, K.; Walter, S.; Papanagiotou, P.; Krick, C. Proximal protection with the Gore PAES can reduce DWI lesion size in high-grade stenosis during carotid stenting. *EuroIntervention* **2014**, *10*, 271–276. [CrossRef]

31. Akioka, N.; Takaiwa, A.; Kashiwazaki, D.; Kuwayama, N.; Endo, S.; Kuroda, S. Clinical Significance of Hemodynamic Cerebral Ischemia on Cognitive Function in Carotid Artery Stenosis—A Prospective Study Before and After Revascularization. *Q. J. Nucl. Med. Mol. Imaging* **2015**, *61*, 323–330.

32. Sasoh, M.; Ogasawara, K.; Kuroda, K.; Okuguchi, T.; Terasaki, K.; Yamadate, K.; Ogawa, A. Effects of EC-IC bypass surgery on cognitive impairment in patients with hemodynamic cerebral ischemia. *Surg. Neurol.* **2003**, *59*, 455–460. [CrossRef]

33. Circo, S.; Gossage, J.R. Pulmonary vascular complications of hereditary haemorrhagic telangiectasia. *Curr. Opin. Pulm. Med.* **2014**, *20*, 421–428. [CrossRef]

34. Hsu, C.C.-T.; Kwan, G.N.; Evans-Barns, H.; Van Driel, M.L. Embolisation for pulmonary arteriovenous malformation. *Cochrane Database Syst. Rev.* **2018**, CD008017. [CrossRef] [PubMed]

35. Hsu, C.C.; Kwan, G.N.; Thompson, S.A.; Evans-Barns, H.; van Driel, M.L. Embolisation for pulmonary arteriovenous malformation. *Cochrane Database Syst. Rev.* **2012**, *1*. [CrossRef]

36. Faughnan, M.E.; Mager, J.J.; Hetts, S.W.; Palda, V.A.; Lang-Robertson, K.; Buscarini, E.; Deslandres, E.; Kasthuri, R.S.; Lausman, A.; Poetker, D.; et al. Second International Guidelines for the Diagnosis and Management of Hereditary Hemorrhagic Telangiectasia. *Ann. Intern. Med.* **2020**, *173*, 989–1001. [CrossRef] [PubMed]

37. Faughnan, M.E.; Palda, V.A.; Garcia-Tsao, G.; Geisthoff, U.W.; McDonald, J.; Proctor, D.D.; Spears, J.; Brown, D.H.; Buscarini, E.; Chesnutt, M.S.; et al. International guidelines for the diagnosis and management of hereditary haemorrhagic telangiectasia. *J. Med. Genet.* **2009**, *48*, 73–87. [CrossRef] [PubMed]

38. Majumdar, S.; McWilliams, J.P. Approach to Pulmonary Arteriovenous Malformations: A Comprehensive Update. *J. Clin. Med.* **2020**, *9*, 1927. [CrossRef] [PubMed]
39. Cho, Y.D.; Kim, S.-E.; Lim, J.W.; Choi, H.J.; Cho, Y.J.; Jeon, J.P. Protected versus Unprotected Carotid Artery Stenting: Meta-Analysis of the Current Literature. *J. Korean Neurosurg. Soc.* **2018**, *61*, 458–466. [CrossRef]
40. Macdonald, S.; Evans, D.H.; Griffiths, P.D.; McKevitt, F.M.; Venables, G.S.; Cleveland, T.J.; Gaines, P.A. Filter-Protected versus Unprotected Carotid Artery Stenting: A Randomised Trial. *Cerebrovasc. Dis.* **2010**, *29*, 282–289. [CrossRef] [PubMed]

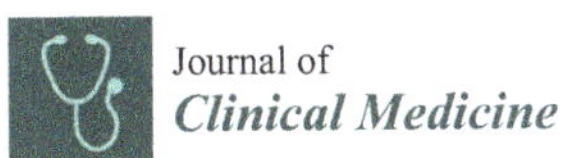 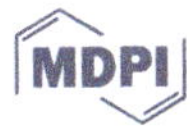

Journal of
Clinical Medicine

Review

Review of Pharmacological Strategies with Repurposed Drugs for Hereditary Hemorrhagic Telangiectasia Related Bleeding

Virginia Albiñana [1,2], Angel M. Cuesta [1,2], Isabel de Rojas-P [1], Eunate Gallardo-Vara [3], Lucía Recio-Poveda [1,2], Carmelo Bernabéu [1,2] and Luisa María Botella [1,2,*]

[1] Centro de Investigaciones Biológicas Margarita Salas, Consejo Superior de Investigaciones Científicas (CSIC), 9 Ramiro de Maeztu Street, 28040 Madrid, Spain; vir_albi_di@yahoo.es (V.A.); acme@cib.csic.es (A.M.C.); iderojas@ucm.es (I.d.R.-P.); lrecio@cib.csic.es (L.R.-P.); bernabeu.c@cib.csic.es (C.B.)
[2] Centro de Investigación Biomédica en Red de Enfermedades Raras (CIBERER), Institute of Health Carlos III, 28040 Madrid, Spain
[3] Yale Cardiovascular Research Center, Section of Cardiovascular Medicine, Department of Internal Medicine, Yale University School of Medicine, 300 George Street, New Haven, CT 06511, USA; eunate.gallardo@yale.edu
* Correspondence: cibluisa@cib.csic.es

Received: 24 April 2020; Accepted: 3 June 2020; Published: 6 June 2020

Abstract: The diagnosis of hereditary hemorrhagic telangiectasia (HHT) is based on the Curaçao criteria: epistaxis, telangiectases, arteriovenous malformations in internal organs, and family history. Genetically speaking, more than 90% of HHT patients show mutations in *ENG* or *ACVRL1/ALK1* genes, both belonging to the TGF-β/BMP9 signaling pathway. Despite clear knowledge of the symptoms and genes of the disease, we still lack a definite cure for HHT, having just palliative measures and pharmacological trials. Among the former, two strategies are: intervention at "ground zero" to minimize by iron and blood transfusions in order to counteract anemia. Among the later, along the last 15 years, three different strategies have been tested: (1) To favor coagulation with antifibrinolytic agents (tranexamic acid); (2) to increase transcription of *ENG* and *ALK1* with specific estrogen-receptor modulators (bazedoxifene or raloxifene), antioxidants (N-acetylcysteine, resveratrol), or immunosuppressants (tacrolimus); and (3) to impair the abnormal angiogenic process with antibodies (bevacizumab) or blocking drugs like etamsylate, and propranolol. This manuscript reviews the main strategies and sums up the clinical trials developed with drugs alleviating HHT.

Keywords: HHT; ALK1; endoglin; raloxifene; bazedoxifene; tranexamic acid; propranolol; FK506; etamsylate; N-acetylcysteine

---

1. Introduction

Hereditary hemorrhagic telangiectasia (HHT) or Rendu-Osler-Weber syndrome is a genetic dominant autosomal multisystemic vascular disease, whose penetrance increases with age. The Curaçao criteria were designed to diagnose HHT, and include its clinical symptoms which are spontaneous and recurrent epistaxis (nose bleeds), mucocutaneous telangiectases, visceral localization (gastrointestinal telangiectases and/or arteriovenous malformations (AVMs), mainly in lung, brain or liver), and a first degree family member with a definite diagnosis of HHT (Figure 1A) [1–3]. The prevalence of HHT varies between 1:5000 and 1:8000 on average, although because of the "founder effect" and "insulation effect," the prevalence is higher in some regions such as the Jura region in France, Funen Island in Denmark and the Caribbean Dutch Antilles [3–5]. Heterozygous mutations in either *ENDOGLIN (ENG)* or *ACVRL1/ALK1* genes trigger the pathogenesis of HHT in over 90% of HHT patients [6,7]. Less common mutations, responsible for 2% of HHT cases, appear in the *SMAD4* gene, leading to a combined syndrome of Juvenile Polyposis HHT (JPHT) [8] consisting of HHT symptoms, colon polyps and thoracic aneurysms [9]. Furthermore, chromosomes 5 and 7 have been described to possess two *loci* with unknown genes, that cause HHT3 [10] and HHT4, respectively [11]. An HHT-like syndrome called HHT5 has been linked to mutations in *BMP9* [12]. All mutations leading to HHT are found in genes belonging to the family of BMP9/TGF-β signaling pathway (Figure 1B).

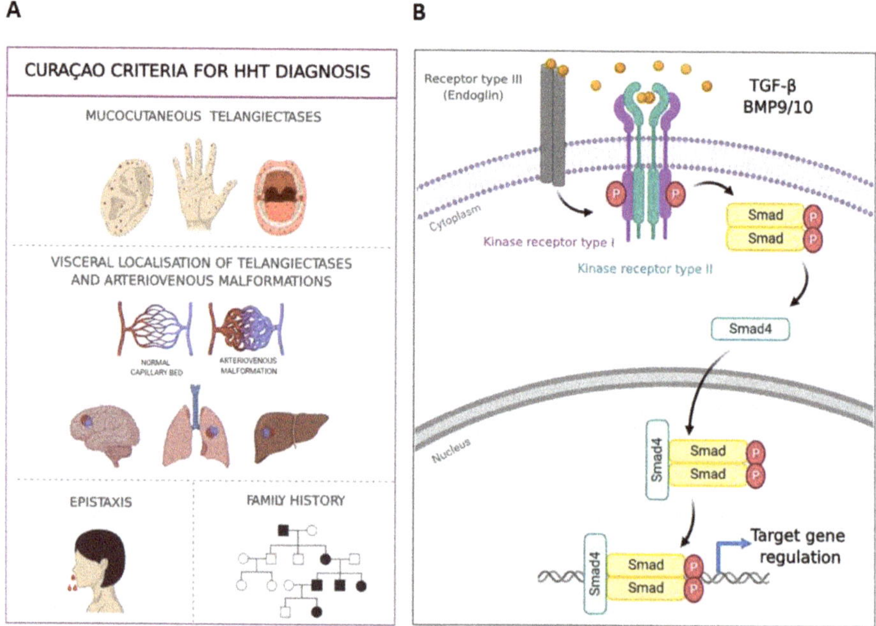

Figure 1. Hereditary Hemorrhagic Telangiectasia. (**A**). Clinical manifestations of HHT, Curaçao criteria. Telangiectasias in ear, hands, tongue, and lips; arteriovenous malformations in internal organs, epistaxis and family history. (**B**). TGF-β/BMP9/10 signaling pathway in endothelial cells. Once the ligand binds to its receptor complex formed by the kinase receptors I and II, and the auxiliary receptor III (endoglin), the signaling cascade leads to the phosphorylation of Smad proteins. The translocation of the Smad protein complex into the nucleus results in transcriptional regulation on target genes. Endothelial cells (EC) express two types of type I kinase Receptors: ALK1 and ALK5.

Moreover, the capillary malformation (CM)/AVM syndrome is phenotypically similar to HHT, and is characterized by the appearance of multiple CMs that are small and red, round to oval shaped with a peripheral white halo and randomly distributed. These are linked to heterozygous pathogenic variants in *EPHB4* or *RASA1* identified by molecular genetic testing [13].

This review will focus on the pharmacological treatment for bleeding in HHT patients. With 93% of patients suffering light to moderate bleedings, epistaxis presents as the most frequent clinical manifestation of HHT [14,15]. It affects over 90% of patients before the age of 21, normally interfering with their quality of life [16]. Epistaxis are due to the telangiectases of the nasal mucosa, focally dilated venules, often connected directly with dilated arterioles [17]. Directly related to epistaxis is gastrointestinal (GI) bleeding, because of telangiectases in the digestive tract and observed in up to 80% of HHT patients [18]. However, GI bleeding becomes more frequent with age [19]. Although currently there is no optimal available treatment for either epistaxis or GI bleeding, the systemic pharmacological treatments that are used for epistaxis might also be useful to manage GI bleedings.

The pharmaceutical therapies which that are discussed in the following sections address therapies wherein the disease is due to heterozygous germ-line mutations in all cells of the HHT patient. These therapies may not be effective for some cutaneous telangiectases, wherein endothelial cells (EC) may have homozygous mutants for *ALK1/ENG* according to a recent publication of Snellings et al. [20].

2. General Care and Control of Anemia

To prevent crusting and allow the nasal mucosa to be correctly hydrated in HHT patients, local moisturizing treatments such as humidification, nasal cleaning with a saline solution and lipid-based topical ointments are used [18]. Despite these options, it is challenging to completely avoid nasal or GI bleeding in HHT, often leading to iron deficiency and anemia in these patients. For this reason, the first line treatment of HHT is focused on managing the anemia resulting from bleeding. Iron-enriched diets and iron supplements are cost-effective steps that significantly reduce the need of blood transfusions although the latter may be necessary in severely affected patients [2,21].

3. Therapeutic Pathways/Strategies of Pharmacological Treatments for HHT

The following section focuses on reviewing the pharmacological treatments, from a preclinical perspective. Robert et al. have also recently reviewed this topic [22].

Options to control nose and GI bleeding could be used, according to the following strategies (Table 1). It should be commented that the drugs were included into each group, according to the main mechanism observed in vitro and/or in vivo experiments, yet in some cases other additional mechanisms maybe contributing to the therapeutic effect.

Table 1. Therapeutic strategies to decrease epistaxis in HHT.

1	Decrease hemorrhages stabilizing the fibrin network with antifibrinolytics ➢ Tranexamic acid ➢ ε-aminocaproicacid
2	Stimulate *ENG* and *ALK1* transcription to increase protein expression to partially overcome haploinsufficiency ➢ SERMs: raloxifene, bazedoxifene ➢ Tacrolimus
3	Decrease the abnormal excessive vasculature of the nose mucosa through antiangiogenesis ➢ By inactivating the VEGF signaling pathway • Bevacizumab, propranolol, timolol, thalidomide or pazopanib ➢ By blocking the FGF-R signaling pathway • Etamsylate

- **Strategy 1**. Although HHT does not result from a clotting failure, the use of antifibrinolytics to restore the balance between coagulation versus fibrinolysis would help to promote a quicker coagulation and to stabilize the fibrin network. Among the antifibrinolytics used for epistaxis treatment, tranexamic acid (TA) and ε-aminocaproic acid (AC) stand out [23,24].
- **Strategy 2**. HHT is associated with haploinsufficiency in *ENG* or *ALK1* genes, therefore stimulating their protein expression is thought to revert the HHT phenotype. At this point, raloxifene hydrochloride and bazedoxifene acetate, two specific estrogen receptor modulators (SERMs), have proven efficiency and safety, and have been designated as orphan drugs for HHT (2010 EU/3/10/730 and 2014 EU/3/14/1367; respectively) [25,26].
- **Strategy 3**. Antiangiogenic therapies tackle the excess of abnormal vasculature present on the nasal mucosa in HHT. Therefore, bevacizumab (BZ) (Avastin®), a humanized monoclonal antibody

against the main angiogenic factor, the vascular endothelial growth factor (VEGF), has been widely used and tested on HHT. Its systemic administration has improved hepatic function, delaying the liver transplant [27] but it has not shown consistent results when tested to decrease epistaxis events by topical spray administration [28,29].

Following the same antiangiogenic strategy, pazopanib, thalidomide, and more recently pomalidomide, have been used to inhibit the VEGF pathway.

Similarly, other cardiovascular drugs such as propranolol and timolol (non-specific β-blockers) have shown their benefits in nose bleeding when administered topically (both) and systemically (propranolol) [30] in HHT patients. Recently, the use of the fibroblast growth factor receptor (FGFR) blocker etamsylate, by local spray administration has been proven effective and has been designated as orphan drug for HHT in 2018 (EU/3/18/2087) [31].

Tables 2 and 3, respectively, summarize the ongoing and finished clinical trials, conducted in HHT with the different drugs, most of them mentioned in this review. In addition, some other recent candidates like Vitamin D, itraconazole and doxycyclin are in ongoing clinical trials.

Table 2. Compilation of the HHT interventional clinical trials (Recruiting, Ongoing, or Unknown status).

Trial Registration #	Country	Phase	Title	Intervention	Number of Patients	Trial Design	Outcome	Start Date	Status
EudraCT 2010-020545-26	IT	2	Bevacizumab, an anti-angiogenic monoclonal antibody effective for prevention of hemorrhage in patients with HHT: possible regression of visceral arteriovenous malformations	Bevacizumab	18	Single-arm, controlled	Frequency of Epistaxis	2008	O
EudraCT 2008-006755-44	FR	2	METAFORE: Maladie de Rendu-Osler: Etude de l'Efficacité et de la tolérance du Bevacizumab utilisé pour le traitement des formes hépatiques sévères. Etude de phase II	Bevacizumab	25	Information not available	Effect on cardiac output in patients with severe liver damage	2009	O
NCT02389959	US	4	Intranasal Bevacizumab for HHT-Related Epistaxis	Bevacizumab	40	Two-arm, randomized, double-blind, placebo-controlled	Improvement in ESS	2014	R
NCT02287558	US	1	Pomalidomide in HHT and Transfusion-Dependent Vascular Ectasia: a Phase I Study	Pomalidomide	9	Single-arm, open-label	Transfusion requirement measure	2015	R
NCT04167085	US	4	NOrth American Study for the Treatment of Recurrent epIstaxis With DoxycycLine: The NOSTRIL Trial	Doxycycline	24	Two-arm, randomized, double-blind, crossover	Frequency of epistaxis	2017	A
NCT02963129	AR	3	Treatment of Nasal Staphylococcus Aureus Colonization in Patients With HHT	Mupirocin	40	Two-arm, randomized, triple-blind, placebo	Nosebleed by Sadick scale	2017	U
NCT03981562	CA	2	Vitamin D and HHT	Vit D	60	Three-arm, randomized, double-blind, placebo	Change in ESS	2018	R
EudraCT z017-003272-31	NL	2	Efficacy and safety of oral itraconazole in the reduction of epistaxis severity in HHT	Itraconazole	25	Single-arm, open-label	Change in epistaxis severity	2018	O
NCT03397004	CA	2	Doxycycline for HHT	Doxycycline Hyclate	30	Two-arm, randomized, double-blind, placebo-controlled, crossover	Reduction in epistaxis (nose bleeding) severity over 96 weeks	2018	R
NCT04113187	FR	3	Propranolol for Epistaxis in HHT a Patients	Propranolol	38	Two-arm, double-blind	Cumulative duration of epistaxis (in minutes)	2019	NR
NCT04139018	US	2	Timolol Gel for Epistaxis in HHT	Timolol Gel	30	Two-arm, double-blind, randomized controlled	ESS	2019	R
NCT03910244	US	2	Pomalidomide for the Treatment of Bleeding in HHT	Pomalidomide	159	Two-arm, placebo-controlled, double-blind	Change in ESS	2019	R
NCT03850730	US	1–2	Pazopanib for the Treatment of Epistaxis in HHT	Pazopanib	30	Single-arm, open-label	Percent change in epistaxis duration in minutes	2019	NR

Table 2. *Cont.*

Trial Registration #	Country	Phase	Title	Intervention	Number of Patients	Trial Design	Outcome	Start Date	Status
NCT03850964	US	2–3	Pazopanib Effects on Bleeding in HHT	Pazopanib	45	Two-arm, double-blind, placebo controlled	Change in epistaxis duration in minutes	2019	NR
EudraCT 2019-003585-40	NL	NA	An uncontrolled, open label pilot-study assessing the efficacy in reducing bleeding severity, and the safety of oral tacrolimus in patients with HHT	Tacrolimus	20	Uncontrolled, single-arm, open-label	Change in the epistaxis and/or gastrointestinal severity	2019	O
EudraCT 2019-002593-31	FR	2	Efficacy of Nintedanib per os as a treatment for epistaxis in HHT disease. A national, randomized, multicenter phase II study EPICURE	Nintedanib	60	Two-arm, double-blind, randomized controlled, placebo	Frequency of Epistaxis	2019	O
EudraCT 2018-004179-11	NL	2	Effectiveness of Somatostatin Analogues in patients with HHT and symptomatic gastrointestinal bleeding, the SAIPAN-trial: a multicenter, randomized, open-label, parallel group, superiority trial	Somatostatin Analogues	38	Two-arm, open-label, randomized controlled	Decreasing the transfusion requirements	2019	O
ACTRN 12619001020178	AU	2	A pilot study assessing the effectiveness of oral Propranolol in preventing epistasis in patients with HHT	Propranolol	15	Single-arm, open-label, non-randomized	Change in Epistasis	2019	NR
NCT03954782	FR	2	Efficacy of Nintedanib Per os as a Treatment for Epistaxis in HHT Disease	Nintedanib	60	Two-arm, triple-blind, randomized	Epistaxis duration assessed on epistaxis grids completed by the patients	2020	O

Table 2. Compilation of the Recruiting, Ongoing, or Unknown HHT interventional clinical trials registered at the EU Clinical Trials Register (EudraCT) (https://www.clinicaltrialsregister.eu), the U.S. National Library of Medicine (NCT) (https://clinicaltrials.gov), and the Australian New Zealand Clinical Trials Registry (ACTRN) (http://www.anzctr.org.au/Default.aspx). Only interventional trials where a therapeutic drug was tested are listed. Abbreviations: Countries: AR (Argentina); AU (Australia); CA (Canada); FR (France); IT (Italy); NL (Netherlands); US (United States of America). Phase: NA (Not Applicable). Status: R (Recruiting); O (Ongoing); U (Unknown). Outcome: ESS (Epistaxis Severity Score).

Table 3. Compilation of the HHT interventional clinical trials (Completed or Terminated status).

Trial Registration #	Country	Phase	Title	Intervention	Number of Patients	Trial Design	Outcome (Summary of Statistically Significant Outcomes)	Start Date	Status	Link to Results
NCT00004327	US	2	Phase II Pilot Study of Octreotide, a Somatostatin Octapeptide Analog, for Gastrointestinal Hemorrhage in Hormone-Refractory HHT and Senile Ectasia	Octreotide	8	Information not available	-	1995	C	-
NCT00004654	US	3	Phase III Randomized, Placebo-Controlled, Crossover Study of Soy Protein Isolate for HHT	Soy protein	60	Randomized	-	1996	C	-
NCT01031992	GE	3	Tranexamic Acid and Epistaxis in HHT	Tranexamic acid	23	Two-arm, double-blind, controlled	No changes in hemoglobin levels. Significant reduction in ESS	2002	C	Article [32]
NCT00375622	IL	2	Anti-Estrogen Therapy for HHT A Double-Blind Placebo-Controlled Clinical Trial	Tamoxifen	25 (60) *	Double-blind, placebo-controlled	Significant reduction in ESS (frequency and severity).	2005	C	Article [39]
NCT00355108	FR	3	ATERO: A Randomized Study with Tranexamic Acid in Epistaxis of Rendu Osler Syndrome	Tranexamic acid	118 (170) *	Single-arm, double-blind, randomized, crossover	Significant decrease in the duration of epistaxis	2006	C	Article [34]
NCT00389935	US	2	Thalidomide Reduces Arteriovenous Malformation Related Gastrointestinal Bleeding	Thalidomide	14	Single-arm, open-label	-	2006	C	-
NCT00588146	US	2	Phase 2 Study of PEG-Intron in HHT	Pegylated IFN-α2B	10	Two-arm, open-label, randomized	Adverse events plus discontinuation of the study supply	2007	T	Trial file
NCT01397695	US	2	Topical Bevacizumab for the Management of Recurrent Epistaxis in Patients with HHT	Bevacizumab	20	Single-arm, open-label, non-randomized	-	2009	T	Trial file
NCT01402531	US	2	Submucosal Bevacizumab for the Management of Recurrent Epistaxis in Patients with HHT	Bevacizumab	10	Single-arm, open-label, non-randomized	-	2010	T	Trial file
EudraCT2009-018049-	AT	2	A randomized double-blind placebo-controlled trial of intranasal submucosal bevacizumab in hereditary hemorrhagic telangiectasia	Bevacizumab	30	Two-arm, double-blind, randomizedcontrolled	-	2010	C	-
NCT01408030	US	2	North American Study of Epistaxis in HHT (NOSE)	Bevacizumab-Estriol-Tranexamic Acid	121	Four-arm, double-blind, placebo-controlled, randomized	No significant differences on epistaxis frequency	2011	C	Article [28]
NCT01408732	US	1	Office-sclerotherapy for Epistaxis Due to HHT	Sclerotherapy with sodium tetradecyl sulfate	18	Two-arm, open-label, randomized-controlled	No significant differences on severity of epistaxis	2011	C	Trial file
NCT01485224	IT	2	Efficacy of Thalidomide in the Treatment of HHT	Thalidomide	31	Single-arm, open-label, non-randomized	100% showed a complete or partial response to epistaxis	2011	C	Article [35]
NCT01314274	AT	2	Intranasal Submucosal Bevacizumab for Epistaxis in HHT	Bevacizumab	15	Two-arm, double-blind, randomized, placebo-controlled	No significant differences on epistaxis frequency	2011	C	Article [36]

Table 3. *Cont.*

Trial Registration #	Country	Phase	Title	Intervention	Number of Patients	Trial Design	Outcome (Summary of Statistically Significant Outcomes)	Start Date	Status	Link to Results
NCT01507480	FR	1	The ELLIPSE Study: A Phase-1 Study Evaluating the Tolerance of Bevacizumab Nasal Spray to Treat Epistaxis in HHT	Bevacizumab	42	Single-arm, double-blind, randomized, placebo-controlled	Bevacizumab nasal spray is safe	2011	C	Article [37]
EudraCT 2011-004096-36	IT	2	Efficacy of thalidomide in the treatment of severe recurrent epistaxis in HHT	Thalidomide	31	Single-arm, non-controlled	-	2011	C	-
NCT01908543	UK	NA	Iron Deficiency and HHT	Ferrous sulphate	3	Single-arm, open-label	-	2013	T	Article [38]
NCT01752049	CA	NA	Topical Anti-angiogenic Therapy for Telangiectasia in HHT: Proof of Concept	Timolol maleate	5	Two-arm, double-blind, placebo-controlled	-	2013	C	-
EudraCT 2013-004204-19 & NCT02157987	FR	1-2	Treatment of HHT of the Nasal Mucosa by Intranasal Bevacizumab: Search for Effective Dose	Bevacizumab	30	Four-arm, double-blind, randomized, controlled	-	2014	C	-
NCT02638012	CA	NA	Prospective Pilot Study of Floseal for the Treatment of Anterior Epistaxis in Patients With HHT	Floseal	10	Two-arm, open-label, non-randomized	No statistically significant difference noted in ESS	2015	C	Article [39]
NCT02204371	US & CA	2	Evaluation of Pazopanib on Bleeding in Subjects with HHT	Pazopanib	7	Two-arm, open-label, non-randomized	No statistically significant difference noted in ESS	2015	T	Trial file
EudraCT 2015-000385-55 & NCT02484716	FR	2	Efficacy of a Timolol Nasal Spray as a Treatment for Epistaxis in Hereditary Hemorrhagic Telangiectasia (HHT)—(TEMPO)	Timolol	58	Two-arm, double-blind, randomized	No statistically significant difference noted in ESS	2015	C	Article [40]
EudraCT 2016-003982-24	ES	4-2	A phase IV-II, single-center, open, single arm treatment, low level of intervention, to assess the efficacy clinical trial and safety of intranasal administration of ethamsylate in the treatment of HHT, during for 4 weeks	Ethamsylate	12	Single-arm, open-label, non-randomized	Statistically significant difference noted in ESS	2016	C	Article [31]
EudraCT 2016-001340-19 & NCT02874326	NL	2	Octreotide in Patients With GI Bleeding Due to Rendu-Osler-Weber	Octreotide LAR	15	Single-arm, open-label	The median number of RBC units needed decreased significantly.	2016	C	Article [41]
NCT03152019	FR	2	Efficacy and Safety of a 0.1% Tacrolimus Nasal Ointment as a Treatment for Epistaxis in Hemorrhagic Hereditary Telangiectasia (HHT) (TACRO)	Tacrolimus	50	Two-arm, double-blind, randomized	No statistically significant difference noted in ESS	2017	C	Article [42]

Table 3. Compilation of the Completed or Terminated HHT interventional clinical trials registered at the EU Clinical Trials Register (EudraCT) (https://www.clinicaltrialsregister.eu), the U.S. National Library of Medicine (NCT) (https://clinicaltrials.gov). Only interventional trials where a therapeutic drug was tested are listed. Abbreviations: Countries: AT (Austria); CA (Canada); ES (Spain); FR (France); IL (Israel); IT (Italy); NL (Netherlands); UK (United Kingdom); US (United States of America). Phase: NA (Not Applicable). Status: C (Completed) and T (Terminated). Outcome: ESS (Epistaxis Severity Score). * The Study Record Detail from the website refers to the number of patients in parenthesis.

All the above-mentioned drugs used were repurposed medicines, which have the added value of an immediate use in clinical trials since their safety is already confirmed from their first indication. As stated by Masoudi et al. (2020) [43], "Drug repurposing is a powerful strategy in the discovery scope because of the time and cost savings". Furthermore, it is an appropriate method for finding therapies for orphan and rare diseases.

3.1. Strategy 1. Antifibrinolysis: ε-Aminocaproic and Tranexamic Acids

Antifibrinolytics block the plasminogen to plasmin conversion by inhibition of its enzymatic disaggregation and consequently, stabilization of the fibrin clot. Accordingly, these drugs are expected to target the wall of the telangiectases where fibrinolysis is activated [44,45].

TA and AC are antifibrinolytic agents used for HHT epistaxis. Both may be administered topically (with the agent embedded in gauze) or systemically by oral intake (500 mg/8 h or even up to 2 g/day) or intravenous administration. AC was the first antifibrinolytic used but showed thrombosis as a side effect and is therefore not recommended in patients prone to thrombosis [46–49]. In addition, TA has shown longer half-life and higher potency (10-fold) than AC [23,24].

In addition to several case reports with successful results, a study with a total of 14 patients with low risk of thrombosis and for whom their quality of life was poor due to epistaxis, were selected to take TA (500 mg/8 h) orally. TA treatment showed a decrease of nose bleedings and increase of hemoglobin levels in all patients, almost avoiding the transfusion necessity, indicating an overall improvement and no side effects of TA treatment [24]. Although the study was not a formal clinical trial, TA was safe and effective at the doses applied. To highlight, TA administered up to 3 g/day was successful in controlling a massive and life-threatening hemorrhage in an HHT patient [23]. Moreover, some published data from in vitro experiments demonstrated on ECs that TA led to increased mRNA and protein levels of endoglin and ALK1, and improved endothelial functions as tubulogenesis and migration [24]. Thus, elevated endoglin or ALK1 expression may act concomitantly to the main antifibrinolytic action, although the proposed mechanism is only based on in vitro evidence.

Nevertheless, some concern must be taken in HHT patients with the elevated levels of the coagulation protein factor VIII (FVIII) and factor V Leiden, since some reports show an HHT-related increment of these protein levels that favor thrombotic risk in these patients. Another putative risk factor is the presence of high levels of factor V Leiden. Therefore, personalized risk-benefit considerations are demanded for HHT management [50].

Generally, clotting factors levels are not altered in HHT patients (excluding patients with altered factor V or VIII expression). However, one way of shortening the time and frequency of bleeding is by displacing the balance between coagulation and anticoagulation process toward a more quick and stable clotting when the abnormal vessels (mucosa telangiectases) break. This is enhanced by the antifibrinolytics, which prompt the clotting and delay its fibrinolysis. Moreover, telangiectases have been reported to have high fibrinolytic activity by Sabbà et al. [51].

In addition, two clinical trials were performed in HHT centers to assess the benefits of TA in HHT patients with reports published in 2014. In the French ATERO assay, TA was shown effective in a multinational center study [34], while Geisthoff et al. [32], demonstrated efficacy in a double-blind clinical trial phase III-B. However, while TA has demonstrated efficiency by systemic use, when topically used by a nasal spray, it did not significantly decrease nose bleeds when compared to placebo in a clinical trial (NOSE study) conducted by Cure HHT in 2016 [28].

3.2. Strategy 2. Upregulating ENG and ACVRL1

3.2.1. Hormonal Therapy: Specific Estrogen Receptor Modulators (SERMs)

The incidence of epistaxis has been observed to be increased in women after they have reached menopausal age, suggesting that estrogens might play a protective role in HHT-derived bleeding in women. Post-menopausal women are also affected by osteoporosis, the imbalance in the rate of bone remodeling/resorption that predisposes elders to higher chances of bone fracture. NFκB, RANK and its ligand RANKL, as well as osteoprotegerin (OPG) play major roles in this pathogenesis [52] (Figure 2). Based on the observation that pre-menopausal HHT women had fewer epistaxis, a study developed by the Yale University's Vascular Malformation Centre attempted to treat GI bleeding of 40 transfusion-dependent HHT patients, with a mean age of 57 years, by means of estradiol treatment. Men, to avoid estradiol feminizing effects, were also treated with ethinylestradiol/norethindrone and danazol. The results were satisfactory as most of the 40 patients showed an improvement in hemoglobin levels and needed fewer blood transfusions [53].

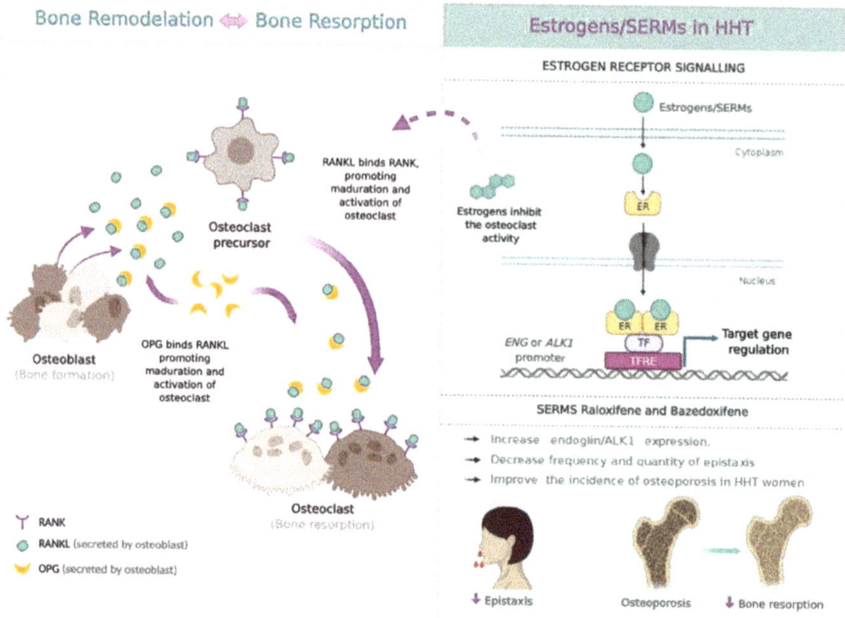

Figure 2. Scheme of Bone formation vs. Bone resorption (**left**). Bone remodeling is promoted by the activity of osteoclasts and osteoblasts. RANKL is a protein expressed by osteoblasts which, upon binding to its RANK receptor on the cell surface of osteoclasts and their precursors, causes RANK to stimulate and promote the adhesion of osteoclasts to bone, thus activating their function and preventing apoptosis. OPG is synthesized by the osteoblasts and acts as a decoy receptor, preventing the binding of RANKL to RANK, therefore decreasing the activity of the osteoclast and its survival [52]. For this reason, for years post-menopausal patients with diagnosed osteoporosis have been receiving estrogenic treatment, which, while correcting this imbalance in bone remodeling, also reduces the activity of the osteoclast and activates the expression of OPG. This is also capable of reducing the epistaxis of these patients [25,33,53,54]. Scheme of Estrogen Receptor (ER) signaling (**right**). Mechanism of action of ER on EC, in the case of the SERMs raloxifene and bazedoxifene. Upon ligand binding, the ER dimer interacts with different transcription factors (TF), promoting gene expression by binding to the TFRE (Transcription Factor Regulatory Element) in the promoter of its target genes. The expression of endoglin and ALK1 increases as a result of the interaction of the ER with Sp1, an essential factor for the expression of both genes. In women, SERMs promote a decrease in the frequency and amount of epistaxis, normalizing the nasal vasculature with concomitant improvement in osteoporosis [25,26].

The use of hormones to treat HHT-induced bleedings was published later in the form of case reports, but mostly without controls [55]. The main conclusion obtained from these studies was that estrogen-progesterone administered at the doses typically used for oral contraception might reduce bleedings in symptomatic HHT women, becoming a reasonable option for fertile HHT female patients. Zacharski et al. published in 2001 a case report in which the use of tamoxifen had ceased epistaxis in the long term in a post-menopausal patient, concluding for the first time that SERM was properly used to treat epistaxis in an HHT patient [56]. According to this, tamoxifen was used in two clinical trials where it again successfully decreased epistaxis. The first of these two consisted of a placebo controlled clinical trial that included both men and women, while the second comprised a long-term monitored clinical trial in which patients were administered 20 mg tamoxifen [33,54].

In the line of using SERMs to decrease HHT-related bleedings, the safety and efficiency of raloxifene hydrochloride was tested by a Spanish HHT reference unit IDIVAL (Sierrallana/Valdecilla). Raloxifene hydrochloride shows similarities with tamoxifen, also presenting beneficial effects on bone mineralization and on prevention of cardiovascular and gynecological cancer. This study included 19 post-menopausal women, previously diagnosed with osteoporosis, and compared the amount of bleeding before and after 6 months of treatment (no placebo was included in the study). Oral intake of raloxifene (60 mg/day) showed a significant reduction in both the frequency and the amount of epistaxis after 6 months of treatment, also revealing an increase in hemoglobin levels [25]. Raloxifene has been shown to be a transcriptional activator of *ENG* and *ACVRL1/ALK1* promoters, binding to their proximal regions and subsequently increasing these genes' transcription rate in a context of in vitro experiments on ECs [25]. As a consequence, the protein levels of endoglin and ALK1 increased, thus compensating partially the haploinsufficiency suffered by HHT patients in this study [25]. In 2010, these studies resulted in the European Medicine Agency (EMA) and Food and Drug Administration (FDA) designation of raloxifene hydrochloride as the first orphan drug to treat bleedings in HHT patients (EU/3/10/730). Bazedoxifene acetate, another SERM, significantly decreased the frequency and intensity of epistaxis, while also improving hemoglobin levels as early as one month after treatment with 20 mg/day [26]. In this case, the increase of *ENG* and *ALK1* was not only observed in experiments in vitro with ECs treated with bazedoxifene, but also, in vivo, by measuring *ENG* and *ALK1* levels in macrophages derived from patients before and after bazedoxifene treatment. Bazedoxifene was also designed as orphan drug for HHT in 2014 by the EMA (EU/3/14/1367).

Of note, estrogens and SERMs, as hormonal receptor ligands, increase the transcription of different promoters, among them, those of coagulation factor genes. Thus, *ENG* and *ACVRL1* are among the stimulated genes, but are not the only targets. In relation to this fact, especially when the treatment with SERMs may upregulate coagulation factors' genes, blood tests should be performed periodically for HHT patients under SERM treatment in order to screen for prothrombotic markers and prevent thrombotic events [57].

Finally, phytoestrogens, compounds of plant origin with structural similarities with the natural estrogen 17β-estradiol, deserve some words in this section as natural plant estrogen related products. Among them, the isoflavone genistein and the coumestan resveratrol are the most relevant in studies related to HHT. Genistein is found in numerous plant species such as soy and red clover and resveratrol in grape skin and in dried fruits and nuts. These phytoestrogens show high affinity for estrogenic receptors. Genistein and resveratrol are involved in reducing inflammation, stimulating apoptosis and inhibiting angiogenesis [58,59], and might present therapeutic benefits in HHT patients as natural analogues to SERMs and estrogens.

3.2.2. Immunosuppressor Tacrolimus (FK506)

Albiñana et al. reported the efficacy of tacrolimus (FK506) in increasing endoglin and ALK1 expression [60,61]. The reason to test this drug came from a case report of an HHT patient who was administered the immunosuppressor FK506 in low doses, in combination with Aspirin and sirolimus to avoid rejection of a liver transplant. One month after the start of this treatment, it was observed that his telangiectases (both internal and external), epistaxis and anemia had all been cured [62]. Based on this report, cultured ECs were treated with tacrolimus and an increase on the protein and mRNA expression of endoglin and ALK1 and enhancement of the TGF-β1/ALK1 signaling pathway and EC functions like tubulogenesis and cell migration were observed [60,61]. These results would explain the improvement in the above-mentioned patient, by means of a partial compensation of endoglin and ALK1 haploinsufficiency. Supporting this view, five years later, Ruiz et al. reported increased ALK1 signaling pathway in HHT patient-derived EC. In an HHT animal model, tacrolimus also inhibited VEGF signaling, decreasing hypervascularization [63].

In a more clinical context, Sommer et al. published in 2019 that low doses of FK506/Advagraf decreased bleeding in an HHT patient presenting also pulmonary arterial hypertension [64]. This case report points to low doses of tacrolimus (0.5–1.5 mg/day) as the optimal range for patients with nose or GI refractory bleeding, rather than high doses (5–10 mg/day) normally used for immunosuppression in transplants [64]. An additional report by Hosman et al., including two patients dependent on HHT transfusions due to severe bleeding, demonstrates improvement after treatment with low-dose tacrolimus [65]. Currently, and according to the HHT European Federation, around 24 HHT patients are being treated "off label" with low tacrolimus doses, prescribed by HHT reference doctors, to control epistaxis and GI bleeding.

Finally, the results regarding efficacy and safety of 0.1% tacrolimus topically applied as nasal ointment of the clinical trial named TACRO have just been published. Tacrolimus nasal ointment did not result in improvement 6 weeks after finishing treatment, but the good tolerance and the significant improvement in epistaxis duration during treatment invited the researchers for a phase 3 trial on a larger patient population and a longer treatment time, with a main outcome of epistaxis duration during treatment [42].

3.2.3. N-Acetylcysteine

Based on the premise that free O_2-radicals might cause precapillary sphincter abnormalities, resulting in epistaxis, Gussem et al. in 2009 wondered whether antioxidants like N-acetylcysteine (NAC) could neutralize those free O_2-radicals and reduce or avoid nose bleedings. Thus, 43 HHT patients were followed-up for frequency, severity, and duration of epistaxis after a daily treatment of 600 mg NAC for 12 weeks. There was a reduction in frequency and severity of nosebleed during the day. Male patients with *ENG* mutations experienced a significant improvement. Only an improvement trend was found in women and patients with an *ALK1* mutation [66].

Based on these results, Albiñana et al. studied the in vitro effects of NAC on endoglin and ALK1 expression levels in ECs. After NAC incubation, mRNA and protein levels of endoglin increased up to 1.5–2 folds, although there were no changes on ALK1 levels [67]. These data could suggest that the improvement experienced with their symptoms in HHT1 patients might be due, in part, due to the increase of endoglin levels after NAC treatment, which could be normalizing the nasal mucosa [66].

3.3. Strategy 3. Antiangiogenesis

Antiangiogenic strategies on HHT act on the mucosa to decrease or normalize its abnormal excessive vasculature. Two key angiogenic pathways in ECs are those triggered by VEGF and FGF.

3.3.1. Anti-VEGF and Tyrosine Kinase Inhibitors (TKI)

VEGFs specifically act on vascular EC and are a key stone in the angiogenic and lymphangiogenic process in both physiological and pathological conditions such as tumors or wound healing [68]. VEGFs play an important role in HHT since high protein levels have been reported in HHT patients [69–72].

Avastin ranks the first antiangiogenic therapeutic agent approved for advanced colorectal cancer [73]. Since then, BZ has been widely administered in other pathologies such as non-small cell lung cancer diabetic retinopathy or age-related macular degeneration [74].

The antiangiogenic properties of Avastin were successfully tested in isolated cases of HHT patients. BZ reverted the need for transplantation in a patient with HHT1 [75]. It also decreased the transfusion requirements and cardiac output in a patient with GI [76]. Thus, the French HHT Network designed a single center phase II clinical trial to address the delay in liver transplantation on HHT patients with serious liver complication [27]. BZ significantly decreased the cardiac output and reduced episodes of epistaxis. Nevertheless, symptoms did not disappear after withdrawal of the drug, making Avastin unsuitable as a surrogated alternative for orthotopic liver transplant (OLT) in HHT. These results supported the designation of BZ as orphan drug for HHT in 2014 (EU/3/14/1390).

It is very difficult to determine the optimum time to perform OLT in severe complicated liver venous malformations (VMs) in HHT. OLT is a radical cure for liver VMs and it should be the therapeutic choice in patients under the age of 65 years due to its excellent outcomes, being BZ probably a better option for patients over 65, much more susceptible to higher risk derived from surgery [77].

BZ has been also administered for very severe epistaxis. Despite of its good results decreasing epistaxis and GI after intravenous administration, it has also serious side effects. Therefore, in those patients where no other option is available, an individualized BZ treatment should be supplied; since HHT is a chronic disease [27,77,78]. This individualized re-dosing strategy will not compromise the patient's safety or quality of life and will significantly reduce the costs [79].

BZ has also been assayed topically as nasal spray for epistaxis. The NOSE assay (under the Cure HHT support in USA, 2011–2015) and the French Ellipse clinical trial (2011–2012) ran in parallel. Unfortunately, no significant improvement could be demonstrated for the BZ vs. saline solution spray [28,29].

An alternative therapeutic approach for reducing epistaxis and GI bleeding caused by the over activated VEGF pathway is the blockade of the tyrosine-kinase activity of the VEGF receptor. As a proof of concept, the therapeutic effect of the TKI GW771806 (a pazopanib analogue), was tested in an Alk1-inducible knockout (iKO) murine HHT2 model. The oral administration of GW771806 significantly improved anemia and GI bleeding in HHT2 mice [80]. Unfortunately, its corresponding phase II human trial designed to follow-up adult HHT patients with significant epistaxis, anemia, or with transfusions could not be completed. A prospective, multi-center, open-label, dose-escalating study on pazopanib has also been published and the results show promising improvements in hemoglobin levels and epistaxis in treated patients [81].

Related to pazopanib and in a further step, nintedanib, a TKI targeting growth factor receptors involved in angiogenesis: platelet-derived growth factor receptor (PDGFR), FGFR and VEGFR, will be assayed as a therapeutic drug in a clinical trial. Nintedanib treatment in combination with rapamycin, synergizes to completely block the AVMs in HHT mice pre-clinical models [82]. This has been the main rationale to continue with nintedanib in clinical trials. In that sense, Epicure, a randomized, multicenter, phase II, double-blind placebo-controlled study promoted by the French Hospices Civils de Lyon, has started its recruitment in 2019. Epicure will test the antiangiogenic benefits of the TKI nintedanib in epistaxis. Initially, patients will be monitored for 24 weeks: 12-weeks of oral treatment plus 12-weeks of follow-up. Theoretically, nintedanib, as a non-specific/wide range TKI, should allow a reduction of epistaxis in HHT [83].

Lastly, in this section dealing with drugs interfering with the VEGF signaling pathway, thalidomide deserves special mention, since it has been used for epistaxis and GI bleeding in HHT. Its mechanism of action was published in 2010 [35] and since then, several case reports and clinical trials have been performed (Tables 2 and 3) prior to its designation as an orphan drug (Table 4). Evidence supporting thalidomide compares favorably in cases of serious and refractory GI and nosebleeds. However, risk vs. benefit should be carefully studied, because of the reported side effects for thalidomide [78]. A derivative of thalidomide with potentially fewer side effects, pomalidomide, has been promoted for a multicenter randomized double-blind placebo controlled clinical trial currently ongoing sponsored by the NIH (Table 2).

3.3.2. Non-Selective Adrenergic β-blockers

Non-selective adrenergic β-blockers of receptors β1 and β2 such as the known propranolol and timolol, have shown antiangiogenic properties related to vasoconstriction, inhibition of EC migration and proliferation and reduced VEGF expression [30,84–86]. Given that an excessive activation of the VEGF pathway is involved in the development of abnormal telangiectases, the properties of these non-selective adrenergic β-blockers may be useful topically. Propranolol and timolol have been used as effective therapies to treat superficial infantile hemangiomas [84–86] and could be considered as a potential treatment option for HHT patients.

The use of topical timolol has been described in some case reports as well as in clinical trials/studies of HHT. According to several reports, topical timolol (0.5% ophthalmic solution) clearly improved the frequency and severity of epistaxis [87,88]. Those studies were done in individual patients as well as in larger groups of HHT patients, with clear positive results in all cases. Even though no secondary adverse effects were observed in these cases, there are some contraindications for its applications which should be kept in mind when prescribing, because β-blockers can cause respiratory and cardiovascular problems. In fact, β-blockers are metabolized in the liver by CYP2D6 and a decreased expression of this enzyme, either by concomitant treatment with CYP2D6 inhibitors or by genetic variants, may lead to strong sinus bradycardia [89,90]. Timolol has also been proved to be an efficient treatment at lower doses (0.1% ophthalmic solution-timogel) in decreasing the extension and appearance of mucocutaneous telangiectases in an HHT clinical study, showing 100% and 75% improvement in HHT2 and HHT1 patients, respectively [91].

Propranolol has also been administred topically in gel formulation and systemically in tablets with very promising results, although the last method could be associated with the above-mentioned side effects, which must be considered before prescribing.

There are several studies supporting the improvement in HHT patients after propranolol topical administration. In a pilot study done with six patients, in which 1.5% propranolol gel was applied on the nasal mucosa (0.5 mL/day per nostril) the severity of epistaxis and the number of blood transfusions pre and post-administration were reduced fast and significantly [92]. As continuation of this study, the same group recently finished a double-blind placebo-controlled study to assess the efficacy and safety of topical propranolol for moderate–severe epistaxis in 24 patients with HHT [93]. The combination of sclerotherapy with polydocanol 1% and the use of propranolol cream at 0.5% prepared in a hospital pharmacy was evaluated in a cross-sectional study of 38 HHT patients. This combined therapy significantly reduced the frequency and severity of epistaxis, with an Epistaxis Severity Score (ESS) improvement of 5 points (from 6.9 $\pm$ 2.6 at the beginning to 1.9 $\pm$ 1.3 after the therapy, $p < 0.05$); and increased the quality of life of these patients (in a 5D scale, from 0.66 $\pm$ 0.27 before therapy to 0.93 $\pm$ 0.12 after the therapy $p < 0.05$) [94].

On the other hand, systemic uptake of propranolol has some side effects such as bradycardia and hypotension. Therefore, propranolol could be used in a systemic way only in HHT patients who do not have a low blood pressure. A clinical study with oral propranolol (40–120 mg/day) was done in seven hypertensive HHT patients. Among them, HHT epistaxis disappeared completely in five out of seven, while in the other two the bleeding reduction was highly significant [95].

3.3.3. Antiangiogenesis by FGF Ligand Blocking

The FGF family is considered one of the largest families of polypeptide growth factors. FGFs interact with membrane tyrosine kinase receptors (FGF Receptors, FGFRs) through which they signal and exert their diverse biological functions. FGF-1 and FGF-2 were the first two pure polypeptides discovered among all FGFs and are considered one of the most potent factors promoting angiogenesis [96,97]. Later on, more factors promoting angiogenesis were described. FGFs constitutively cooperate with VEGF promoting the proliferation of EC [98] and inducing angiogenesis [99]. Consequently, FGF inhibition constitutes an alternative to the antiangiogenic effect of VEGF, becoming an interesting new therapeutic approach to treat diseases caused by uncontrolled angiogenesis. Many of the characteristics summarized previously suggest that the inhibition of the FGF signaling pathways could be an appropriate treatment to inhibit the abnormal vascularization of HHT patients [100].

FGF signaling may be inhibited in vitro and in vivo with chemical compounds. One of these products is the anion dihydroxy benzene sulfonate (2,5, DHBS), also known as dobesilate. Dobesilate is commercially available as tablets of its calcium and N-ethylene ethanamine salts (Doxium and Dicynone, respectively), or as injectable solution (Dicynone or etamsylate). Experiments done in vitro with primary cultures from healthy and HHT derived EC, show that etamsylate acts as an antiangiogenic factor, inhibiting wound healing and EC tubulogenesis [31]. A pilot clinical trial (EudraCT: 2016–003982–24, see Table 3) was performed with 12 HHT patients treated with a topical spray of etamsylate twice a day for 4 weeks. The HHT-ESS and other pertinent parameters were analyzed and registered. The significant reduction in the HHT-ESS scale (pre-treatment 4.1 vs. post-treatment 2.8), together with the lack of significant side effects, allowed the designation of topical etamsylate as a new orphan drug for epistaxis in HHT patients in 2018 (EU/3/10/18/2087) [31].

Table 4. Orphan drugs approved by the EMA for HHT.

Active Substance	Date	EU-Designated Number	Sponsor	Degree of Evidence Clinical Trial
Etamsylate	11/2018	EU/3/10/18/2087	CSIC, Spain	EudraCT: 2016–003982–24
Thalidomide	02/2017	EU/3/17/1845	PlumeStars, S.R.L., Italy	Several clinical trials, Table 3
Bevacizumab	12/2014	EU/3/14/1390	Dupuis-Girod, France	Several clinical trials, Table 3
Bazedoxifene	11/2014	EU/3/14/1367	CSIC, Spain	Observational study, 5 patients
Raloxifene	06/2010	EU/3/10/730	CSIC, Spain	Observational study, 19 patients

4. Conclusions

The currently available pharmacological treatments for HHT are summarized according to their mechanism of action on Figure 3. The drugs here included may be used on an individual level; treatment for rare diseases should follow the premises of personalized medicine, relying on the reference doctor expertise. A first-line treatment to avoid or decrease epistaxis or GI bleeding is to reinforce the speed and stability of coagulation with antifibrinolytics, preferentially TA. The only contraindication may apply to patients with risk of thrombosis. Doses vary from 1.5 g/day up to 3 g/day in episodes of severe bleeding. In countries where TA is not commercially available, AC could be used instead.

For bleedings interfering with normal life, currently the best treatment option for women in fertile age are feminine hormones used for contraception. Women in peri- or post-menopausal age can benefit from the use of SERMs. Although SERMs are primarily used to prevent or treat osteoporosis, they have shown to be effective in HHT compensating partially, the haploinsufficiency present in HHT patients by increasing the protein levels of endoglin and ALK1. Raloxifene hydrochloride was designated as orphan drug by the EMA and by the FDA. Bazedoxifene acetate was also designated as orphan drug by the EMA but it is not commercialized in United States.

Among the list of drugs that increase the expression levels of endoglin and ACVRL1/ALK1, tacrolimus was demonstrated to activate the signaling of endoglin/ALK1 in ECs. It would be the treatment of choice for immunosuppression in transplanted patients. However, recent case reports have opened the possibility of using systemic tacrolimus at low, non-immunosuppressive doses, to treat HHT bleeding. Currently, around 25 patients are using tacrolimus as an "off-label" treatment and it will be very interesting to hear about the outcome of these patients. Other treatment includes NAC which increases the endoglin RNA and protein levels and can be used as an anti-inflammatory and antioxidant drug without any side effects.

BZ is used (off-label) for antiangiogenic strategy in HHT patients with severe bleeding or symptomatic liver AVMs, in order to reduce bleedings and excessive number of abnormal mucosa vessels. TKIs (pazopanib, nintenadib, sunitinib or buparlisib) and thalidomide have also been used or are planned to be used in clinical trials [22,83,101,102] (Table 3).

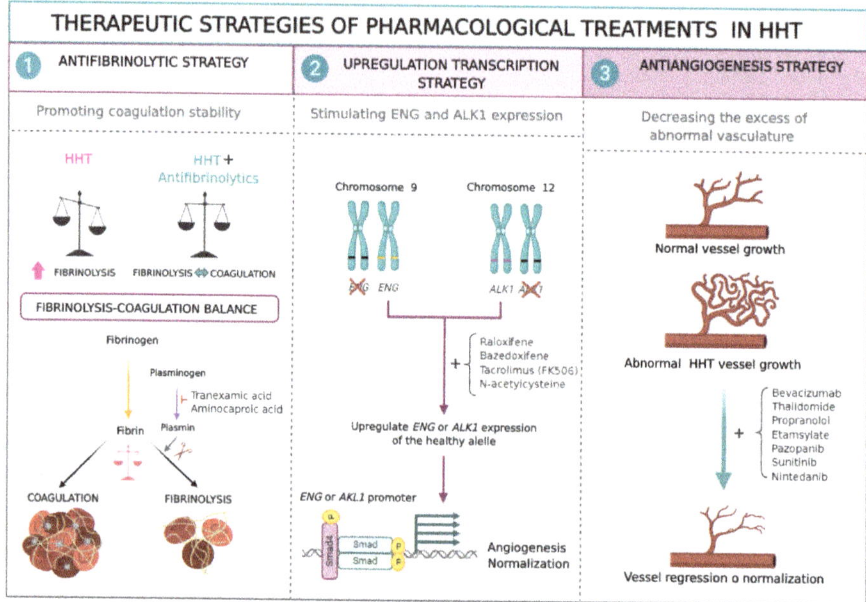

Figure 3. Therapeutic strategies of pharmacological treatments in HHT. (1) Antifibrinolytic strategy; prevents the conversion of plasminogen to plasmin, thus delaying the lysis of the fibrin clot, and therefore the bleeding. (2) Upregulation strategy. The drug works by increasing the expression of the *ENG* or *ALK1* genes, and thus resulting in increased amount of proteins, improving the BMP/TGF-β signaling and normalizing the formation of new vessels. (3) Antiangiogenesis strategy; makes disappear the excess of existing abnormal vasculature or normalizes it.

Another group of antiangiogenic drugs comprises the non-selective adrenergic β-blockers like propranolol and timolol. These drugs are preferentially used topically, as creams or gels. They reduce nose bleedings by decreasing and delaying the formation of telangiectases on the mucosa. Propranolol can also be used systemically, but special attention is indicated with regards to blood pressure and heart rate.

Lastly, as emerging treatments, the orphan drug designation of etamsylate for topical treatment of epistaxis opens a new perspective following the antiangiogenic strategy.

This review has delved into the various treatment strategies of HHT and the clinical trials that support these treatments. The repurposing strategy has led to the formal approval of several orphan drugs for HHT (Table 4).

Author Contributions: L.M.B. designed the project. L.M.B. wrote the manuscript with the contribution of V.A., A.M.C., E.G.-V., I.d.R.-P., and L.R.-P., V.A. and A.M.C. designed the figures. V.A., A.M.C., E.G.-V., I.d.R.-P., L.R.-P., proofread the text. C.B. revised the manuscript and provided funding. L.M.B. supervised the project and provided funding. All authors discussed the results and contributed to the final manuscript. All authors have read and agreed to the published version of the manuscript.

Funding: This research was funded by Ministry of Economy and Competitivity, grant number SAF2017-83351-R to L.M.B.

Acknowledgments: In memoriam of José Sánchez Andújar, who passed away on 22 May 2020. He was a founder member and the first President of the Spanish Association of HHT patients.

Conflicts of Interest: The authors declare no conflict of interest.

Abbreviations

AC	Aminocaproic acid
ACVRL1/ALK1	Activin Receptor-Like Kinase 1
AVM	Arteriovenous Malformation
BMP9	Bone Morphogenetic Protein 9
BZ	Bevacizumab
CM	Capillary Malformation
CYP2D6	Cytochrome P450 2D6
ECs	Endothelial Cells
EMA	European Medicine Agency
ENG	Endoglin
EPHB4	Ephrin Type-B Receptor 4
ER	Estrogen Receptor
ESS	Epistaxis Severity Score
FDA	Food and Drug Administration
FGF	Fibroblast Growth Factor
FK506	Tacrolimus
GI	Gastrointestinal
HHT	Hereditary Hemorrhagic Telangiectasia
iKO	inducible Knockout
JPHT	Juvenile Polyposis/HHT
MADH4/Smad4	Mothers Against Decapentaplegic Homolog 4
mRNA	messenger Ribonucleic Acid
NAC	N-acetylcysteine
OLT	Orthotopic Liver Transplant
OPG	Osteoprotegerin
PDGF	Platelet Derived Growth Factor
RANK	Receptor Activator of Nuclear Factor κ B
RANK-L	Receptor Activator of Nuclear Factor κ B Ligand
RASA1	RAS P21 Protein Activator 1
SERMs	Selective Estrogen Receptor Modulator
TA	Tranexamic Acid
TFRE	Transcription Factor Regulatory Element
TGF-β	Transforming Growth Factor β
VEGF	Vascular Endothelial Growth Factor
VM	Venous Malformation

References

1. Shovlin, C.L.; Guttmacher, A.E.; Buscarini, E.; Faughnan, M.E.; Hyland, R.H.; Westermann, C.J.J.; Kjeldsen, A.D.; Plauchu, H. Diagnostic criteria for Hereditary Hemorrhagic Telangiectasia (Rendu-Osler-Weber Syndrome). *Am. J. Med. Genet.* **2000**, *91*, 66–67. [CrossRef]
2. Shovlin, C.L. Hereditary haemorrhagic telangiectasia: Pathophysiology, diagnosis and treatment. *Blood Rev.* **2010**, *24*, 203–219. [CrossRef]
3. Shovlin, C.L. Pulmonary arteriovenous malformations. *Am. J. Respir. Crit. Care Med.* **2014**, *190*, 1217–1228. [CrossRef] [PubMed]
4. Kjeldsen, A.D.; Vase, P.; Green, A. Hereditary haemorrhagic telangiectasia: A population-based study of prevalence and mortality in Danish patients. *J. Intern. Med.* **1999**, *245*, 31–39. [CrossRef] [PubMed]
5. Jessurun, G.A.J.; Kamphuis, D.J.; Van der Zande, F.H.R.; Nossent, J.C. Cerebral arteriovenous malformations in the Netherlands Antilles. High prevalence of hereditary hemorrhagic telangiectasia-related single and multiple cerebral arteriovenous malformations. *Clin. Neurol. Neurosurg.* **1993**, *95*, 193–198. [CrossRef]
6. McAllister, K.A.; Grogg, K.M.; Johnson, D.W.; Gallione, C.J.; Baldwin, M.A.; Jackson, C.E.; Helmbold, E.A.; Markel, D.S.; McKinnon, W.C.; Murrel, J.; et al. Endoglin, a TGF-β binding protein of endothelial cells, is the gene for hereditary haemorrhagic telangiectasia type 1. *Nat. Genet.* **1994**, *8*, 345–351. [CrossRef]
7. Johnson, D.W.; Berg, J.N.; Baldwin, M.A.; Gallione, C.J.; Marondel, I.; Yoon, S.J.; Stenzel, T.T.; Speer, M.; Pericak-Vance, M.A.; Diamond, A.; et al. Mutations in the activin receptor-like kinase 1 gene in hereditary haemorrhagic telangiectasia type. *Nat. Genet.* **1996**, *13*, 189–195. [CrossRef]

8. Gallione, C.J.; Repetto, G.M.; Legius, E.; Rustgi, A.K.; Schelley, S.L.; Tejpar, S.; Mitchell, G.; Drouin, É.; Westermann, C.J.J.; Marchuk, D.A. A combined syndrome of juvenile polyposis and hereditary haemorrhagic telangiectasia associated with mutations in MADH4 (SMAD4). *Lancet.* **2004**, *363*, 852–859. [CrossRef]

9. Duan, X.Y.; Guo, D.C.; Regalado, E.S.; Shen, H.; Coselli, J.S.; Estrera, A.L.; Safi, H.J.; Bamshad, M.J.; Nickerson, D.A.; LeMaire, S.A.; et al. SMAD4 rare variants in individuals and families with thoracic aortic aneurysms and dissections. *Eur. J. Hum. Genet.* **2019**, *27*, 1054–1060. [CrossRef]

10. Cole, S.G.; Begbie, M.E.; Wallace, G.M.F.; Shovlin, C.L.L. A new locus for hereditary haemorrhagic telangiectasia (HHT3) maps to chromosome 5. *J. Med. Genet.* **2005**, *42*, 577–582. [CrossRef]

11. Bayrak-Toydemir, P.; McDonald, J.; Akarsu, N.; Toydemir, R.M.; Calderon, F.; Tuncali, T.; Tang, W.; Miller, F.; Mao, R. A fourth locus for hereditary hemorrhagic telangiectasia maps to chromosome 7. *Am. J. Med. Genet. A* **2006**, *140*, 2155–2162. [CrossRef] [PubMed]

12. Wooderchak-Donahue, W.L.; McDonald, J.; O'Fallon, B.; Upton, P.D.; Li, W.; Roman, B.L.; Young, S.; Plant, P.; Fülöp, G.T.; Langa, C.; et al. BMP9 mutations cause a vascular-anomaly syndrome with phenotypic overlap with hereditary hemorrhagic telangiectasia. *Am. J. Hum. Genet.* **2013**, *93*, 530–537. [CrossRef] [PubMed]

13. Bayrak-Toydemir, P.; Stevenson, D. Capillary Malformation-Arteriovenous Malformation Syndrome. In *GeneReviews®*; Adam, M.P., Ardinger, H.H., Pagon, R.A., Wallace, S.E., Eds.; University of Washington: Seattle, WA, USA, 1993. [PubMed]

14. Morales-Angulo, C.; Del Valle-Zapico, A. Hereditary hemorrhagic telangiectasia. *Otolaryngol. Head Neck Surg.* **1998**, *119*, 293. [PubMed]

15. AAssar, O.S.; Friedman, C.M.; White, R.I. The Natural History of Epistaxis in Hereditary Hemorrhagic Telangiectasia. *Laryngoscope* **1991**, *101*, 977–980. [CrossRef] [PubMed]

16. Geisthoff, U.W.; Schneider, G.; Fischinger, J.; Plinkert, P.K. Hereditäre hämorrhagische teleangiektasie (Morbus Osler). Eine interdisziplinäre herausforderung. *HNO* **2002**, *50*, 114–128. [CrossRef] [PubMed]

17. Guttmacher, A.E.; Marchuk, D.A.; White, R.I. Hereditary hemorrhagic telangiectasia. *N. Engl. J. Med.* **1995**, *333*, 918–924. [CrossRef]

18. Ingrosso, M.; Sabbà, C.; Pisani, A.; Principi, M.; Gallitelli, M.; Cirulli, A.; Francavilla, A. Evidence of small-bowel involvement in hereditary hemorrhagic telangiectasia: A capsule-endoscopic study. *Endoscopy* **2004**, *36*, 1074–1079. [CrossRef]

19. Vase, P.; Grove, O. Gastrointestinal Lesions in Hereditary Hemorrhagic Telangiectasia. *Gastroenterology* **1986**, *91*, 1079–1083. [CrossRef]

20. Snellings, D.A.; Gallione, C.J.; Clark, D.S.; Vozoris, N.T.; Faughnan, M.E.; Marchuk, D.A. Somatic Mutations in Vascular Malformations of Hereditary Hemorrhagic Telangiectasia Result in Bi-allelic Loss of ENG or ACVRL1. *Am. J. Hum. Genet.* **2019**, *105*, 894–906. [CrossRef]

21. Kasthuri, R.S.; Montifar, M.; Nelson, J.; Kim, H.; Lawton, M.T.; Faughnan, M.E. Prevalence and predictors of anemia in hereditary hemorrhagic telangiectasia. *Am. J. Hematol.* **2017**, *92*, E591–E593. [CrossRef]

22. Robert, F.; Desroches-Castan, A.; Bailly, S.; Dupuis-Girod, S.; Feige, J.J. Future treatments for hereditary hemorrhagic telangiectasia. *Orphanet J. Rare. Dis.* **2020**, *15*, 4. [CrossRef] [PubMed]

23. Pérez Del Molino, A.; Zarrabeitia, R.; Fernández-L, A.; Botella, L.M. Efficacy of tranexamic acid in a patient with hereditary haemorrhagic telangiectasia and massive epistaxis. *Med. Clin. (Barc.)* **2004**, *123*, 118–119. [CrossRef]

24. Fernandez-L, A.; Garrido-Martin, E.M.; Sanz-Rodriguez, F.; Ramirez, J.R.; Moralez-Angulo, C.; Zarrabeltia, R.; Perez-Molino, A.; Bernabéu, C.; Botella, L.M. Therapeutic action of tranexamic acid in hereditary haemorrhagic telangiectasia (HHT): Regulation of ALK-I/endoglin pathway in endothelial cells. *Thromb. Haemost.* **2007**, *97*, 254–262. [CrossRef] [PubMed]

25. Albiñana, V.; Bernabeu-Herrero, M.E.; Zarrabeitia, R.; Bernabeu, C.; Botella, L.M. Estrogen therapy for hereditary haemorrhagic telangiectasia (HHT): Effects of raloxifene, on Endoglin and ALK1 expression in endothelial cells. *Thromb. Haemost.* **2010**, *103*, 525–534. [CrossRef] [PubMed]

26. Zarrabeitia, R.; Ojeda-Fernandez, L.; Recio, L.; Bernabéu, C.; Parra, J.A.; Albiñana, V.; Botella, L.M. Bazedoxifene, a new orphan drug for the treatment of bleeding in hereditary haemorrhagic telangiectasia. *Thromb. Haemost.* **2016**, *115*, 1167–1177. [CrossRef]

27. Dupuis-Girod, S.; Ginon, I.; Saurin, J.C.; Marion, D.; Guillot, E.; Decullier, E.; Roux, A.; Carette, M.F.; Gilbert-Dussardier, B.; Hatron, P.Y.; et al. Bevacizumab in patients with hereditary hemorrhagic telangiectasia and severe hepatic vascular malformations and high cardiac output. *JAMA J. Am. Med. Assoc.* **2012**, *307*, 948–955. [CrossRef]

28. Whitehead, K.J.; Sautter, N.B.; McWilliams, J.P.; Chakinala, M.M.; Merlo, C.A.; Johnson, M.H.; James, M.; Everett, E.M.; Clancy, M.S.; Faughnan, M.E.; et al. Effect of topical intranasal therapy on epistaxis frequency in patients with hereditary hemorrhagic telangiectasia: A randomized clinical trial. *JAMA J. Am. Med. Assoc.* **2016**, *316*, 943–951. [CrossRef]

29. Dupuis-Girod, S.; Ambrun, A.; Decullier, E.; Fargeton, A.E.; Roux, A.; Bréant, V.; Colombet, B.; Rivière, S.; Cartier, C.; Lacombe, P.; et al. Effect of bevacizumab nasal spray on epistaxis duration in hereditary hemorrhagic telangectasia: A randomized clinical trial. *JAMA J. Am. Med. Assoc.* **2016**, *316*, 934–942. [CrossRef]

30. Albiñana, V.; Recio-Poveda, L.; Zarrabeitia, R.; Bernabéu, C.; Botella, L.M. Propranolol as antiangiogenic candidate for the therapy of hereditary haemorrhagic telangiectasia. *Thromb. Haemost.* **2012**, *108*, 41–53. [CrossRef]

31. Albiñana, V.; Giménez-Gallego, G.; García-Mato, A.; Palacios, P.; Recio-Poveda, L.; Cuesta, A.-M.; Patier, J.-L.; Botella, L.-M. Topically Applied Etamsylate: A New Orphan Drug for HHT-Derived Epistaxis (Antiangiogenesis through FGF Pathway Inhibition). *TH Open* **2019**, *3*, e230–e243. [CrossRef]

32. Geisthoff, U.W.; Seyfert, U.T.; Kübler, M.; Bieg, B.; Plinkert, P.K.; König, J. Treatment of epistaxis in hereditary hemorrhagic telangiectasia with tranexamic acid—A double blind placebo-controlled cross-over phase IIIB study. *Thromb. Res.* **2014**, *134*, 565–571. [CrossRef] [PubMed]

33. Yaniv, E.; Preis, M.; Hadar, T.; Shvero, J.; Haddad, M. Antiestrogen therapy for Hereditary hemorrhagic telangiectasia: A double-blind placebo-controlled clinical trial. *Laryngoscope* **2009**, *119*, 284–288. [CrossRef] [PubMed]

34. Gaillard, S.; Dupuis-Girod, S.; Boutitie, F.; Rivière, S.; Morinière, S.; Hatron, P.Y.; Manfredi, G.; Kaminsky, P.; Capitaine, A.L.; Roy, P.; et al. Tranexamic acid for epistaxis in hereditary hemorrhagic telangiectasia patients: A European cross-over controlled trial in a rare disease. *J. Thromb. Haemost.* **2014**, *12*, 1494–1502. [CrossRef] [PubMed]

35. Lebrin, F.; Srun, S.; Raymond, K.; Martin, S.; Van Den Brink, S.; Freitas, C.; Bréant, C.; Mathivet, T.; Larrivée, B.; Thomas, J.L.; et al. Thalidomide stimulates vessel maturation and reduces epistaxis in individuals with hereditary hemorrhagic telangiectasia. *Nat. Med.* **2010**, *16*, 420–428. [CrossRef]

36. Riss, D.; Burian, M.; Wolf, A.; Kranebitter, V.; Kaider, A.; Arnoldner, C. Intranasal submucosal bevacizumab for epistaxis in hereditary hemorrhagic telangiectasia: A double-blind, randomized, placebo-controlled trial. *Head Neck.* **2015**, *37*, 783–787. [CrossRef]

37. Dupuis-Girod, S.; Ambrun, A.; Decullier, E.; Samson, G.; Roux, A.; Fargeton, A.E.; Rioufol, C.; Schwiertz, V.; Disant, F.; Chapuis, F.; et al. ELLIPSE Study: A Phase 1 study evaluating the tolerance of bevacizumab nasal spray in the treatment of epistaxis in hereditary hemorrhagic telangiectasia. *MAbs* **2014**, *6*, 794–799. [CrossRef]

38. Shovlin, C.L.; Gilson, C.; Busbridge, M.; Patel, D.; Shi, C.; Dina, R.; Abdulla, F.N.; Awan, I. Can Iron Treatments Aggravate Epistaxis in Some Patients With Hereditary Hemorrhagic Telangiectasia? *Laryngoscope* **2016**, *126*, 2468–2474. [CrossRef]

39. Lee, J.M.; Wu, V.; Faughnan, M.E.; Lasso, A.; Figol, A.; Kilty, S.J. Prospective pilot study of Floseal® for the treatment of anterior epistaxis in patients with hereditary hemorrhagic telangiectasia (HHT). *J. Otolaryngol. Head Neck Surg.* **2019**, *48*, 48. [CrossRef]

40. Dupuis-Girod, S.; Pitiot, V.; Bergerot, C.; Fargeton, A.E.; Beaudoin, M.; Decullier, E.; Bréant, V.; Colombet, B.; Philouze, P.; Faure, F.; et al. Efficacy of TIMOLOL nasal spray as a treatment for epistaxis in hereditary hemorrhagic telangiectasia. A double-blind, randomized, placebo-controlled trial. *Sci. Rep.* **2019**, *9*, 1986. [CrossRef]

41. Kroon, S.; Snijder, R.J.; Mager, J.J.; Post, M.C.; Tenthof van Noorden, J.; Van Geenen, E.J.M.; Drenth, J.P.H.; Grooteman, K.V. Octreotide for gastrointestinal bleeding in hereditary hemorrhagic telangiectasia: A prospective case series. *Am. J. Hematol.* **2019**, *94*, E247–E249. [CrossRef]

42. Dupuis-Girod, S.; Fargeton, A.-E.; Grobost, V.; Rivière, S.; Beaudoin, M.; Decullier, E.; Bernard, L.; Bréant, V.; Colombet, B.; Philouze, P.; et al. Efficacy and Safety of a 0.1% Tacrolimus Nasal Ointment as a Treatment for Epistaxis in Hereditary Hemorrhagic Telangiectasia: A Double-Blind, Randomized, Placebo-Controlled, Multicenter Trial. *J. Clin. Med.* **2020**, *9*, 1262. [CrossRef] [PubMed]

43. Masoudi-Sobhanzadeh, Y.; Omidi, Y.; Amanlou, M.; Masoudi-Nejad, A. Drug databases and their contributions to drug repurposing. *Genomics* **2020**, *112*, 1087–1095. [CrossRef] [PubMed]

44. Kwaan, H.C.; Silverman, S. Fibrinolytic Activity in Lesions of Hereditary Hemorrhagic Telangiectasia. *Arch. Dermatol.* **1973**, *107*, 571–573. [CrossRef] [PubMed]

45. Watanabe, M.; Hanawa, S.; Morishima, T. Fibrinolytic activity in cutaneous lesions of hereditary hemorrhagic telangiectasia. *Nippon Hifuka Gakkai Zasshi. Jpn. J. Dermatol.* **1985**, *95*, 11–16.

46. Saba, H.I.; Morelli, G.A.; Logrono, L.A. Treatment of bleeding in hereditary hemorrhagic telangiectasia with aminocaproic acid. *N. Engl. J. Med.* **1994**, *330*, 1789–1790. [CrossRef]

47. Annichino-Bizzacchi, J.M.; Facchini, R.M.; Torresan, M.Z.; Arruda, V.R. Hereditary hemorrhagic telangiectasia response to aminocaproic acid treatment. *Thromb. Res.* **1999**, *96*, 73–76. [CrossRef]

48. Korzenik, J.R.; Topazian, M.D.; White, R.; Saba, H.I.; Morelli, G.; Logrono, L. Treatment of bleeding in hereditary hemorrhagic telangiectasia with aminocaproic acid. *N. Engl. J. Med.* **1994**, *331*, 1236.

49. Mannucci, P.M. Hemostatic drugs. *N. Engl. J. Med.* **1998**, *339*, 245–253. [CrossRef]

50. Shovlin, C.L.; Sulaiman, N.L.; Govani, F.S.; Jackson, J.K.; Begbie, M.E. Elevated factor VIII in hereditary haemorrhagic telangiectasia (HHT): Association with venous thromboembolism. *Thromb. Haemost.* **2007**, *98*, 1031–1039.

51. Sabba, C.; Gallitelli, M.; Palasciano, G. Efficacy of unusually high doses of tranexamic acid for the treatment of epistaxis in hereditary hemorrhagic telangiectasia. *N. Engl. J. Med.* **2001**, *345*, 926. [CrossRef]

52. Kearns, A.E.; Khosla, S.; Kostenuik, P.J. Receptor activator of nuclear factor κB ligand and osteoprotegerin regulation of bone remodeling in health and disease. *Endocr. Rev.* **2008**, *29*, 155–192. [CrossRef] [PubMed]

53. Longacre, A.V.; Gross, C.P.; Gallitelli, M.; Henderson, K.J.; White, R.I.; Proctor, D.D. Diagnosis and management of gastrointestinal bleeding in patients with hereditary hemorrhagic telangiectasia. *Am. J. Gastroenterol.* **2003**, *98*, 59–65. [CrossRef] [PubMed]

54. Yaniv, E.; Preis, M.; Shvero, J.; Nageris, B.; Hadar, T. Anti-estrogen therapy for hereditary hemorrhagic telangiectasia—A long-term clinical trial. *Rhinology* **2011**, *49*, 214–216. [CrossRef] [PubMed]

55. Haq, A.U.; Glass, J.; Netchvolodoff, C.V.; Bowen, L.M. Hereditary hemorrhagic telangiectasia and danazol. *Ann. Intern. Med.* **1988**, *109*, 171. [CrossRef]

56. Zacharski, L.R.; Dunbar, S.D.; Newsom, W.A. Hemostatic effects of tamoxifen in hereditary hemorrhagic telangiectasia. *Thromb. Haemost.* **2001**, *85*, 371–372. [PubMed]

57. Nelson, E.R.; Wardell, S.E.; McDonnell, D.P. The molecular mechanisms underlying the pharmacological actions of estrogens, SERMs and oxysterols: Implications for the treatment and prevention of osteoporosis. *Bone* **2013**, *53*, 42–50. [CrossRef]

58. Athar, M.; Back, J.H.; Kopelovich, L.; Bickers, D.R.; Kim, A.L. Multiple molecular targets of resveratrol: Anti-carcinogenic mechanisms. *Arch. Biochem. Biophys.* **2009**, *486*, 95–102. [CrossRef]

59. Park, E.; Lee, S.M.; Jung, I.K.; Lim, Y.; Kim, J.H. Effects of genistein on early-stage cutaneous wound healing. *Biochem. Biophys. Res. Commun.* **2011**, *410*, 514–519. [CrossRef]

60. Albiñana, V.; Sanz-Rodríguez, F.; Recio-Poveda, L.; Bernabéu, C.; Botella, L.M. Immunosuppressor FK506 increases endoglin and activin receptor-like kinase 1 expression and modulates transforming growth factor-β1 signaling in endothelial cells. *Mol. Pharmacol.* **2011**, *79*, 833–843. [CrossRef]

61. Albiñana, V.; Velasco, L.; Zarrabeitia, R.; Botella, L.M. Tacrolimus as a therapeutic drug in hereditary hemorrhagic telangiectasia (HHT). In *Tacrolimus: Effectiveness, Safety and Drug Interactions*; Nova Science Publishers: Hauppauge, NY, USA, 2013; pp. 163–172, ISBN 9781628083668.

62. Skaro, A.I.; Marotta, P.J. Regression of cutaneous and gastrointestinal telangiectasia with sirolimus and aspirin in a patient with hereditary hemorrhagic telangiectasia. *Ann. Intern. Med.* **2006**, *144*, 226–227.

63. Ruiz, S.; Chandakkar, P.; Zhao, H.; Papoin, J.; Chatterjee, P.K.; Christen, E.; Metz, C.N.; Blanc, L.; Campagne, F.; Marambaud, P. Tacrolimus rescues the signaling and gene expression signature of endothelial ALK1 loss-of-function and improves HHT vascular pathology. *Hum. Mol. Genet.* **2017**, *26*, 4786–4798. [CrossRef] [PubMed]

64. Sommer, N.; Droege, F.; Gamen, K.E.; Geisthoff, U.; Gall, H.; Tello, K.; Richter, M.J.; Deubner, L.M.; Schmiedel, R.; Hecker, M.; et al. Treatment with low-dose tacrolimus inhibits bleeding complications in a patient with hereditary hemorrhagic telangiectasia and pulmonary arterial hypertension. *Pulm. Circ.* **2019**, *9*, 2045894018805406. [CrossRef] [PubMed]

65. Hosman, A.; Kroon, S.; Vorselaars, V.; Doef, H.; Post, M.; Snijder, R.; Mager, J. Tacrolimus treatment for two rare complications caused by hereditary haemorrhagic telangiectasia: A description of two cases. *Angiogenesis* **2019**, *22*, 629.

66. De Gussem, E.M.; Snijder, R.J.; Disch, F.J.; Zanen, P.; Westermann, C.J.J.; Mager, J.J. The effect of N-acetylcysteine on epistaxis and quality of life in patients with HHT: A pilot study. *Rhinology* **2009**, *47*, 85–88. [PubMed]

67. Albiñana, V. Ensayos Preclínicos In Vitro con Células Endoteliales, Como Aproximaciones Terapéuticas Farmacológicas Para la Telangiectasia Hemorrágica Hereditaria (HHT). Ph.D. Thesis, Universidad Complutense, Madrid, Spain, 28 June 2012.

68. Roy, H.; Bhardwaj, S.; Ylä-Herttuala, S. Biology of vascular endothelial growth factors. *FEBS Lett.* **2006**, *580*, 2879–2887. [CrossRef]

69. Cirulli, A.; Liso, A.; D'Ovidio, F.; Mestice, A.; Pasculli, G.; Gallitelli, M.; Rizzi, R.; Specchia, G.; Sabbà, C. Vascular endothelial growth factor serum levels are elevated in patients with hereditary hemorrhagic telangiectasia. *Acta Haematol.* **2003**, *110*, 29–32. [CrossRef]

70. Sadick, H.; Riedel, F.; Naim, R.; Goessler, U.; Hörmann, K.; Hafner, M.; Lux, A. Patients with hereditary hemorrhagic telangiectasia have increased plasma levels of vascular endothelial growth factor and transforming growth factor-β1 as well as high ALK1 tissue expression. *Haematologica* **2005**, *90*, 818–828.

71. Peng, H.L.; Hu, G.Y.; Zhang, G.S.; Gong, F.J. Analysis of angiogenesis related proteins and its implication in type-2 hereditary hemorrhagic telangiectasia. *Zhonghua Xue Ye Xue Za Zhi* **2006**, *27*, 616–620.

72. Botella, L.M.; Albiñana, V.; Ojeda-Fernandez, L.; Recio-Poveda, L.; Bernabéu, C. Research on potential biomarkers in hereditary hemorrhagic telangiectasia. *Front. Genet.* **2015**, *6*, 115. [CrossRef]

73. Hurwitz, H.; Fehrenbacher, L.; Novotny, W.; Cartwright, T.; Hainsworth, J.; Heim, W.; Berlin, J.; Baron, A.; Griffing, S.; Holmgren, E.; et al. Bevacizumab plus irinotecan, fluorouracil, and leucovorin for metastatic colorectal cancer. *N. Engl. J. Med.* **2004**, *350*, 2335–2342. [CrossRef]

74. Michels, S.; Rosenfeld, P.J.; Puliafito, C.A.; Marcus, E.N.; Venkatraman, A.S. Systemic bevacizumab (Avastin) therapy for neovascular age-related macular degeneration: Twelve-week results of an uncontrolled open-label clinical study. *Ophthalmology* **2005**, *112*, 1035–1047. [CrossRef] [PubMed]

75. Mitchell, A.; Adams, L.A.; MacQuillan, G.; Tibballs, J.; Vanden Driesen, R.; Delriviere, L. Bevacizumab reverses need for liver transplantation in hereditary hemorrhagic telangiectasia. *Liver Transplant.* **2008**, *14*, 210–213. [CrossRef] [PubMed]

76. Flieger, D.; Hainke, S.; Fischbach, W. Dramatic improvement in hereditary hemorrhagic telangiectasia after treatment with the vascular endothelial growth factor (VEGF) antagonist bevacizumab. *Ann. Hematol.* **2006**, *85*, 631–632. [CrossRef] [PubMed]

77. Dupuis-Girod, S.; Buscarini, E. Hereditary hemorrhagic telangiectasia: To transplant or not to transplant? *Liver Int.* **2016**, *36*, 1741–1744. [CrossRef] [PubMed]

78. Buscarini, E.; Botella, L.M.; Geisthoff, U.; Kjeldsen, A.D.; Mager, H.J.; Pagella, F.; Suppressa, P.; Zarrabeitia, R.; Dupuis-Girod, S.; Shovlin, C.L.; et al. Safety of thalidomide and bevacizumab in patients with hereditary hemorrhagic telangiectasia. *Orphanet. J. Rare Dis.* **2019**, *14*, 28. [CrossRef]

79. Albitar, H.A.; Choby, G.; Pruthi, R.; O'Brien, E.; Stokken, J.; Kamath, P.; Leise, M.; Gallo De Moraes, A.; Cajigas, H.; Dubrock, H.; et al. Intravenous bevacizumab in HHT-related bleeding: Significant inter-individual variability in the need for maintenance therapy. *Angiogenesis* **2019**, *22*, 589–590.

80. Kim, Y.H.; Kim, M.J.; Choe, S.W.; Sprecher, D.; Lee, Y.J.; Oh, S.P. Selective effects of oral antiangiogenic tyrosine kinase inhibitors on an animal model of hereditary hemorrhagic telangiectasia. *J. Thromb. Haemost.* **2017**, *15*, 1095–1102. [CrossRef]

81. Faughnan, M.E.; Gossage, J.R.; Chakinala, M.M.; Oh, S.P.; Kasthuri, R.; Hughes, C.C.W.; McWilliams, J.P.; Parambil, J.G.; Vozoris, N.; Donaldson, J.; et al. Pazopanib may reduce bleeding in hereditary hemorrhagic telangiectasia. *Angiogenesis* **2019**, *22*, 145–155. [CrossRef]

82. Ruiz, S.; Zhao, H.; Chandakkar, P.; Papoin, J.; Choi, H.; Nomura-Kitabayashi, A.; Patel, R.; Gillen, M.; Diao, L.; Chatterjee, P.K.; et al. Correcting Smad1/5/8, mTOR, and VEGFR2 treats pathology in hereditary hemorrhagic telangiectasia models. *Clin. Investig.* **2020**, *130*, 942–957. [CrossRef]

83. Kovacs-Sipos, E.; Holzmann, D.; Scherer, T.; Soyka, M.B. Nintedanib as a novel treatment option in hereditary haemorrhagic telangiectasia. *BMJ. Case. Rep.* **2017**, *2017*, bcr2017219393. [CrossRef]

84. Léauté-Labrèze, C.; De La Roque, E.D.; Hubiche, T.; Boralevi, F.; Thambo, J.B.; Taïeb, A. Propranolol for severe hemangiomas of infancy. *N. Engl. J. Med.* **2008**, *358*, 2649–2651. [CrossRef] [PubMed]

85. Storch, C.H.; Hoeger, P.H. Propranolol for infantile haemangiomas: Insights into the molecular mechanisms of action. *Br. J. Dermatol.* **2010**, *163*, 269–274. [CrossRef] [PubMed]

86. Sánchez-Carpintero, I.; Ruiz-Rodriguez, R.; López-Gutiérrez, J.C. Propranolol in the treatment of infantile hemangioma: Clinical effectiveness, risks, and recommendations. *Actas Dermosifiliogr.* **2011**, *102*, 766–779. [CrossRef] [PubMed]

87. Olitsky, S.E. Topical timolol for the treatment of epistaxis in hereditary hemorrhagic telangiectasia. *Am. J. Otolaryngol. Head Neck Med. Surg.* **2012**, *33*, 375–376. [CrossRef]

88. Ichimura, K.; Kikuchi, H.; Imayoshi, S.; Dias, M.S. Topical application of timolol decreases the severity and frequency of epistaxis in patients who have previously undergone nasal dermoplasty for hereditary hemorrhagic telangiectasia. *Auris Nasus Larynx.* **2016**, *43*, 429–432. [CrossRef]

89. Epperla, N.; Brilliant, M.H.; Vidaillet, H. Topical timolol for treatment of epistaxis in hereditary haemorrhagic telangiectasia associated with bradycardia: A look at CYP2D6 metabolising variants. *BMJ Case. Rep.* **2014**, *2014*, bcr2013203056. [CrossRef]

90. Volotinen, M.; Hakkola, J.; Pelkonen, O.; Vapaatalo, H.; Mäenpää, J. Metabolism of ophthalmic timolol: New aspects of an old drug. *Basic Clin. Pharmacol. Toxicol.* **2011**, *108*, 297–303. [CrossRef]

91. Botella, L.M.; Zarrabeitia, R.; Albinana, V.; Ojeda-Fernández, M.L.; Diez-Gonzalez, V.; Parra-Blanco, J.A. Efficacy of topical timolol for the treatment of mucocutaneous telangiectasias in patients with hereditary haemorrhagic telangiectasia. *Angiogenesis* **2015**, *18*, 594.

92. Mei-Zahav, M.; Blau, H.; Bruckheimer, E.; Zur, E.; Goldschmidt, N. Topical propranolol improves epistaxis in patients with hereditary hemorrhagic telangiectasia—A preliminary report. *J. Otolaryngol. Head Neck Surg.* **2017**, *46*, 58. [CrossRef]

93. Mei-Zahav, M.; Goldschmidt, N.; Bruckheimer, E.; Soudri, E. A double-blind placebo-controlled study assessing the safety and efficacy of topical propranolol for moderate–severe epistaxis in patients with hereditary hemorrhagic telangiectasia (HHT). *Angiogenesis* **2019**, *22*, 597–598.

94. Esteban-Casado, S.; Martín de Rosales Cabrera, A.M.; Usarralde Pérez, A.; Martínez Simón, J.J.; Zhan Zhou, E.; Marcos Salazar, M.S.; Pérez Encinas, M.; Botella Cubells, L. Sclerotherapy and Topical Nasal Propranolol: An Effective and Safe Therapy for HHT-Epistaxis. *Laryngoscope* **2019**, *129*, 2216–2223. [CrossRef] [PubMed]

95. Patier, J.L.; Camacho Aguirre, A.; Sirgo, N.; Gonzalez Nino, I.; Suárez Carantoña, C.; Gonzalez Garcia, A.; López Rodriguez, M.; Botella, L.M. Effectiveness and safety of the treatment with oral propranolol in patients with hereditary hemorrhagic telangiectasia and bloodhypertension or atrial fibrillation: A possible anti-angiogenictreatment in epistaxis. *Angiogenesis* **2019**, *22*, 628.

96. Thomas, K.A.; Rios-Candelore, M.; Gimenez-Gallego, G.; DiSalvo, J.; Bennett, C.; Rodkey, J.; Fitzpatrick, S. Pure brain-derived acidic fibroblast growth factor is a potent angiogenic vascular endothelial cell mitogen with sequence homology to interleukin 1. *Proc. Natl. Acad. Sci. USA* **1985**, *82*, 6409–6413. [CrossRef] [PubMed]

97. Esch, F.; Baird, A.; Ling, N.; Ueno, N.; Hill, F.; Denoroy, L.; Klepper, R.; Gospodarowicz, D.; Böhlen, P.; Guillemin, R. Primary structure of bovine pituitary basic fibroblast growth factor (FGF) and comparison with the amino-terminal sequence of bovine brain acidic FGF. *Proc. Natl. Acad. Sci. USA* **1985**, *82*, 6507–6511. [CrossRef] [PubMed]

98. Hanahan, D.; Weinberg, R.A. Hallmarks of cancer: The next generation. *Cell* **2011**, *144*, 646–674. [CrossRef] [PubMed]

99. Cross, M.J.; Claesson-Welsh, L. FGF and VEGF function in angiogenesis: Signalling pathways, biological responses and therapeutic inhibition. *Trends. Pharmacol. Sci.* **2001**, *22*, 201–207. [CrossRef]

100. Loges, S.; Mazzone, M.; Hohensinner, P.; Carmeliet, P. Silencing or Fueling Metastasis with VEGF Inhibitors: Antiangiogenesis Revisited. *Cancer Cell* **2009**, *15*, 167–170. [CrossRef]

101. Droege, F.; Thangavelu, K.; Lang, S.; Geisthoff, U. Improvement in hereditary hemorrhagic telangiectasia after treatment with the multi-kinase inhibitor Sunitinib. *Ann. Hematol.* **2016**, *95*, 2077–2078. [CrossRef]

102. Geisthoff, U.W.; Nguyen, H.L.P.; Hess, D. Improvement in hereditary hemorrhagic telangiectasia after treatment with the phosphoinositide 3-kinase inhibitor BKM120. *Ann. Hematol.* **2014**, *93*, 703–704. [CrossRef]

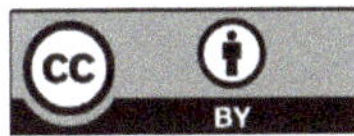

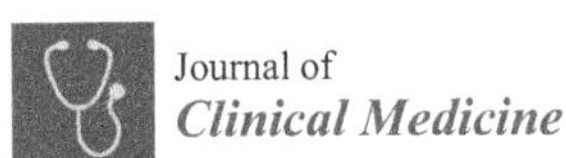

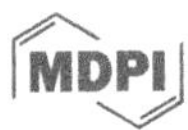

Journal of
Clinical Medicine

Article

Efficacy and Safety of a 0.1% Tacrolimus Nasal Ointment as a Treatment for Epistaxis in Hereditary Hemorrhagic Telangiectasia: A Double-Blind, Randomized, Placebo-Controlled, Multicenter Trial

Sophie Dupuis-Girod [1,2,*], Anne-Emmanuelle Fargeton [1], Vincent Grobost [3], Sophie Rivière [4], Marjolaine Beaudoin [1], Evelyne Decullier [5,6], Lorraine Bernard [5], Valentine Bréant [7], Bettina Colombet [7], Pierre Philouze [8], Sabine Bailly [2], Frédéric Faure [9] and Ruben Hermann [9]

[1] Hospices Civils de Lyon, Hôpital Femme-Mère-Enfants, Centre de Référence pour la Maladie de Rendu-Osler, F-69677 Bron, France; anne-emmanuelle.fargeton@chu-lyon.fr (A.-E.F.); marjolaine.beaudoin@chu-lyon.fr (M.B.)

[2] Inserm, CEA, Laboratory Biology of Cancer and Infection, University Grenoble Alpes, F-38000 Grenoble, France; sabine.bailly@cea.fr

[3] Service de Médecine Interne, CHU Estaing, 63100 Clermont-Ferrand, France; vgrobost@chu-clermontferrand.fr

[4] Service de Médecine Interne CHU de Montpellier, Hôpital St Eloi, and Centre d'Investigation Clinique, Inserm, CIC 1411, F-34295 Montpellier CEDEX 7, France; s-riviere@chu-montpellier.fr

[5] Hospices Civils de Lyon, Pôle Santé Publique, F-69003 Lyon, France; evelyne.decullier@chu-lyon.fr (E.D.); lorraine.bernard01@chu-lyon.fr (L.B.)

[6] EA 4129, Faculté de Médecine, Université Lyon 1, 69008 Lyon, France

[7] Hospices Civils de Lyon, Pharmacie, Hôpital Louis Pradel, F-69677 Bron, France; valentine.breant@chu-lyon.fr (V.B.); bettina.colombet@ghnd.fr (B.C.)

[8] Hospices Civils de Lyon, Hôpital de la Croix Rousse, Service ORL, F-69317 Lyon, France; pierre.philouze@chu-lyon.fr

[9] Hospices Civils de Lyon, Hôpital E. Herriot, Service ORL, F-69437 Lyon, France; frederic.faure@chu-lyon.fr (F.F.); ruben.hermann@chu-lyon.fr (R.H.)

*   Correspondence: sophie.dupuis-girod@chu-lyon.fr

Received: 6 April 2020; Accepted: 20 April 2020; Published: 26 April 2020

Abstract: Hereditary hemorrhagic telangiectasia is a rare but ubiquitous genetic disease. Epistaxis is the most frequent and life-threatening manifestation and tacrolimus, an immunosuppressive agent, appears to be an interesting new treatment option because of its anti-angiogenic properties. Our objective was to evaluate, six weeks after the end of the treatment, the efficacy on the duration of nosebleeds of tacrolimus nasal ointment, administered for six weeks to patients with hereditary hemorrhagic telangiectasia complicated by nosebleeds, and we performed a prospective, multicenter, randomized, placebo-controlled, double-blinded, ratio 1:1 phase II study. Patients were recruited from three French Hereditary Hemorrhagic Telangiectasia (HHT) centers between May 2017 and August 2018, with a six-week follow-up, and we included people aged over 18 years, diagnosed with hereditary hemorrhagic telangiectasia and epistaxis (total duration > 30 min/6 weeks prior to inclusion). Tacrolimus ointment 0.1% was self-administered by the patients twice daily. About 0.1 g of product was to be administered in each nostril with a cotton swab. A total of 50 patients was randomized and treated. Mean epistaxis duration before and after treatment in the tacrolimus group were 324.64 and 249.14 min, respectively, and in the placebo group 224.69 and 188.14 min, respectively. Epistaxis duration improved in both groups, with no significant difference in our main objective comparing epistaxis before and after treatment ($p = 0.77$); however, there was a significant difference in evolution when comparing epistaxis before and during treatment ($p = 0.04$). Toxicity was low and no severe adverse events were reported. In conclusion, tacrolimus nasal ointment, administered for six weeks, did not improve epistaxis in HHT patients after the end of the treatment. However, the

J. Clin. Med. **2020**, *9*, 1262

good tolerance, associated with a significant improvement in epistaxis duration during treatment, encouraged us to perform a phase 3 trial on a larger patient population with a main outcome of epistaxis duration during treatment and a longer treatment time.

Keywords: hereditary hemorrhagic telangiectasia; epistaxis; nosebleeds; tacrolimus; nasal ointment; genetic disease; rare disease

1. Introduction

HHT is a rare but ubiquitous hereditary vascular disease, with an estimated prevalence of 1/5000 to 1/8000. The ENG (endoglin) and ACVRL1 encoding ALK1 (activin receptor-like kinase 1) genes are responsible for 90% of cases of HHT [1]. These genes both intervene in the BMP9/ALK1/ENG/SMAD pathway in endothelial cells, and it has been hypothesized that HHT is related to disequilibrium in the angiogenic balance, resulting from an increase in the factors involved in the activation phase and a decrease in those involved in the maturation phase of angiogenesis [2].

The recognized manifestations of HHT are all due to abnormalities in vascular structure. Lesions may be cutaneous and/or mucosal telangiectases or visceral arteriovenous malformations (AVMs) in the lungs, liver, and central nervous system [3]. Telangiectases and AVMs vary widely between individuals and even within the same family. Nosebleeds are the most frequent complication in HHT and may occur as often as several times per day. They are spontaneous, very variable in time and from one patient to another, but recurrent in 90% of patients. They can be associated with severe anemia in 2–10% of patients, and blood transfusions are required sometimes or regularly (every 2 or 3 weeks) in 2–5% of patients [4]. These nosebleeds thus significantly reduce quality of life [5].

The incomplete and transient efficacy of nasal surgical therapies has inspired a new search for adjuvant medical treatments which would greatly diminish daily iron loss [6]. For this reason, anti-angiogenic treatments such as intra-venous anti-VEGF treatment (bevacizumab) and thalidomide have been evaluated in clinical studies [7,8], but their use is limited to severe forms of the disease. Furthermore, local bevacizumab administration (nasal spray) recently evaluated in 2 phase 2 studies was not efficient [9,10]. We thus decided to investigate the feasibility and efficacy on epistaxis in HHT of other known anti-angiogenic drugs with a possible nasal administration and absorption that would target and reactivate the altered BMP9/ALK1/ENG/SMAD pathway.

Based on our collaboration with Bailly's group, and on the results obtained by Ruiz et al. [11], working on the repositioning approach developed by screening the libraries of Food and Drug Administration approved drugs that could potentiate the BMP9 signaling response, we concluded that the most promising activating drug was tacrolimus, a potent activator of the BMP9-ALK1-BMPR2-Smad1/5/9 signaling cascade. How tacrolimus activates this pathway is still not completely understood. Tacrolimus (FK506) can bind to FKBP12 (FK-506-binding protein-12), a protein known to interact with the TGF-ß family type I receptors [12]. Tacrolimus binding to FKBP12 leads to FKBP12 dissociation from the type 1 receptors, which can then activate the Smad transcription factors. Alternatively, tacrolimus has also been reported to stimulate endoglin and ALK-1 expression in endothelial cells, and to enhance the TGF-β1/ALK1 signaling pathway and endothelial cell functions such as tubulogenesis and migration [13]. In parallel, preclinical models have shown that injections of tacrolimus decreased the number of retinal arteriovenous malformations induced by BMP9/10-immunodepletion in a mouse HHT model [11]. These results suggest that the mechanism of action of FK506 involves a partial correction of endoglin and ALK1 haplosufficiency, and may therefore be an interesting drug for use in patients with HHT. Furthermore, improvement in epistaxis has been shown in HHT patients after a liver transplant [14], and it has been hypothesized that the immunosuppressive treatment (FK506) used to prevent rejection may have an anti-angiogenic effect.

Topical nasal administration of tacrolimus may be an easy-to-use and non-invasive treatment. In addition, tacrolimus ointment is available on the market as a treatment for eczema and can therefore readily be used for nasal administration. Its tolerability on mucosae has been evaluated in the treatment of chronic plaque psoriasis and oral lichen planus [15–18]. Transient burning sensations have been described in tacrolimus patient groups, but no serious adverse effects necessitating stopping treatment have been recorded. Furthermore, none of the patients showed any abnormality in hematological or biochemical parameters. Data from healthy human subjects indicate that there is little or no systemic exposure to tacrolimus following repeated topical application of tacrolimus ointment. Several studies in infants [19,20] on the pharmacokinetics of tacrolimus after first and repeated application showed minimal systemic exposure (less than 1 ng per mL in all cases) and there was no evidence of systemic accumulation. Further to administration on mucosae, the pharmacokinetics were evaluated in two clinical trials and no systemic absorption was detected [16,18].

For all these reasons, tacrolimus ointment was a good candidate treatment for HHT. Our objective was to evaluate the efficacy on the duration of nosebleeds of tacrolimus nasal ointment in patients with hereditary hemorrhagic telangiectasia complicated by nosebleeds.

2. Materials and Methods

2.1. Trial Design and Treatment

The study was a prospective, phase II multicenter, randomized study, ratio 1:1, carried out in a double-blind setting. It was approved by the local research ethics committee and by the French Medical Products Agency (ANSM) in March 2017. Written informed consent was obtained from all patients in accordance with national regulations. The trial was conducted in accordance with the principles of the Declaration of Helsinki [21] and Good Clinical Practice guidelines. All the authors were involved in designing or conducting the study, and preparing the manuscript, including the decision to submit it for publication. This trial was registered with the ClinicalTrials.gov Identifier #NCT03152019.

The nasal ointment was self-administered by patients, twice daily, for 6 weeks. About 0.1 g of product was to be administered in each nostril. The tube was gently squeezed to extract an amount roughly equivalent to the size of the head of a cotton swab. The ointment was then introduced into each nostril with a cotton swab, and extended into the nostril with a cotton swab or/and by external pressure on the nostril.

Marketed 30 g tubes of Protopic® 0.1% (Léo Pharma, Voisins le Bretonneux, France) were used for this study. For the placebo, the manufacturing and filling were managed by an external pharmaceutical laboratory with GMP accreditation. The placebo formulation was similar to the active ointment; it contained all the ingredients except the active one: tacrolimus. The product was provided in strictly identical tubes. The same masked label was placed on both batches in order to respect the blind.

2.2. Participants

This study enrolled patients over the age of 18 years, with clinically confirmed HHT suffering from epistaxis (more than 30 min during the 6 weeks prior to the time of inclusion justified by completed follow-up grids), and who had not undergone nasal surgery in the 6 weeks prior to inclusion. We did not include women who were pregnant or those likely to become so during the study, or patients with known hypersensitivity to macrolides in general, to tacrolimus or to any of the excipients, or patients who had incompletely filled in the nosebleed grids, or patients with an inherited skin barrier, or with CYP3A4 inhibitor treatment (erythromycin, itraconazole, ketoconazole, and diltiazem), or patients with ongoing immunosuppressive treatment, or with known and symptomatic immune deficiency.

2.3. Patient Information and Follow-Up

Patients were informed and recruited during a standard consultation with the ENT doctor or doctor responsible in the reference center or skill center for HHT, and informed of the study and the need to complete nosebleed grids for ENT monitoring for the 6 weeks prior to the start of the treatment. Patients were included during a consultation at the reference center or skill center for HHT and the treatment was prescribed during the same consultation.

The follow-up consisted of 2 phone calls on days 15 and 31 (i.e., 14 and 30 days after the beginning of the treatment) in order to collect information regarding tolerance and observance, and in visits (with medical and ENT consultations) at the end of the 6 weeks of treatment, and at 6 weeks after the end of the treatment.

2.4. Study End Points

The main outcome was the percentage of patients experiencing an improvement in their nosebleeds. An improvement was defined as a 30% reduction in the total duration of nosebleeds over the 6 weeks following treatment, compared with the duration of the nosebleeds in the 6 weeks before the treatment.

Secondary outcomes were total duration of nosebleeds, number of nosebleeds, and number of red blood cell transfusions before, during, and after treatment, progress in the scores obtained in the SF36 quality of life questionnaire and in the ESS (Epistaxis Severity Score) using data from the specific questionnaire and biological efficacy criteria (hemoglobin and serum ferritin). All were recorded before treatment and at 6 and 12 weeks after the end of the treatment.

2.5. Safety

Safety was evaluated at each visit by means of a physical examination (monitoring of blood pressure, clinical ear, nose, and throat examination to check the nasal septum and other side effects on nasal mucosa), and assessment for adverse events (AE). All AE were coded using the Medical Dictionary for Regulatory Activities (MedDRA). Adverse events were classified by the investigators as unrelated, dubitable, or possibly, probably or certainly related to the treatment. Monitoring the safety of administration of the product, motivated by the iatrogenic risks, justified the setting up of a specific independent monitoring and safety committee. The committee met in particular in the case of the occurrence of serious adverse events and gave its recommendations on the continuation of the study after collection of adverse events and observance of the treatment after 30 days for the first 8 patients included. It was composed of a specialist of the disease not involved in the study, an ENT specialist, and a statistician specialized in the methodology of clinical trials.

Systemic absorption of tacrolimus was evaluated by means of FK506 dosages in blood samples 8, 22, and 43 days after the beginning of the treatment. No systemic absorption and effects were expected, but, in case of a positive dosage of 5 ng/mL or more, it was decided that the laboratory would immediately inform the investigator in order to ask the patient to stop the treatment.

2.6. Sample Size Calculation

We hypothesized that 60% of patients would be improved in the treatment group against 15% in the placebo group. It was therefore necessary to include 22 patients in each group to reach an 80% power with a 5% alpha (bilateral), leading to 44 patients overall (Fisher exact test).

Taking into account early withdrawal and patients who may be lost to follow-up, we planned to include 24 patients in each group, that is to say, a total of 48 patients.

2.7. Randomization

The randomization process was centralized. Patients were randomized by blocks of 4 and unstratified. Allocation of a randomization arm to an included patient was made by IWRS (Interactive Web Response System), on the basis of a unique randomization list for all investigation centers. The randomization list was pre-established, by the "Pole IMER" at the Hospices Civils de Lyon–Clinical Research Unit. Clinsight software version 7.1 (Ennov Clinical®, Paris, France) was used to manage this study. After verifying the inclusion criteria, the investigator connected to the platform to create the list of patients. Once the inclusion criteria had been validated, the patient was randomized and a treatment code was allocated by the system. The treatment was then dispensed by the pharmacy at the Hospital Center. This was a double-blind study in which neither the patient nor the investigator was aware of the nature of the treatment administered.

2.8. Statistical Methods

Populations: 2 populations were defined. The per protocol population, which was set at 70% adherence, consisted of all patients receiving at least 60 ointment treatments of the 84 planned. The intention-to-treat (ITT) population consisted of all randomized patients starting the treatment, and patients were considered in their randomization group. All analyses were performed on the ITT populations; the main outcome was also analyzed on the per protocol population.

Initial characteristics of the patients were summarized by means of descriptive statistics (number, average, standard deviation, median, minimum, and maximum for the quantitative variables, and numbers and percentages for the qualitative variables).

Analysis of the main outcome: the percentage of patients experiencing improvement in their nosebleeds was computed in each group. The percentage was compared between groups using a Chi^2 test (or Fisher exact test if the conditions for Chi^2 were not fulfilled), and the analysis was performed on the intention-to-treat population and on the per protocol population. Patients who stopped the treatment but who had filled in epistaxis grids were analyzed using their data. Patients who withdraw from the study before completing the follow-up were considered as failures.

Analysis of the secondary outcomes: the percentage of patients with at least one adverse event was computed and compared between the 2 groups. Quantitative parameters were presented as mean ± standard deviation and median (minimum and maximum) for all groups and were compared using the Student *t*-test (or Mann–Whitney test in case of non-normality). Qualitative parameters at inclusion were presented in terms of number (percentage) and compared using the Chi^2 test (or Fisher exact test where conditions for the Chi^2 test were not fulfilled). Mixed models were produced to compare evolution between the groups.

All analyses were performed using SAS software version 9.4 (SAS Institute Inc., Cary, NC, USA). Effect sizes were computed as risk difference (Chan–Zhan 95% CI) and relative risks for binary outcomes, and as Cohen's d for quantitative outcomes.

2.9. Missing Data

The main outcome was based on grids that were filled in daily. If one day was missing, the value was replaced by an average of the 4 values before and the 4 values after the missing value. This strategy was applied up to 7 missing values over 6 weeks (i.e., 10%). If more than 7 days and less than 21 days (included) were missing, a daily average was computed from the data available (from the 6-week period evaluated) and multiplied by 42 to estimate epistaxis duration. If a patient was lost to follow-up or refused to communicate his nosebleed grids or had more than 21 days missing on his grids, the result for the patient concerned was considered as a failure.

3. Results

3.1. Trial Population

After screening 155 patients, 50 patients were included and randomized between May 2017 and August 2018 in three different centers (Lyon, Clermont-Ferrand, and Montpellier). The baseline characteristics are summarized in Table 1. All individuals except one met the inclusion criteria and were enrolled in the study. Due to one wrong allocation in the placebo group and to one wrong inclusion, the independent committee recommended that it was necessary to include two more patients (50 instead of the 48 patients initially scheduled) (Figure 1). One patient in the placebo group discontinued his follow-up due to a severe adverse event. All patients in the tacrolimus group filled in the epistaxis grids and completed six weeks of treatment. Twenty-five patients in the placebo group filled in the epistaxis grids and out of them 24 completed six weeks of placebo treatment.

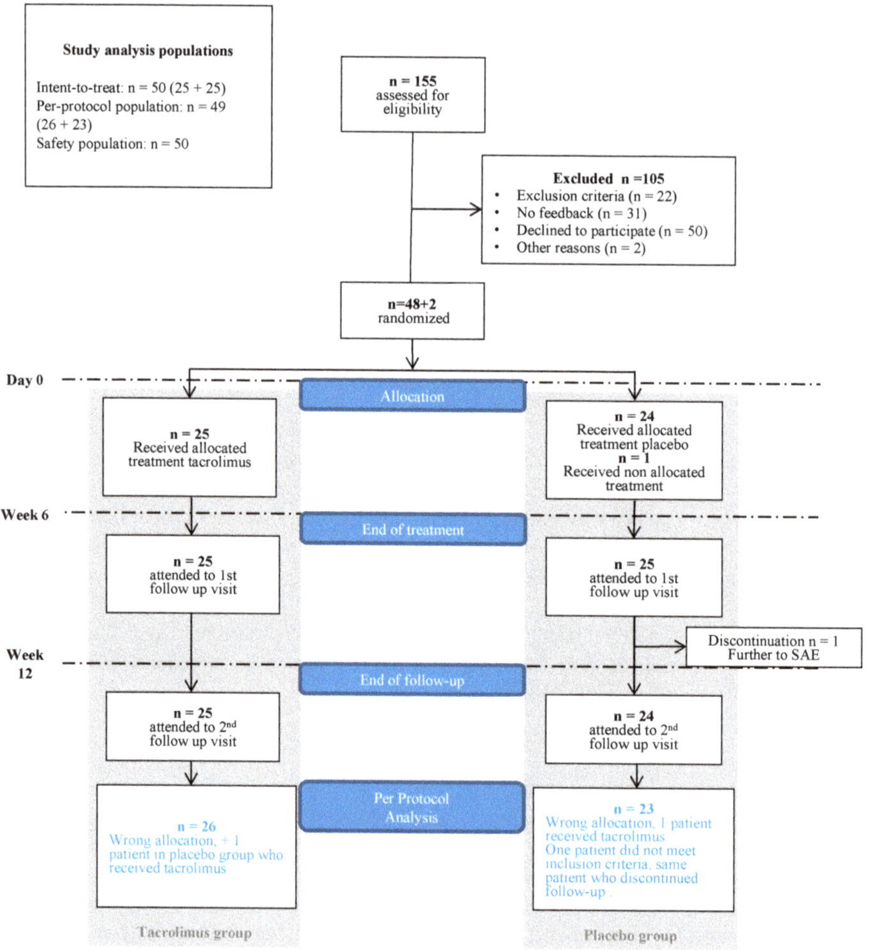

Figure 1. Flow chart.

Table 1. Patient characteristics before treatment.

Variable	Modality	All	Tacro Group n (%)	Placebo Group n (%)
Number	n	50	25	25
Age (years)	Median (min–max) Mean (SD)	62 (27–85) 60.92 (11.26)	60 (27–81) 59.04 (12.26)	64 (39–85) 62.8 (10.06)
Females	n (%)	23 (46)	9 (36)	14 (56)
Mutated gene ALK1 ENG On-going Not known	n (%)	36 (72) 10 (20) 2 (4) 2 (4)	20 (80) 5 (20)	16 (64) 5 (20) 2 (8) 2 (8)
Blood transfusions in the last 6 weeks before inclusion	n (%)	2 (4)	0 (0)	2 (8)
Parameters on inclusion (D0)				
Nasal surgery	n (%)	35 (70)	21 (84)	14 (56)
Nasal septum perforation	n (%)	7 (14.3)	3 (12.5)	4 (16)
Hemoglobin level (g/dL)	Mean ± SD Median (Min–Max)	126.62 (22.66) 130 (66–163)	127.6 (20.82) 129 (90–163)	125.64 (24.75) 130 (66–158)
Ferritin level (ng/mL)	Mean ± SD Median (Min–Max)	50.12 (73.7) 28 (4–458)	51.28 (94.79) 23 (4–458)	48.96 (45.83) 33 (6–174)
Systolic blood pressure (mmHg)	Mean ± SD Median (Min–Max)	130.7 (20.98) 126.5 (100–181)	133.16 (16.5) 130 (110–163)	128.24 (24.78) 124 (100–181)
Diastolic blood pressure (mmHg)	Mean ± SD Median (Min–Max)	80.24 (16.32) 80 (28–129)	82.2 (11.42) 80 (60–105)	78.28 (20.13) 80 (28–129)

3.2. Response to Treatment

3.2.1. Primary Outcome

All patients in the intention-to-treat population were analyzed ($n = 50$). The results are summarized in Table 2. According to our main outcome (30% reduction in the total duration of epistaxis over six weeks after treatment), no statistical difference was observed in the tacrolimus groups compared to the placebo group. Analysis of the per protocol population led to the same conclusions.

Table 2. Main outcome ($n = 50$) analysis: Efficacy of tacrolimus ointment on mean epistaxis duration six weeks before and after treatment.

Variable	Modality	All	Tacro Group n (%)	Placebo Group n (%)	p-Value	Effect Size *
Epistaxis duration decrease > 30% (ITT)	No Yes	31 (62) 19 (38)	15 (60) 10 (40)	16 (64) 9 (36)	0.77	RD 4.0 (−23.4–31.2) RR 1.11 (0.55–2.26)
Epistaxis duration decrease > 30% (PP)	No Yes	30 (61.2) 19 (38.8)	16 (61.5) 10 (38.5)	14 (60.9) 9 (39.1)	0.96	RD −1.0 (−28.2–28.0) RR 0.98 (0.49–1.99)
Other data related to primary outcome						
Epistaxis total duration 6 weeks before treatment (min)	n median (min–max) Mean (SD)	50 226.5 (11–1116) 274.67 (239.24)	25 240 (46–1116) 324.64 (292.06)	25 226 (11–510.8) 224.69 (162.35)	0.34	−0.42 (−1.00–0.15)
Epistaxis total duration 6 weeks immediately after the end of the treatment (min)	n median (min–max) Mean (SD)	49 170 (1–1058) 219.26 (213.72)	25 177 (16–1058) 249.14 (252.7)	24 114.5 (1–547) 188.14 (163.43)	0.42	−0.29 (−0.86–0.29)

Legends: * risk difference (RD) and relative risks (RR) for binary outcomes; and Cohen's d for quantitatives.

3.2.2. Secondary Outcomes

Duration and number of nosebleeds before, during, and after treatment are presented in Figure 2. As for percentage of improvement, there was no difference between the tacrolimus group and the placebo group regarding evolution in the parameters during the six weeks following treatment. However, there was a difference in evolution when comparing epistaxis before and during treatment in terms of epistaxis duration ($p = 0.04$, Cohen's d: 0.53 (–0.04–1.11) and epistaxis number ($p = 0.04$, Cohen's d: 0.39 (–0.19–0.96)) (Figure 2).

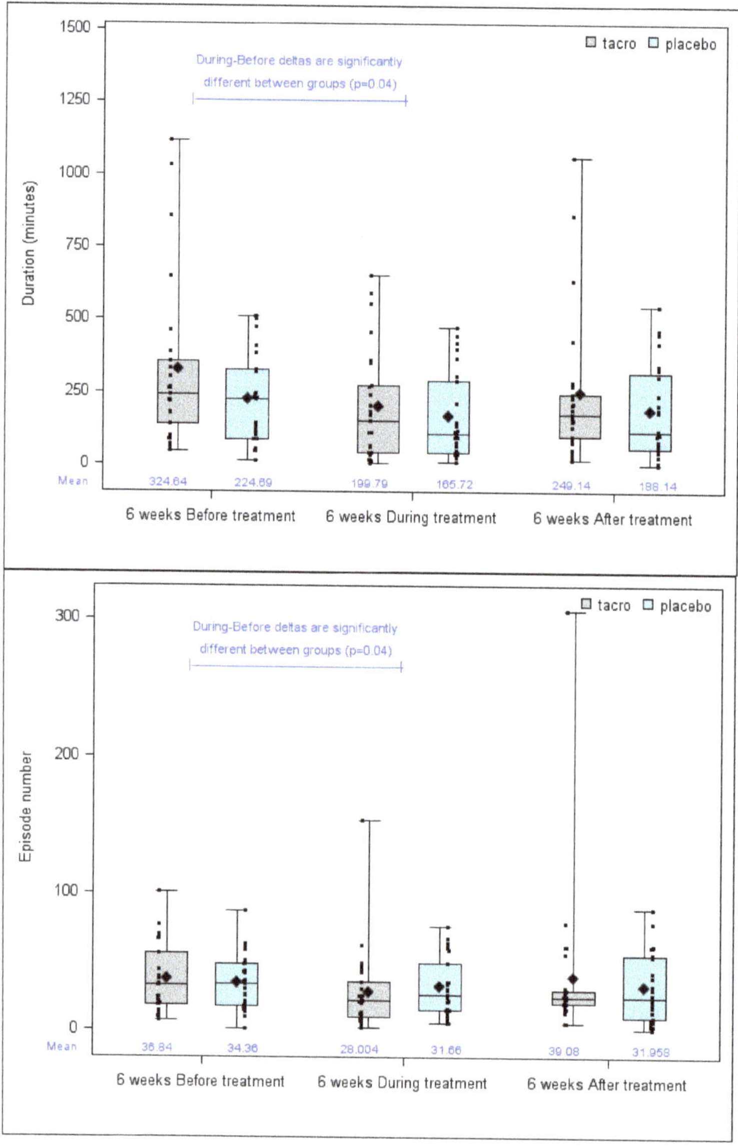

Figure 2. Mean epistaxis duration and number on six weeks before, during and after treatment. Legends: Lines from bottom to top: minimum, 25th percentile, median, 75th percentile and maximum. Diamond: mean. Small squares: individual data.

The number of red blood cell transfusions did not differ before and during treatment ($p = 0.57$, Cohen's d: -0.21 (-0.77–0.36)), or before and after treatment ($p = 0.69$, Cohen's d: -0.23 (-0.8–0.34)). Three patients had blood transfusions before treatment and all of them were in the placebo group. Of them, two patients also had blood transfusions during treatment.

The SF-36 questionnaire revealed no differences in the dimensions of quality of life before, during, and after treatment (Table 3).

The difference in the ESS after and before treatment in the tacrolimus group (mean = -0.43 (SD = 1.47)) and the placebo group (mean = -0.26 (SD = 0.99)) ($p = 0.69$, Cohen's d: 0.13 (-0.53–0.8)), and during and before treatment in the tacrolimus group (mean = -1.47 (SD = 1.55)) and the placebo group (-0.96 (SD = 1.26)) ($p = 0.31$, Cohen's d: 0.36 (-0.35–1.07)) were not significantly different.

The biological criteria (hemoglobin and ferritin levels) did not significantly improve during or after treatment. The effect sizes for evolution in these parameters were 0.38 (-0.2–0.95) and 0.11 (-0.46–0.69) during treatment, and were even lower after treatment (0.19 (-0.38–0.76) and -0.32 (-0.9–0.26)), respectively. Mean levels on inclusion, six weeks after the beginning of the treatment, and six weeks after the end of the treatment in both the tacrolimus and placebo groups were 12.8, 13.3, 13.0 and 12.6, 12.6, and 12.6 for hemoglobin (g/dL), and 51.3, 75.6, 43.9 and 49.0, 59.9, and 69.3 for ferritin (μg/L), respectively. Using mixed models, we did not find a significant trend over time for hemoglobin levels ($p = 0.61$) or ferritin levels ($p = 0.36$), and no difference in evolution between groups was observed ($p = 0.59$ for hemoglobin and 0.60 for ferritin).

Table 3. Evolution of SF36 scores before and during treatment (B/D) and before and after treatment (B/A).

Variable			All	Tacro Group	Placebo Group	*p*-Value *	Effect Size **
Physical functioning	B/D	*n*	46	22	24	0.89	0.04 (−0.55–0.63)
		median (min–max)	0 (−25–40)	0 (−15–20)	0 (−25–40)		
		Mean (SD)	0.43 (11.44)	0.68 (9.55)	0.21 (13.14)		
	B/A	*n*	49	25	24	0.38●	0.07 (−0.5–0.64)
		median (min–max)	0 (−35–55)	0 (−35–20)	0 (−30–55)		
		Mean (SD)	−0.51 (14.62)	0 (10.99)	−1.04 (17.88)		
Physical role	B/D	*n*	45	22	23	0.28●	0.39 (−0.21–0.99)
		median (min–max)	0 (−50–125)	0 (−50–125)	0 (−50–75)		
		Mean (SD)	5 (37.91)	12.5 (42.08)	−2.17 (32.78)		
	B/A	*n*	46	23	23	0.78●	0.3 (−0.29–0.9)
		median (min–max)	0 (−75–125)	0 (−50–125)	0 (−75–50)		
		Mean (SD)	2.17 (35.68)	7.61 (40.19)	−3.26 (30.44)		
Bodily pain	B/D	*n*	46	22	24	0.53	0.19 (−0.41–0.78)
		median (min–max)	0 (−59–38)	0 (−59–38)	0 (−29–22)		
		Mean (SD)	−0.02 (17.36)	1.68 (20.24)	−1.58 (14.51)		
	B/A	*n*	49	25	24	0.88●	−0.12 (−0.69–0.45)
		median (min–max)	0 (−43–22)	0 (−38–22)	0 (−43–22)		
		Mean (SD)	−0.49 (15.66)	−1.4 (17.14)	0.46 (14.26)		
General health	B/D	*n*	46	22	24	0.36	0.27 (−0.32–0.87)
		median (min–max)	0 (−20–25)	2.75 (−20–23.75)	0 (−20–25)		
		Mean (SD)	2.06 (10.06)	3.5 (11.35)	0.74 (8.75)		
	B/A	*n*	49	25	24	0.59	0.15 (−0.42–0.73)
		median (min–max)	0 (−17–28.25)	0 (−15–28.25)	0 (−17–25)		
		Mean (SD)	0.14 (10.01)	0.9 (10.23)	−0.65 (9.93)		
Vitality	B/D	*n*	46	22	24	0.45	0.23 (−0.37–0.82)
		median (min–max)	0 (−25–30)	3.34 (−10–25)	0 (−25–30)		
		Mean (SD)	2.32 (11.81)	3.71 (9.64)	1.04 (13.59)		
	B/A	*n*	49	25	24	0.64	−0.13 (−0.71–0.44)
		median (min–max)	−3.33 (−35–35)	−3.33 (−35–35)	−2.5 (−20–20)		
		Mean (SD)	−2.11 (12.54)	−2.93 (14.06)	−1.25 (10.96)		
Social functioning	B/D	*n*	46	22	24	0.67	0.13 (−0.47–0.72)
		median (min–max)	0 (−37.5–37.5)	12.5 (−25–37.5)	0 (−37.5–37.5)		
		Mean (SD)	5.16 (16.37)	6.25 (15.79)	4.17 (17.16)		
	B/A	*n*	49	25	24	0.93	0.02 (−0.55–0.6)
		median (min–max)	0 (−25–37.5)	0 (−25–37.5)	0 (−25–37.5)		
		Mean (SD)	2.81 (16.39)	3 (16.65)	2.6 (16.48)		
Emotional role	B/D	*n*	46	22	24	0.69●	0.21 (−0.38–0.8)
		median (min–max)	0 (−100–100)	0 (−66.67–100)	0 (−100–100)		
		Mean (SD)	5.8 (43.49)	10.61 (44.11)	1.39 (43.38)		
	B/A	*n*	49	25	24	0.42●	0.18 (−0.39–0.75)
		median (min–max)	0 (−66.67–100)	0 (−66.67–100)	0 (−33.33–100)		
		Mean (SD)	7.48 (35.53)	10.67 (41.63)	4.17 (28.34)		
Mental health	B/D	*n*	46	22	24	0.1	−0.5 (−1.1–0.1)
		median (min–max)	1 (−19–28)	0 (−19–24)	4 (−16–28)		
		Mean (SD)	2.59 (9.9)	0.05 (9.54)	4.92 (9.83)		
	B/A	*n*	49	25	24	0.03●	−0.65 (−1.24–0.06)
		median (min–max)	0 (−44–24)	0 (−44–24)	8 (−12–24)		
		Mean (SD)	1.33 (11.68)	−2.24 (13.27)	5.04 (8.52)		

* Student *t*-test (or Mann–Whitney in case of non-normality, signaled by "●") ** Effect size: Cohen's d.

3.3. Safety Outcomes

A total of 51 AE (25 in the tacrolimus group and 26 in the placebo group) and three severe adverse events (SAE) (one in the tacrolimus group and two in the placebo group) were recorded without differences between the groups. No SAE certainly or probably related to the treatment were recorded.

Of the 29 possibly or probably related AE, 13 patients had nose burning or a tingling sensation (10 in the tacrolimus group and three in the placebo group), two had infection, both in the tacrolimus group (genital HSV infection ($n = 1$), intercostal VZV infection ($n = 1$)), seven had a local sensation (burning eyes ($n = 1$), burning throat ($n = 2$), sneezing ($n = 1$), rhinitis ($n = 1$) and nose smell ($n = 2$) (four in the tacrolimus group and three in the placebo group) and five had other symptoms (thoracic pain ($n = 1$), back pain ($n = 2$), diarrhea ($n = 1$) and headache ($n = 1$), all in the placebo group.

Systemic absorption of tacrolimus: as expected, all FK506 dosages were < 5.0 ng/mL on day 8 ($n = 48$), day 22 ($n = 46$) and day 43 ($n = 46$) after the beginning of the treatment. Tacrolimus was detected in two patients (4.3%), both in the tacrolimus group on day 8 (1.2 and 1.02 ng/mL), four patients (8.3%) on day 22 (1.03, 1.02, 1.2 and 1.05 ng/mL), and not detected on day 43 (0%).

4. Discussion

To our knowledge, this was the first phase II, double-blind, multicenter, randomized, placebo-controlled trial evaluating the efficacy of tacrolimus nasal ointment on epistaxis in HHT. In the present study, there was no significant benefit to using tacrolimus ointment administered twice a day on the nasal mucosa for six weeks after the end of the treatment, compared with placebo. We chose this time point for our main outcome (before treatment vs. after the end of the treatment) on the basis of physiology and on our previous studies using anti-angiogenic drugs which usually improved patients many weeks after the beginning of the treatment. Tacrolimus enhanced the ALK-1 signaling pathway in the endothelial cells of HHT patients, and inhibited increased VEGF signaling and hypervascularization in an HHT animal model [11], and we hypothesized that the effect which involved "blood vessel remodeling" would not be immediate. Furthermore, recent clinical data in one patient treated with low oral doses of tacrolimus showed that ESS improvement was observed three months after the beginning of the treatment [22]. However, we did not take into account that this treatment was local and with good local absorption, as confirmed by blood dosages which were very low but positive in four cases, and maybe had a quick effect during treatment which stopped after the end of the treatment. Moreover, the vast majority of patients in the tacrolimus group had a prior history of nasal surgery, compared to only half in the placebo group. It can be argued that this disequilibrium may have blunted the apparent effect of tacrolimus during the treatment period and/or contributed to the lack of an obvious effect after tacrolimus was halted. Similarly, fewer women were assigned to the tacrolimus than the placebo group, which may have influenced the results.

Importantly, we observed for our secondary outcome a significant improvement in epistaxis duration and number during the treatment phase in the tacrolimus group. These results suggest that the effect of the drug occurred only during treatment and patients relapsed after they stopped the treatment. However, although this trial was randomized, we know that moistening nasal mucosa improves epistaxis in HHT [10], and we cannot exclude the idea that the efficacy observed in the treatment group was partly related to the effect of the ointment, not to the drug itself. Furthermore, this observation highlighted the fact that prolonged tacrolimus use would be necessary, and we do not have data on the long-term safety on mucosae. The ESS did not improve during treatment; however, even though the ESS has been shown to be a validated tool in the evaluation of epistaxis in HHT [23,24], we chose not to use it as our main outcome. This was firstly because our patients are used to completing epistaxis grids, and secondly because the ESS is self-administered by patients and is more subjective than an epistaxis duration measurement. It effectively includes subjective questions such as intensity, need for medical attention and anemia, not defined by hemoglobin level but by our patients' own evaluation.

Tolerance of the nasal ointment was good after a 6-week treatment. No severe adverse events were observed. The most frequent related adverse event was a sensation of burning in the nose in 34.5% of patients in the tacrolimus group, but it was transient in most cases. None of the patients stopped the treatment for this reason. This result was similar in non-HHT patients receiving tacrolimus ointment on mucosae (oral lichen planus) in randomized studies. Corrocher et al. [16] and Vohra et al. [17] observed a burning sensation in 56% and 35% of patients, respectively, treated for oral lichen planus, and, similarly, this event resolved rapidly within four to five days. In the present study, we observed two infections in the tacrolimus group but not locally, one genital and one skin infection, and the pharmacokinetics monitoring performed revealed moderate systemic absorption, almost undetectable in most cases. It is thus unlikely that these complications were related to an immunosuppressive effect of tacrolimus. Other adverse events were observed with the same frequency in both groups. Nasal cartilaginous septum perforation was followed closely and not observed in either group after treatment.

This trial had several significant limitations. First, patients completed epistaxis grids and noted epistaxis duration, which are not directly observed outcomes, partly subjective and imprecise, and are subject to error. Second, we included all HHT patients with nosebleeds and did not take into account a history of nasal surgery or nasal crusts or septal perforation, which may change mucosal drug absorption. Almost all patients had undergone different types of surgery and most of the mucosa of the nasal cavity cannot be touched by a cotton swab, thus possibly resulting in under treatment. Third, the blinding process was successful in most cases; however, burning sensations were more frequent in the tacrolimus group. This could lead to underestimation of the placebo effect and overestimation of the relative treatment effect because patients can deduce that they are in the placebo arm and may be less likely to report improvement [25]. Finally, we observed a decrease in epistaxis duration in the placebo group, during and after treatment, which could be partly due to a Hawthorne effect. While nasal moisturizing is a recommended treatment for preventing HHT bleeding, participating in a study would probably improve the way it was done.

5. Conclusions

In HHT patients with epistaxis, tacrolimus nasal ointment, administered twice daily compared with a placebo, did not reduce monthly epistaxis duration in the six consecutive weeks after treatment compared to the six weeks immediately before the start of treatment. However, good tolerance associated with a significant improvement in epistaxis duration during treatment encouraged us to perform a phase 3 trial on a larger patient population with a main outcome of epistaxis duration during treatment and a longer treatment time.

Author Contributions: Conceptualization, S.D.-G., E.D., and A.-E.F.; methodology, E.D. and L.B.; software, E.D. and L.B.; validation, S.D.-G., A.-E.F., and R.H.; formal analysis, S.D.-G., E.D., and L.B.; investigation, S.D.G., A.-E.F., M.B., V.G., and S.R.; resources, E.D.; data curation, S.D.-G., E.D., M.B., and A.-E.F.; writing—original draft preparation, S.D.-G.; writing—review and editing, S.D.-G., A.E.F., M.B., V.G., S.R., E.D., L.B., V.B., B.C., R.H., F.F., P.P., and S.B.; visualization, S.D.-G., A.-E.F., M.B., V.G., S.R., E.D., L.B., V.B., B.C., R.H., F.F., P.P., and S.B.; supervision, S.D.-G.; project administration, S.D.-G., A.-E.F., and M.B.; funding acquisition, S.D.-G. and R.H.; All authors have read and agreed to the published version of the manuscript.

Funding: This work was financed by the institution (Hospices Civils de Lyon) grant supported by the National Research Programme (PHRC 2016) and by the patients' association (AMRO-France). Neither the funding organization (National Research Program) nor the patients' association (AMRO) played any role in designing or conducting the study; collecting, managing, analyzing, or interpreting the data; or preparing, reviewing, or approving the manuscript.

Acknowledgments: We would like to thank all the patients who participated in this study, the Association of patients, and all the members of the French HHT Network, particularly Nicolas Saroul (CHU Clermont-Ferrand) and Cesar Cartier (CHU Montpellier). We would also like to thank the members of the independent data and safety monitoring committee (IDMC), Yves Donazzolo (EUROFINS/OPTIMED Clinical Research, Gières, France), Elisabetta Buscarini (HHT center, Crema, Italy), and Xavier Lassartesse (ENT surgeon, Avignon, France). They did not receive any compensation for this contribution.

Conflicts of Interest: The authors declare no conflict of interest.

Trial Registration: ClinicalTrials.gov Identifier #NCT 03152019 (TACRO study).

References

1. Lesca, G.; Olivieri, C.; Burnichon, N.; Pagella, F.; Carette, M.F.; Gilbert-Dussardier, B.; Goizet, C.; Roume, J.; Rabilloud, M.; Saurin, J.C.; et al. Genotype-phenotype correlations in hereditary hemorrhagic telangiectasia: Data from the French-Italian HHT network. *Genet. Med.* **2007**, *9*, 14–22. [CrossRef] [PubMed]
2. Tillet, E.; Bailly, S. Emerging roles of BMP9 and BMP10 in hereditary hemorrhagic telangiectasia. *Front. Genet.* **2014**, *5*, 456. [CrossRef] [PubMed]
3. Guttmacher, A.E.; Marchuk, D.A.; White, R.I., Jr. Hereditary hemorrhagic telangiectasia. *N. Engl. J. Med.* **1995**, *333*, 918–924. [CrossRef] [PubMed]
4. Dupuis-Girod, S.; Bailly, S.; Plauchu, H. Hereditary hemorrhagic telangiectasia: From molecular biology to patient care. *J. Thromb. Haemost.* **2010**, *8*, 1447–1456. [CrossRef] [PubMed]
5. Geisthoff, U.W.; Heckmann, K.; D'Amelio, R.; Grunewald, S.; Knobber, D.; Falkai, P.; Konig, J. Health-related quality of life in hereditary hemorrhagic telangiectasia. *Otolaryngol. Head Neck Surg.* **2007**, *136*, 726-e1. [CrossRef]
6. Robert, F.; Desroches-Castan, A.; Bailly, S.; Dupuis-Girod, S.; Feige, J.J. Future treatments for hereditary hemorrhagic telangiectasia. *Orphanet J. Rare Dis.* **2020**, *15*, 4. [CrossRef]
7. Dupuis-Girod, S.; Ginon, I.; Saurin, J.C.; Marion, D.; Guillot, E.; Decullier, E.; Roux, A.; Carette, M.F.; Gilbert-Dussardier, B.; Hatron, P.Y.; et al. Bevacizumab in patients with hereditary hemorrhagic telangiectasia and severe hepatic vascular malformations and high cardiac output. *JAMA* **2012**, *307*, 948–955. [CrossRef]
8. Lebrin, F.; Srun, S.; Raymond, K.; Martin, S.; van den Brink, S.; Freitas, C.; Breant, C.; Mathivet, T.; Larrivee, B.; Thomas, J.L.; et al. Thalidomide stimulates vessel maturation and reduces epistaxis in individuals with hereditary hemorrhagic telangiectasia. *Nat. Med.* **2010**, *16*, 420–428. [CrossRef]
9. Dupuis-Girod, S.; Ambrun, A.; Decullier, E.; Fargeton, A.E.; Roux, A.; Breant, V.; Colombet, B.; Riviere, S.; Cartier, C.; Lacombe, P.; et al. Effect of bevacizumab nasal spray on epistaxis duration in hereditary hemorrhagic telangectasia: a randomized clinical trial. *JAMA* **2016**, *316*, 934–942. [CrossRef]
10. Whitehead, K.J.; Sautter, N.B.; McWilliams, J.P.; Chakinala, M.M.; Merlo, C.A.; Johnson, M.H.; James, M.; Everett, E.M.; Clancy, M.S.; Faughnan, M.E.; et al. Effect of topical intranasal therapy on epistaxis frequency in patients with hereditary hemorrhagic telangiectasia: A randomized clinical trial. *JAMA* **2016**, *316*, 943–951. [CrossRef]
11. Ruiz, S.; Chandakkar, P.; Zhao, H.; Papoin, J.; Chatterjee, P.K.; Christen, E.; Metz, C.N.; Blanc, L.; Campagne, F.; Marambaud, P. Tacrolimus rescues the signaling and gene expression signature of endothelial ALK1 loss-of-function and improves HHT vascular pathology. *Hum. Mol. Genet.* **2017**, *26*, 4786–4798. [CrossRef]
12. Spiekerkoetter, E.; Tian, X.; Cai, J.; Hopper, R.K.; Sudheendra, D.; Li, C.G.; El-Bizri, N.; Sawada, H.; Haghighat, R.; Chan, R.; et al. FK506 activates BMPR2, rescues endothelial dysfunction, and reverses pulmonary hypertension. *J. Clin. Investig.* **2013**, *123*, 3600–3613. [CrossRef]
13. Albinana, V.; Sanz-Rodriguez, F.; Recio-Poveda, L.; Bernabeu, C.; Botella, L.M. Immunosuppressor FK506 increases endoglin and activin receptor-like kinase 1 expression and modulates transforming growth factor-beta1 signaling in endothelial cells. *Mol. Pharmacol.* **2011**, *79*, 833–843. [CrossRef]
14. Dupuis-Girod, S.; Chesnais, A.L.; Ginon, I.; Dumortier, J.; Saurin, J.C.; Finet, G.; Decullier, E.; Marion, D.; Plauchu, H.; Boillot, O. Long-term outcome of patients with hereditary hemorrhagic telangiectasia and severe hepatic involvement after orthotopic liver transplantation: A single-center study. *Liver Transplant.* **2010**, *16*, 340–347.
15. Liao, Y.H.; Chiu, H.C.; Tseng, Y.S.; Tsai, T.F. Comparison of cutaneous tolerance and efficacy of calcitriol 3 microg g(-1) ointment and tacrolimus 0.3 mg g(-1) ointment in chronic plaque psoriasis involving facial or genitofemoral areas: A double-blind, randomized controlled trial. *Br. J. Dermatol.* **2007**, *157*, 1005–1012. [CrossRef]
16. Corrocher, G.; Di Lorenzo, G.; Martinelli, N.; Mansueto, P.; Biasi, D.; Nocini, P.F.; Lombardo, G.; Fior, A.; Corrocher, R.; Bambara, L.M.; et al. Comparative effect of tacrolimus 0.1% ointment and clobetasol 0.05% ointment in patients with oral lichen planus. *J. Clin. Periodontol.* **2008**, *35*, 244–249. [CrossRef]
17. Vohra, S.; Singal, A.; Sharma, S.B. Clinical and serological efficacy of topical calcineurin inhibitors in oral lichen planus: A prospective randomized controlled trial. *Int. J. Dermatol.* **2016**, *55*, 101–105. [CrossRef]

18. Arduino, P.G.; Carbone, M.; Della Ferrera, F.; Elia, A.; Conrotto, D.; Gambino, A.; Comba, A.; Calogiuri, P.L.; Broccoletti, R. Pimecrolimus vs. tacrolimus for the topical treatment of unresponsive oral erosive lichen planus: A 8 week randomized double-blind controlled study. *J. Eur. Acad. Dermatol. Venereol.* **2014**, *28*, 475–482. [CrossRef]

19. Reitamo, S.; Mandelin, J.; Rubins, A.; Remitz, A.; Makela, M.; Cirule, K.; Rubins, S.; Zigure, S.; Ho, V.; Dickinson, J.; et al. The pharmacokinetics of tacrolimus after first and repeated dosing with 0.03% ointment in infants with atopic dermatitis. *Int. J. Dermatol.* **2009**, *48*, 348–355. [CrossRef]

20. Harper, J.; Smith, C.; Rubins, A.; Green, A.; Jackson, K.; Zigure, S.; Bourke, J.; Alomar, A.; Stevenson, P.; Foster, C.; et al. A multicenter study of the pharmacokinetics of tacrolimus ointment after first and repeated application to children with atopic dermatitis. *J. Investig. Dermatol.* **2005**, *124*, 695–699. [CrossRef]

21. World Medical Association. World Medical Association Declaration of Helsinki: Ethical principles for medical research involving human subjects. *JAMA* **2013**, *310*, 2191–2194. [CrossRef] [PubMed]

22. Sommer, N.; Droege, F.; Gamen, K.E.; Geisthoff, U.; Gall, H.; Tello, K.; Richter, M.J.; Deubner, L.M.; Schmiedel, R.; Hecker, M.; et al. Treatment with low-dose tacrolimus inhibits bleeding complications in a patient with hereditary hemorrhagic telangiectasia and pulmonary arterial hypertension. *Pulm. Circ.* **2019**, *9*, 2045894018805406. [CrossRef] [PubMed]

23. Hoag, J.B.; Terry, P.; Mitchell, S.; Reh, D.; Merlo, C.A. An epistaxis severity score for hereditary hemorrhagic telangiectasia. *Laryngoscope* **2010**, *120*, 838–843. [CrossRef] [PubMed]

24. Yin, L.X.; Reh, D.D.; Hoag, J.B.; Mitchell, S.E.; Mathai, S.C.; Robinson, G.M.; Merlo, C.A. The minimal important difference of the epistaxis severity score in hereditary hemorrhagic telangiectasia. *Laryngoscope* **2016**, *126*, 1029–1032. [CrossRef]

25. Hrobjartsson, A.; Forfang, E.; Haahr, M.T.; Als-Nielsen, B.; Brorson, S. Blinded trials taken to the test: An analysis of randomized clinical trials that report tests for the success of blinding. *Int. J. Epidemiol.* **2007**, *36*, 654–663. [CrossRef]

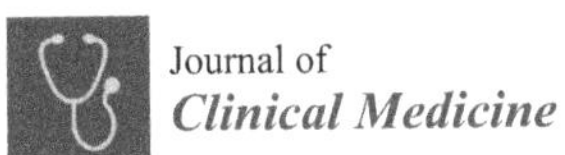 Journal of
Clinical Medicine

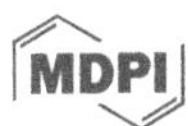

Article

Gastrointestinal Bleeding in Patients with Hereditary Hemorrhagic Telangiectasia: Risk Factors and Endoscopic Findings

José María Mora-Luján [1,2,3], Adriana Iriarte [1,2,3], Esther Alba [1,3,4],
Miguel Ángel Sánchez-Corral [1,3,5], Ana Berrozpe [3,6], Pau Cerdà [1,2,3], Francesc Cruellas [1,3,7],
Jesús Ribas [1,3,8], Jose Castellote [1,3,6] and Antoni Riera-Mestre [1,2,3,9,*]

[1] HHT Unit, Hospital Universitari de Bellvitge, 08907 Barcelona, Spain;
jmora@bellvitgehospital.cat (J.M.M.-L.); adriana.iriarte@bellvitgehospital.cat (A.I.);
estheralba@bellvitgehospital.cat (E.A.); mmena@bellvitgehospital.cat (M.Á.S.-C.);
pau.pauet@gmail.com (P.C.); fcruellas@bellvitgehospital.cat (F.C.); jribass@bellvitgehospital.cat (J.R.);
jcastellote@bellvitgehospital.cat (J.C.)
[2] Internal Medicine Department, Hospital Universitari de Bellvitge, 08907 Barcelona, Spain
[3] Bellvitge Biomedical Research Institute (IDIBELL), L'Hospitalet de Llobregat, 08907 Barcelona, Spain;
aberrozpe@bellvitgehospital.cat
[4] Radiology Department, Hospital Universitari de Bellvitge, 08907 Barcelona, Spain
[5] Cardiology Department, Hospital Universitari de Bellvitge, 08907 Barcelona, Spain
[6] Gastroenterolgy Department, Hospital Universitari de Bellvitge, 08907 Barcelona, Spain
[7] Otorhinolaringology Department, Hospital Universitari de Bellvitge, 08907 Barcelona, Spain
[8] Pneumology Department, Hospital Universitari de Bellvitge, 08907 Barcelona, Spain
[9] Clinical Sciences Department, Faculty of Medicine and Health Sciences, Universitat de Barcelona,
L'Hospitalet de Llobregat, 08907 Barcelona, Spain
[*] Correspondence: ariera@bellvitgehospital.cat; Tel.: +34-93-260-7699

Received: 22 November 2019; Accepted: 25 December 2019; Published: 28 December 2019

Abstract: Background: We aimed to describe risk factors for gastrointestinal (GI) bleeding and endoscopic findings in patients with hereditary hemorrhagic telangiectasia (HHT). Methods: This is a prospective study from a referral HHT unit. Endoscopic tests were performed when there was suspicion of GI bleeding, and patients were divided as follows: with, without, and with unsuspected GI involvement. Results: 67 (27.9%) patients with, 28 (11.7%) patients without, and 145 (60.4%) with unsuspected GI involvement were included. Age, tobacco use, endoglin (ENG) mutation, and hemoglobin were associated with GI involvement. Telangiectases were mostly in the stomach and duodenum, but 18.5% of patients with normal esophagogastroduodenoscopy (EGD) had GI involvement in video capsule endoscopy (VCE). Telangiectases ≤ 3 mm and ≤ 10 per location were most common. Among patients with GI disease, those with hemoglobin < 8 g/dL or transfusion requirements (65.7%) were older and had higher epistaxis severity score (ESS) and larger telangiectases (>3 mm). After a mean follow-up of 34.2 months, patients with GI involvement required more transfusions and more emergency department and hospital admissions, with no differences in mortality. Conclusions: Risk factors for GI involvement have been identified. Patients with GI involvement and severe anemia had larger telangiectases and higher ESS. VCE should be considered in patients with suspicion of GI bleeding, even if EGD is normal.

Keywords: hereditary hemorrhagic telangiectasia; rare diseases; telangiectasis; transforming growth factor-beta (TGF-β); Smad pathway; gastrointestinal bleeding

1. Introduction

Hereditary hemorrhagic telangiectasia (HHT) or Rendu-Osler-Weber syndrome (ORPHA774) is an autosomal dominant rare vascular disease characterized by telangiectases and larger vascular malformations (VMs) [1–3]. HHT can be diagnosed either clinically using the Curaçao criteria (recurrent epistaxis, muco-cutaneous telangiectasia, visceral lesions, and family history) or through a molecular gene test [4–6]. Mutations in endoglin (*ENG*) and activin A receptor type II-like 1 (*ACVRL1*) genes are detected in approximately 90% of cases submitted to molecular diagnosis for clinical suspicion of HHT and cause HHT1 and HHT2, respectively [2,7–9]. Mutations in *SMAD4* (encoding the transcription factor Smad4) have been described in less than 2% of the HHT population [8]. Endoglin (encoded by *ENG*) is an auxiliary co-receptor at the endothelial cell surface that promotes BMP9 signaling through the activin receptor-like kinase 1 (ALK1; encoded by *ACVRL1*) [2]. Both proteins contribute to the signaling hub formed by BMP9-endoglin-ALK1-Smad with a high impact in the angiogenesis process [10].

Telangiectasis is the characteristic lesion in HHT and shows dilated post capillary venules directly connected with dilated arterioles losing the capillary bed [11]. These dilated microvessels are more prone to hemorrhage due to fragile walls and turbulent blood flow, especially those located in mucosae, such as nasal or gastrointestinal (GI). Telangiectasia in nasal mucosae can cause spontaneous, recurrent epistaxis, usually the earliest and most common clinical manifestation of HHT [2,9,12].

Unlike epistaxis or visceral involvement, which occur since adolescence, GI bleeding begins in the fifth or sixth decades of life [4,13]. The prevalence of GI telangiectasia ranges from 13% to 30% in the overall HHT population to more than 90% in HHT patients with anemia [14–20]. In HHT patients, GI bleeding is usually chronic, low degree, and in an intermittent fashion [16,17]. However, clinical presentation can be diverse, with some patients presenting none or mild anemia, while others require periodic transfusions. Although argon plasma coagulation (APC) is the most effective endoscopic therapy for active GI bleeding, some patients have either multiple or non-accessible telangiectases for APC and usually require additional or alternative therapies [4,13,16,21]. Therefore, pharmacological treatment, such as with estrogen/progesterone, somatostatin analog octreotide, and bevacizumab, has been considered in these patients. However, these pharmacological therapies have not been well established and are based on either individual case reports or small case series [4,13,16,21,22].

Though GI telangiectasia is included in the visceral lesions defined in the Curaçao criteria, international guidelines only recommend endoscopic study in adult patients with disproportionate anemia to the severity of epistaxis [4,5]. Unfortunately, there is no clear definition for disproportionate anemia, so indication for endoscopic study often depends on physician experience. Though some studies have suggested an association between age or female gender and GI disease, risk factors predisposing GI disease are currently unknown [4,8,13,15,16]. Identifying possible risk factors associated with GI involvement could be useful for HHT clinical management. The objective of the present study is to describe risk factors for GI involvement and to assess endoscopic findings and outcomes in this scenario.

2. Materials and Methods

2.1. Study Design

This is a prospective, observational study, which includes all consecutive patients attended in a referral HHT unit in a university hospital from September 2011 to June 2019. This HHT unit attends adult patients from all over Catalonia (Spain), which accounts for seven million inhabitants. During this period, a total of 330 patients were visited in our unit. All patients provided oral consent for participation in the study in accordance with local Ethic Committee requirements. Patients with a definite diagnosis according to the Curaçao criteria (meeting ≥ 3 criteria) or a positive genetic study were included [4–6]. We followed the Strengthening the Reporting of Observational Studies in Epidemiology (STROBE) statement guidelines for observational cohort studies [23].

The main objective was to describe risk factors for GI involvement among patients with definite or molecular diagnosis of HHT. Secondary objectives were to compare endoscopic findings among patients with GI involvement according to clinical severity and to assess clinical outcomes according to GI involvement.

2.2. Assessment of Gastrointestinal Involvement

Suggestive symptoms/signs of GI involvement were defined as either the presence of overt upper or lower GI bleeding or the presence of anemia that is disproportionate to the severity of epistaxis [4]. Endoscopic study (GIF-Q165; Olympus, Hamburg, Germany) was performed when suggestive symptoms/signs of GI involvement were present. In patients with active or recently bleeding telangiectases, treatment with APC was performed. A video capsule endoscopy (VCE) (PillCamSB 3; Medtronic, Yokneam, Israel) study was mostly performed in patients with persistent anemia after APC treatment.

Endoscopic study was defined as positive when HHT suggestive telangiectasia was found in the GI tract. Normal endoscopic study or non-suggestive findings of HHT were defined as a negative study. Using these criteria and according to GI disease, three groups were established: (a) GI involvement: patients with positive endoscopic study; (b) no GI involvement: patients with negative endoscopic study; (c) unsuspected GI involvement: patients without suggestive symptoms/signs of GI bleeding and no endoscopic study performed.

Among patients with GI involvement, telangiectases were classified according to their number (few: ≤10 telangiectases or multiple: >10 telangiectases) and size (small: ≤3 mm or large: >3 mm) [13]. Patients with GI involvement were classified into two subgroups according to clinical severity: patients with either hemoglobin levels less than 8 g/dL or red blood cell (RBC) transfusion requirements and patients with none of these conditions. Endoscopic findings were compared between both subgroups.

2.3. Clinical Variables, Screening Tests, and Follow-Up

Baseline demographic characteristics, comorbidities, history of alcohol or tobacco use (previous or currently), hemoglobin levels, genetic study, blood test, and epistaxis severity score (ESS) were collected. ESS is an online tool that quantifies the epistaxis severity considering different parameters during the previous three months [24].

To screen for pulmonary visceral involvement, a contrast transthoracic echocardiography (TTE) was performed [4,25]. The Barzilai scale was used to establish the degree of right-left shunt (R-L) and the need to undergo a thoracic computed tomography (CT) angiography to confirm the presence of pulmonary arteriovenous (AV) fistula [4,26]. In addition, an abdominal CT angiography was performed to study hepatic and/or abdominal VMs. A cerebral CT angiography or brain MRI angiography was carried out in cases of neurological symptoms or a family history of neurological involvement [4,25].

All patients were prospectively followed-up depending on disease severity, at the treating clinician's discretion. The lowest hemoglobin level detected and different treatment strategies used during follow-up were recorded. Patients with objectively confirmed GI involvement and severe anemia despite iron therapy and/or requiring blood transfusions were assessed for treatment with octreotide or bevacizumab. The number of packed RBCs transfused before and during both treatments was recorded. Moreover, the need for visits to the emergency department (ED) and/or hospital admissions, the number of RBC transfusions required, and any mortality during follow-up were also registered. These outcomes were compared between HHT groups according to GI involvement.

2.4. Statistical Analysis

A descriptive statistical analysis was performed for all categorical and continuous variables and expressed as proportions or means with standard deviations (SD), respectively. Categorical variables were compared with the chi-square test or Fisher's exact test, whereas the t-test or the Mann–Whitney U test were used to compare continuous variables.

Logistic regression analyses were performed to identify associated risk factors for GI disease and presented as odds ratios (OR) with 95% confidence intervals (95% CI). Logistic regression was performed in patients with suggestive symptoms/signs of GI involvement. For the manual backward stepwise multivariable logistic regression model, we assessed variables that had a significant level of P less than 0.1 in univariable analyses. To analyze the predictive power of the associated risk factors, a receiver operating characteristic (ROC) curve was performed and the area under the curve (AUC) was calculated. *p* values of <0.05 were considered to be statistically significant. Analyses were performed using SPSS, version 15 for the PC (SPSS Inc., Chicago, IL, USA).

3. Results

3.1. Clinical Characteristics

During the study period, 240 patients met the inclusion criteria. Most patients (57.1%) were female, and mean age was 53.6 ± 13.6 years. Clinical diagnosis of HHT was definitive according to the Curaçao criteria (meeting ≥ 3 criteria) in 229 (95.4%) patients and by a positive molecular test in the remaining 11 (4.6%) patients. A genetic test was carried out in 161 patients: 75 (45.2%) had *ENG* mutation, and 73 (43.9%) had *ACVRL1* mutation, with no mutation found in 13 (7.8%). After screening tests, 176 patients (73.3%) had visceral involvement: 67 (27.9%) with pulmonary AV fistula, 110 (45.8%) with hepatic VMs, 73 (30.4%) with other intraabdominal VM, and 10 (4.2%) with central nervous system involvement.

In 67 (27.9%) patients, GI disease was confirmed with the positive endoscopic study, while 28 (11.7%) patients had suggestive symptoms but a negative endoscopic study, and GI disease was unsuspected in the remaining 145 (60.4%) patients.

3.2. Risk Factors for GI Involvement

Patients with GI involvement were more likely to use tobacco and to have *ENG* mutation, lower hemoglobin values at diagnosis, lower minimal hemoglobin levels during follow-up, lower ferritin levels (<15 ug/L), and higher systolic pulmonary artery pressure (sPAP) at TTE than those with no GI involvement. Compared to patients with unsuspected GI involvement, those with GI involvement were older and were more likely to use tobacco or alcohol and to have more comorbidities, higher ESS, lower ferritin (<15 ug/L), minimal hemoglobin levels, and a higher cardiac index (CI) and sPAP at TTE (Table 1).

Table 1. Clinical characteristics and screening tests according to gastrointestinal involvement in 240 patients with hereditary hemorrhagic telangiectasia (HHT).

	GI Involvement (*n* = 67)	No GI Involvement (*n* = 28)	*p* Value	Unsuspected GI Involvement (*n* = 145)	*p* Value *
Clinical characteristics					
Gender (female), *n* (%)	35 (52.2)	18 (64.3)	0.380	84 (57.9)	0.437
Age years-old, mean (SD)	59.5 (11.1)	56.9 (13.3)	0.332	44.3 (16.3)	<0.001
Epistaxis age of presentation, mean (SD)	16.6 (13.1)	13.8 (7.4)	0.207	16.1 (11.9)	0.813
Underlying conditions, *n* (%)					
Smoking history	38 (56.7)	8 (28.6)	0.012	59 (40.7)	0.029
Alcoholism	15 (22.4)	4 (14.3)	0.368	13 (9)	0.007
Hypertension	25 (37.3)	11 (39.3)	0.857	27 (18.6)	0.003
Diabetes mellitus	14 (20.9)	3 (10.7)	0.238	9 (6.2)	0.001
Dislipemia	24 (35.8)	11 (39.3)	0.750	31 (21.4)	0.026
Ischemic heart disease	15 (22.4)	3 (10.7)	0.186	12 (8.3)	0.004
Lung disease	19 (28.4)	6 (21.4)	0.484	12 (8.3)	<0.001
CNS ischemic disease	13 (19.4)	1 (3.6)	0.059	11 (7.6)	0.012
Heart failure	7 (10.4)	0	0.101	2 (1.4)	0.005
Cancer	9 (13.4)	0	0.054	8 (5.5)	0.048
Atrial fibrillation	9 (13.4)	2 (7.1)	0.498	4 (2.8)	0.005
HHT screening,					
Curaçao criteria ≥ 3, *n* (%)	67 (100)	27 (96.4)	0.295	136 (93.8)	0.060

Table 1. *Cont.*

	GI Involvement (*n* = 67)	No GI Involvement (*n* = 28)	*p* Value	Unsuspected GI Involvement (*n* = 145)	*p* Value *
Epistaxis, *n* (%)	67 (100)	27 (96.4)	0.295	137 (94.5)	0.058
ESS, mean (SD)	4.2 (2.2)	3.5 (1.9)	0.137	3.4 (2.2)	0.019
ESS ≥ 4, *n* (%)	35 (56.5)	10 (37)	0.092	52 (36.4)	0.009
Family history, n (%)	61 (91)	26 (92.9)	1.000	141 (97.2)	0.076
Muco-cutaneous telangiectasia, n (%)	67 (100)	27 (96.4)	0.295	139 (95.9)	0.180
Visceral involvement (excluding GI involvement), *n* (%)	53 (79.1)	19 (67.9)	0.318	89 (61.3)	0.012
Genetic test, *n* (%)					
Undergone	40 (59.7)	20 (71.4)	0.280	106 (73.1)	0.050
ENG	21 (52.5)	4 (20)	0.001	50 (49)	0.709
ACVRL1	17 (42.5)	14 (70)	0.044	42 (41.2)	0.886
Negative	2 (5)	2 (10)	0.595	9 (8.8)	0.728
Blood test,					
Hemoglobin levels (g/dL), mean (SD)	113.1 (24.7)	131.4 (22.6)	0.007	133.9 (22.9)	<0.001
Minimal hemoglobin levels (g/dL), mean (SD)	84.3 (30.8)	108.3 (32.7)	0.002	118.2 (30.5)	<0.001
Ferritin level < 15 ug/L, n (%)	56 (83.6)	15 (55.6)	0.004	76 (55.1)	<0.001
Other tests,					
Positive contrast TTE, *n* (%)	45 (67.1)	13 (46.4)	0.252	94 (64.8)	0.640
CI at TTE (l/min/m^2), mean (SD)	3.4 (0.9)	3.4 (1.2)	0.988	2.9 (0.6)	<0.001
sPAP at TTE (mm Hg), mean (SD)	37.9 (12.3)	31.3 (7.1)	0.024	29.8 (6.9)	<0.001
sPAP > 40mmHg, *n* (%)	12 (32.4)	2 (15.4)	0.303	6 (9.5)	0.004
Pulmonary AVM at CT, *n* (%)	25 (37.3)	3 (10.7)	0.256	39 (26.8)	0.077
Abdominal CT, *n* (%)	62 (92.5)	22 (78.6)	0.077	103 (71)	<0.001
Hepatic involvement	40 (59.7)	17 (60.7)	0.271	53 (36.5)	0.101
Other visceral involvement	34 (50.7)	10 (35.7)	0.487	29 (20)	0.001
CNS involvement, *n* (%)	5 (7.5)	0	0.298	5 (3.4)	0.482

GI: Gastrointestinal; ACVRL1: Activin A receptor type II-like 1 gene; ENG: Endoglin gene; SD: Standard deviation; CI: Cardiac index; sPAP: Systolic pulmonary artery pressure; TTE: Transthoracic echocardiography; CNS: Central nervous system. * Comparison between GI involvement and unsuspected GI involvement groups.

After multivariate analysis, age (OR 1.07, 1.06–1.14, *p* = 0.033), *ENG* mutations (OR 5.7, 1.02–31.93 95% CI, *p* = 0.047), previous/current tobacco use (OR 7.8, 1.37–44.52 95% CI, *p* = 0.020), and hemoglobin values (OR 0.96, 0.93–0.96 95% CI, *p* = 0.033) were associated with GI involvement at endoscopy tests (Table 2). The ROC analysis showed a good predictive power of the associated risk factors for GI involvement (AUC = 0.834).

Table 2. Uni- and multivariable logistic regression analyses for gastrointestinal bleeding in patients with HHT.

	Univariable			Multivariable		
	OR	95% CI	*p*	OR	95% CI	*p*
Male	1.64	0.66–4.08	0.283	0.90	0.15–5.32	0.910
Age, years	1.02	0.98–1.05	0.339	1.07	1.06–1.14	0.033
Age > 50 years	2.30	0.86–6.16	0.095	2.06	0.07–61.42	0.676
Smoking	3.27	1.26–8.48	0.015	7.82	1.37–44.52	0.020
ENG mutations	4.42	1.25–15.57	0.021	5.72	1.02–31.93	0.047
ACVRL1 mutations	0.31	0.10–0.99	0.049	1.99	0.07–54.84	0.685
Ferritin levels < 15 ug/L	4.07	1.5–11.03	0.006	3.09	0.55–17.5	0.202
Hemoglobin, g/dL	0.97	0.95–0.99	0.003	0.96	0.93–0.96	0.033
Hemoglobin levels < 8 g/dL	2.18	0.83–5.76	0.112	0.75	0.09–6.55	0.801
ESS ≥ 4	2.20	0.87–5.57	0.095	1.57	0.26–9.66	0.624

OR: odds ratio; 95% CI: 95% confidence intervals; *ACVRL1*: activin A receptor type II-like 1 gene; *ENG*: endoglin gene; ESS: epistaxis severity score.

3.3. GI Involvement

Telangiectasia was more frequently found in the stomach and duodenum. All but one patient with telangiectasia based on the esophagogastroduodenoscopy (EGD) also showed telangiectases in the colonoscopy (CS). Most patients (81.5%) with gastric or duodenal telangiectasia in EGD also had small intestine involvement at VCE. The size of telangiectases most commonly was ≤3 mm in all locations, and most patients had ≤10 telangiectases per location. Multiple (>10) telangiectases were mostly found in the jejunum and ileum.

Most patients with GI disease had hemoglobin levels < 8 g/dL and/or RBC transfusion requirements during follow-up (n = 44; 65.7%). These patients were older and with a higher ESS than the subgroup of patients without these conditions. No gender, epistaxis, age, or visceral involvement differences were found between any subgroups. Patients with hemoglobin levels < 8 g/dL and/or transfusion requirements had larger telangiectases (>3 mm) and needed APC therapy more often than the remaining patients with GI involvement, with no other differences in location or the number of telangiectases (Table 3).

Table 3. Clinical characteristics and endoscopic findings among patients with gastrointestinal involvement.

	Patients with Hb ≤ 8 or Transfusion (n = 44)	Patients with Hb > 8 and No Transfusion (n = 23)	p Value
Clinical characteristics			
Gender (female), n (%)	22 (50)	13 (56.5)	0.612
Age at presentation, mean (SD)	61.3 (11.2)	53.8 (9.6)	0.006
Epistaxis age at presentation, mean (SD)	16.5 (12.9)	16.7 (13.7)	0.941
ESS, mean (SD)	4.9 (2.2)	2.9 (1.6)	<0.001
ESS > 4, n (%)	27 (69.2)	8 (34.8)	0.008
Visceral involvement (excluding *GI* involvement), n (%)	34 (77.3)	18 (78.3)	0.927
GI tests, n (%)			
Both EGD and CS	30 (68.2)	13 (56.5)	0.345
Video capsule endoscopy	20 (45.5)	7 (30.4)	0.234
APC therapy	25 (64.1)	6 (30%)	0.013
Site of GI telangiectases, n (%)			
Esophagical	7 (15.9)	3 (13)	1.000
>10 telangiectases	0	0	
Size: ≤3 mm	4 (66.7)	3 (100)	
>3 mm	2 (33.3)	0	0.500
Gastric	36 (81.8)	16 (69.6)	0.253
>10 telangiectases	6 (16.7)	2 (12.5)	1.000
Size: ≤3 mm	12 (42.9)	11 (73.3)	
>3 mm	16 (57.1)	4 (26.7%)	0.056
Duodenal	31 (70.5)	13 (56.5)	0.254
>10 telangiectases	6 (19.4)	1 (7.1)	0.407
Size: ≤3 mm	15 (55.6)	10 (83.3)	
>3 mm	12 (44.4)	2 (16.7)	0.151
Jejunal	21 (47.7)	7 (30.4)	0.173
>10 telangiectases (n)	10 (47.6)	3 (42.9)	1.000
Size: ≤3 mm	10 (50)	6 (85.7)	
>3 mm	10 (50)	1 (14.3)	0.183
Ileal	15 (75)	5 (71.4)	0.294
>10 telangiectases	8 (57.1)	1 (20)	0.303
Size: ≤3mm	5 (55.6)	4 (100)	
>3 mm	4 (44.4)	0	0.228
Colonic	16 (39)	5 (23.8)	0.231
>10 telangiectases	1 (6.7)	0	1.000
Size: ≤3 mm	7 (58.3)	2 (66.7)	
>3 mm	5 (41.7)	1 (33.3)	1.000
Patients with large telangiectases (>3 mm) (all tests), n (%)	23 (65.7)	3 (20)	0.003
Patients with >10 telangiectases in any location (all tests), n (%)	20 (46.5)	7 (35)	0.390

APC: argon plasma coagulation; EGD: esophagogastroduodenoscopy; EES: epistaxis severity score; CS: colonoscopy; *GI*: gastrointestinal; Hb: Hemoglobin; SD: standard deviation.

3.4. Outcomes

Overall, mean follow-up was 34.2 ± 22.8 (1–124) months, with no differences between groups according to GI involvement. Patients with GI involvement required significantly more often RBC transfusions, ED attention, and hospital admissions than patients without GI disease or than those with unsuspected GI involvement. Overall, five patients (2.1%) died, with no differences in mortality between groups (Table 4).

Table 4. Clinical outcomes during follow-up according to gastrointestinal involvement.

	GI Involvement (n = 67)	No GI Involvement (n = 28)	p Value	Unsuspected GI Involvement (n = 145)	p Value *
Follow-up (months), mean (SD)	33.6 (21.9)	29.2 (20.5)	0.354	35.4 (23.6)	0.585
Outcomes,					
RBC transfusion, n (%)	41 (61.2)	8 (28.6)	0.004	22 (15.4)	<0.001
Number of transfusions, mean (range)	26.2 (1–218)	8.9 (2–35)	0.042	9.1 (1–50)	0.101
ED visit, n (%)	40 (59.7)	7 (25)	0.002	42 (29)	<0.001
Hospital admission, n (%)	28 (41.8)	5 (17.9)	0.025	16 (11)	<0.001
Mortality, n (%)	2 (3%)	0	1.000	3 (2.1)	0.652

GI: gastrointestinal; SD: standard deviation; RBC: red blood cells; ED: Emergency Department; * Comparison between GI involvement and unsuspected GI involvement groups.

Nine patients received treatment with octreotide: four with 100 mcg bid and five with long-acting release (LAR) octreotide at doses between 10 and 30 mcg monthly. In five of these nine patients, a marked decrease in the number of packed RBC units transfused was observed in the first weeks of treatment. Only one patient presented diarrhea as a side effect with the 100 mcg bid dose, which disappeared after switching to a monthly LAR formulation. Two patients without improvement after octreotide daily doses received bevazicumab at doses of 5 mg/kg every two weeks with tapering frequency to a final maintenance dose every 6–8 weeks. One of these patients needed hypertension therapy adjustment because of bevacizumab-induced hypertension with severe epistaxis and an increase of RBC transfusion requirements during the first six months of treatment. After blood pressure control, both patients experienced a rather marked reduction in the number of packed RBC units transfused under bevacizumab therapy (Table 5).

Table 5. Evolution of patients with gastrointestinal involvement treated with octreotide and bevacizumab.

Patients	Gender	Age (Years)	VCE	Large (>3 mm) Telangiectases	>10 Telangiectases	Site	Before Treatment		Octreotide			Bevacizumab	
							Follow-Up (m)	n° RBC	Follow-Up (m)	n° RBC	Dose	Follow-Up (m)	n° RBC
P.1	Male	68	Yes	Yes	No	G-D-J	66	11	21	4	10 mcg/m	-	-
P.2	Male	71	Yes	Yes	No	G-D	8	22	12	0	100 mcg/12 h	-	-
P.3	Male	55	Yes	Yes	No	G-D	38	8	3	1	20 mcg/m	-	-
P.4	Male	58	No	No	No	G-D	40	20	2	0	100 mcg/12 h	-	-
P.5	Female	55	No	Yes	Yes	G-D-J-I	21	9	16	3	30 mcg/m	-	-
P.6	Male	66	Yes	No	Yes	G-D-J-I	100	>100	15	92	100 mcg/12 h	21	3
P.7	Male	51	Yes	Yes	Yes	G-D-J-I	74	93	6	12	100 mcg/12 h	13	13 *
P.8	Female	51	Yes	Yes	Yes	G-D-J-I	36	36	9	5	10 mcg/m	-	-
P.9	Male	62	Yes	Yes	Yes	G-D-J-I	48	48	4	0	20 mcg/m	-	-

VCE: video capsule endoscopy; G: Gastric; D: Duodenal; I: ileal; J: jejunal; m: month; n° RBC: number of units of packed red blood cells transfused before and during octreotide or bevacizumab treatments. * All during the first six months of bevacizumab treatment because of bevacizumab-induced hypertension and resulting severe epistaxis.

4. Discussion

In our study, age, *ENG* mutation, tobacco use, and hemoglobin levels were associated with GI involvement in HHT patients. We found a 7% increased risk of GI involvement per year of age. These results are consistent with the mean age of GI bleeding onset observed in previous studies [4,13]. However, we have not detected previously described female predominance [4,17,21]. Smoking history has been related to a 7-fold increase risk of GI involvement in our series. Tobacco use has already been associated with an increased risk of upper GI bleeding and gastroduodenal ulcers in non-HHT patients, but no relationship between tobacco and GI telangiectasia has been published [27]. Though this finding strengthens the importance of avoiding tobacco in HHT patients, it also needs to be confirmed in further studies. Canzonieri et al. and van Tuyl et al. systemically studied the extent of GI involvement with EGD, VCE, and CS in 22 and 35 HHT patients, respectively, and found a higher prevalence of telangiectasia in patients with *ENG* mutation [13,19]. However, Berg et al., Sabbà et al., and Letteboer et al. assessing genotype–phenotype relationships in HHT patients, reported similar incidence of GI telangiectasia between HHT1 and HHT2 patients [28–30]. Differently, and according to current guidelines, we studied patients with clinical suspicion of GI bleeding, but not indiscriminately screened [4]. Thus, *ENG* mutation was associated with 5-fold increase risk of GI involvement compared to those with negative endoscopic study. In addition, in our cohort, hemoglobin levels were also associated with GI involvement. These four variables could help physicians experiencing the difficult management of GI involvement in HHT patients.

Many cases of anemia are misattributed to overt epistaxis instead of attributing them to GI bleeding among patients with HHT [16,31]. In fact, we have not found significant differences in epistaxis severity measured by the ESS between patients with and without GI involvement. This finding supports that lower hemoglobin levels found in patients with GI involvement were disproportionate. Moreover, among patients with GI involvement, the ESS was higher in those with hemoglobin levels < 8 g/dL or with transfusion requirements. This relationship could be explained by a microvessel predominant pattern, as telangiectasis is a pathological feature in both nasal and digestive mucosae. Because both types of bleeding can coexist, a high clinical suspicion of GI bleeding in patients with severe anemia, despite a high ESS, is necessary.

In our series, telangiectasia is more frequently found in the stomach or duodenum. This location is highly related to small bowels and colon telangiectasia in VCE. These results are in line with international guidelines, which recommend EGD as the initial screening procedure when GI involvement is suspected [4,13]. However, if the EGD is negative, VCE should be considered in patients with high suspicion of GI involvement and severe anemia to detect telangiectasia within the small intestine, as it occurred in 18.5% of our patients [13,19]. Longrace et al., in 43 consecutive HHT patients with GI bleeding, reported that patients with >20 telangiectases had significantly lower hemoglobin levels and higher transfusion requirements [21]. We found that patients with hemoglobin levels <8 g/dL or RBC transfusion requirements had larger telangiectases. These endoscopic findings strengthen the usefulness and benefits of VCE and should be taken into account in the follow-up and treatment assessment of HHT patients with GI involvement.

Chronic GI bleeding treatment is largely endoscopic and supported by frequent blood transfusions. In our study, patients with GI involvement needed RBC transfusions and medical attention more often than those with no or unsuspected GI involvement. However, no difference in mortality was found between groups. Although severe anemia secondary to GI bleeding can lead to multiple complications, GI bleeding has not been described as a cause of the lower life expectancy of HHT patients [29,32]. HHT patients with GI bleeding usually have telangiectases that are not fit for APC treatment, and require pharmacological treatment, with different and controversial options [4,13,16,21]. Our series included nine patients on octreotide treatment from daily clinical practice. This agent has shown a reduction in digestive bleeding and an anemia improvement in non-HHT patients with intestinal angiodysplasia by reducing splanchnic blood flow, but evidence of its use in HHT patients is scarce [33–36]. A non-randomized prospective clinical trial to assess the efficacy of monthly injection of 20 mg of octreotide LAR has been recently published [36]. Although this study was underpowered (beta of 0.5), RBC transfusion requirements were lower during the six months treatment period than they were prior to treatment, in all 11 patients included. We have observed similar results in five out of nine patients treated with octreotide. Further studies are needed to confirm the efficacy and safety of long-term octreotide therapy. Similarly, the benefit of bevacizumab in patients with GI involvement needs has been poorly described [37,38]. Bevacizumab-induced hypertension is a well-known adverse effect; high blood pressure can make epistaxis worse and provoke RBC transfusion requirements, as it occurred in one of our patients [39]. Other treatments such as talidomide or estrogen/progesterone preparations have also shown improvement in hemoglobin levels or transfusion requirements in case reports or short series [21,22,40,41]. The hypothetical benefit in this scenario of future agents that block or activate pathways involved in HHT pathogenesis, such as sirolimus, tacrolimus, nintedanib, or a combination of them, needs further investigation [42–44].

There are some limitations and strengths of our study that should be mentioned. VCE was not performed in all patients and GI involvement could be underestimated in patients with negative EGD. Additionally, VCE could have influenced the number and size of small bowel telangiectases. Another limitation is that endoscopic study was not performed on all patients. However, this is in agreement with recommendations of current guidelines [4]. Difficulties in attributing low hemoglobin levels to epistaxis or GI bleeding could be another inherent limitation. However, our study represents the largest series of HHT patients with objectively confirmed GI involvement, and is the only one comparing these patients with those with a negative endoscopic study or with unsuspected GI involvement. On top of that, the prospective nature of our study and the broad long-term follow-up reinforce the robustness of the results and allow for a better assessment of outcomes.

5. Conclusions

In conclusion, age, *ENG* mutation, tobacco use, and hemoglobin levels have been associated with GI involvement in HHT patients. Telangiectasia was more frequently found in the stomach and duodenum. Patients with large telangiectases have severe anemia and high RBC transfusion requirements. VCE should be considered in patients with a high suspicion of GI bleeding, even if EGD resulted negative. Among HHT patients, those with GI involvement need medical attention more often, with no differences in mortality.

Author Contributions: Conceptualization: J.M.M.-L. and A.R.-M.; data curation: J.M.M.-L., A.I., A.B., P.C. and A.R.-M.; formal analysis: J.M.M.-L., A.I., P.C. and A.R.-M.; investigation: J.M.M.-L., A.I., E.A., M.Á.S.-C., A.B., P.C., F.C., J.R., J.C. and A.R.-M.; methodology: J.M.M.-L. and A.R.-M.; supervision: J.R., J.C. and A.R.-M.; validation: J.M.M.-L., A.I., E.A., M.Á.S.-C., A.B., P.C., F.C., J.R., J.C. and A.R.-M.; visualization: J.M.M.-L., E.A., F.C. and A.R.-M.; writing—original draft preparation: J.M.M.-L., A.I., E.A., M.Á.S.-C, A.B., P.C., F.C. and A.R.-M.; writing—review and editing: J.M.M.-L., J.R., J.C. and A.R-M; funding acquisition: A.R.-M. All authors have read and agreed to the published version of the manuscript.

Funding: This research was funded by the Instituto de Salud Carlos III, grant number PI17/00669, co-funded by the European Regional Development Fund (ERDF), "A Way to Build Europe".

References

1. The Portal for Rare Diseases and Orphan Drugs. Available online: https://www.orpha.net/consor/cgi-bin/index.php (accessed on 22 July 2019).
2. McDonald, J.; Wooderchak-Donahue, W.; VanSant Webb, C.; Whitehead, K.; Stevenson, D.A.; Bayrak-Toydemir, P. Hereditary hemorrhagic telangiectasia: Genetics and molecular diagnostics in a new era. *Front. Genet.* **2015**, *6*, 1. [CrossRef]
3. Donaldson, J.W.; McKeever, T.M.; Hall, I.P.; Hubbard, R.B.; Fogarty, A.W. The UK prevalence of hereditary haemorrhagic telangiectasia and its association with sex, socioeconomic status and region of residence: A population-based study. *Thorax* **2014**, *69*, 161–167. [CrossRef]

4. Faughnan, M.E.; Palda, V.A.; Garcia-Tsao, G.; Geisthoff, U.W.; McDonald, J.; Proctor, D.D.; Spears, J.; Brown, D.H.; Buscarini, E.; Chesnutt, M.S.; et al. HHT Foundation International Guidelines Working Group. International guidelines for the diagnosis and management of hereditary haemorrhagic telangiectasia. *J. Med. Genet.* **2011**, *48*, 73–87. [CrossRef]

5. Shovlin, C.L.; Guttmacher, A.E.; Buscarini, E.; Faughnan, M.E.; Hyland, R.H.; Westermann, C.J.; Kjeldsen, A.D.; Plauchu, H. Diagnostic criteria for hereditary hemorrhagic telangiectasia (Rendu- Osler-Weber syndrome). *Am. J. Med. Genet.* **2000**, *91*, 66–67. [CrossRef]

6. Shovlin, C.L.; Buscarini, E.; Kjeldsen, A.D.; Mager, H.J.; Sabba, C.; Droege, F.; Geisthoff, U.; Ugolini, S.; Dupuis-Girod, S. European Reference Network for Rare Vascular Diseases (VASCERN) Outcome measures for Hereditary Haemorrhagic Telangiectasia (HHT). *Orphanet J. Rare Dis.* **2018**, *13*, 136. [CrossRef]

7. Abdalla, S.A.; Letarte, M. Hereditary haemorrhagic telangiectasia: Current views on genetics and mechanisms of disease. *J. Med. Genet.* **2006**, *43*, 97–110. [CrossRef]

8. Gallione, C.J.; Repetto, G.M.; Legius, E.; Rustgi, A.K.; Schelley, S.L.; Tejpar, S.; Mitchell, G.; Drouin, E.; Westermann, C.J.; Marchuk, D.A. A combined syndrome of juvenile polyposis and hereditary haemorrhagic telangiectasia associated with mutations in MADH4 (SMAD4). *Lancet* **2004**, *363*, 852–859. [CrossRef]

9. Lesca, G.; Olivieri, C.; Burnichon, N.; Pagella, F.; Carette, M.F.; Gilbert-Dussardier, B.; Goizet, C.; Roume, J.; Rabilloud, M.; Saurin, J.C.; et al. French-Italian-Rendu-Osler Network. Genotype-phenotype correlations in hereditary hemorrhagic telangiectasia: Data from the French-Italian HHT network. *Genet. Med.* **2007**, *9*, 14–22. [CrossRef]

10. Tillet, E.; Bailly, S. Emerging roles of BMP9 and BMP10 in hereditary hemorrhagic telangiectasia. *Front. Genet.* **2015**, *5*, 456. [CrossRef]

11. Braverman, I.M.; Keh, A.; Jacobson, B.S. Ultrastructure and three-dimensional organization of the telangiectases of hereditary hemorrhagic telangiectasia. *J. Investig. Dermatol.* **1990**, *95*, 422–427. [CrossRef]

12. Riera-Mestre, A.; Luján, J.M.M.; Martínez, R.S.; Cabeza, M.A.T.; de la Peña, J.L.P.; Rodrigo, M.C.J.; Wolf, D.L.; Sosa, A.O.; Monserrat, L.; Rodríguez, M.L. Computerized registry of patients with hemorrhagic hereditary telangiectasia (RiHHTa Registry) in Spain: Objectives, methods, and preliminary results. *Rev. Clin. Esp.* **2018**, *218*, 468–476. [CrossRef] [PubMed]

13. Canzonieri, C.; Centenara, L.; Ornati, F.; Pagella, F.; Matti, E.; Alvisi, C.; Danesino, C.; Perego, M.; Olivieri, C. Endoscopic evaluation of gastrointestinal tract in patients with hereditary hemorrhagic telangiectasia and correlation with their genotypes. *Genet. Med.* **2014**, *16*, 3–10. [CrossRef] [PubMed]

14. Smith, C.R., Jr.; Bartholomew, L.G.; Cain, J.C. Hereditary hemorrhagic telangiectasia and gastrointestinal hemorrhage. *Gastroenterology* **1963**, *44*, 1–6. [CrossRef]

15. Vase, P.; Grove, O. Gastrointestinal lesions in hereditary hemorrhagic telangiectasia. *Gastroenterology* **1986**, *91*, 1079–1083. [CrossRef]

16. Kjeldsen, A.D.; Kjeldsen, J. Gastrointestinal bleeding in patients with hereditary hemorrhagic telangiectasia. *Am. J. Gastroenterol.* **2000**, *95*, 415–418. [CrossRef]

17. Proctor, D.D.; Henderson, K.J.; Dziura, J.D.; Longacre, A.V.; White, R.I., Jr. Enteroscopic evaluation of the gastrointestinal tract in symptomatic patients with hereditary hemorrhagic telangiectasia. *J. Clin. Gastroenterol.* **2005**, *39*, 115–119. [PubMed]

18. Ingrosso, M.; Sabbà, C.; Pisani, A.M.; Gallitelli, M.; Cirulli, A.; Francavilla, A. Evidence of small-bowel involvement in hereditary hemorrhagic telangiectasia: A capsule-endoscopic study. *Endoscopy* **2004**, *36*, 1074–1079. [CrossRef]

19. Van Tuyl, S.A.; Letteboer, T.G.; Rogge-Wolf, C.; Kuipers, E.J.; Snijder, R.J.; Westermann, C.J.; Stolk, M.F. Assessment of intestinal vascular malformations in patients with hereditary hemorrhagic teleangiectasia and anemia. *Eur. J. Gastroenterol. Hepatol.* **2007**, *19*, 153–158. [CrossRef]

20. Chamberlain, S.M.; Patel, J.; Carter Balart, J.; Gossage, J.R., Jr.; Sridhar, S. Evaluation of patients with hereditary hemorrhagic telangiectasia with video capsule endoscopy: A single-center prospective study. *Endoscopy* **2007**, *39*, 516–520. [CrossRef]

21. Longacre, A.V.; Gross, C.P.; Gallitelli, M.; Henderson, K.J.; White, R.I., Jr.; Proctor, D.D. Diagnosis and management of gastrointestinal bleeding in patients with hereditary hemorrhagic telangiectasia. *Am. J. Gastroenterol.* **2003**, *98*, 59–65. [CrossRef]

22. Van Cutsem, E.; Rutgeerts, P.; Vantrappen, G. Treatment of bleeding gastrointestinal vascular malformations with oestrogen-progesterone. *Lancet* **1990**, *335*, 953–955. [CrossRef]

23. Von Elm, E.; Altman, D.G.; Egger, M.; Pocock, S.J.; Gøtzsche, P.C.; Vandenbroucke, J.P. STROBE Initiative. The strengthening the reporting of observational studies in epidemiology (STROBE) statement: Guidelines for reporting observational studies. *Ann. Intern. Med.* **2007**, *147*, 573–577. [CrossRef]

24. Hoag, J.B.; Terry, P.; Mitchell, S.; Reh, D.; Merlo, C.A. An epistaxis severity score for hereditary hemorrhagia telangiectasia. *Laryngoscope* **2010**, *120*, 838–843. [CrossRef] [PubMed]

25. Riera-Mestre, A.; Ribas, J.; Castellote, J. Hemorrhagic hereditary telangiectasia in adult patients. *Med. Clin.* **2019**, *152*, 274–280. [CrossRef] [PubMed]

26. Barzilai, B.; Waggoner, A.D.; Spessert, C.; Picus, D.; Goodenberger, D. Two-dimensional contrast echocardiography in the detection and follow-up of congenital pulmonary arteriovenous malformations. *Am. J. Cardiol.* **1991**, *68*, 1507–1510. [CrossRef]

27. Kim, S.H.; Yun, J.M.; Chang, C.B.; Piao, H.; Yu, S.J.; Shin, D.W. Prevalence of upper gastrointestinal bleeding risk factors among the general population and osteoarthritis patients. *World J. Gastroenterol.* **2016**, *22*, 10643–10652. [CrossRef]

28. Berg, J.; Porteous, M.; Reinhardt, D.; Gallione, C.; Holloway, S.; Umasunthar, T.; Lux, A.; McKinnon, W.; Marchuk, D.; Guttmacher, A. Hereditary haemorrhagic telangiectasia: A questionnaire based study to delineate the different phenotypes caused by endoglin and ALK1 mutations. *J. Med. Genet.* **2003**, *40*, 585–590. [CrossRef]

29. Sabbà, C.; Pasculli, G.; Lenato, G.M.; Suppressa, P.; Lastella, P.; Memeo, M.; Dicuonzo, F.; Guant, G. Hereditary hemorrhagic telangiectasia: Clinical features in ENG and ALK1 mutation carriers. *J. Thromb. Haemost.* **2007**, *5*, 1149–1157. [CrossRef]

30. Letteboer, T.G.; Mager, J.J.; Snijder, R.J.; Koeleman, B.P.; Lindhout, D.; Ploos van Amstel, J.K.; Westermann, C.J. Genotype-phenotype relationship in hereditary haemorrhagic telangiectasia. *J. Med. Genet.* **2006**, *43*, 371–377. [CrossRef]

31. Jackson, S.B.; Villano, N.P.; Benhammou, J.N.; Lewis, M.; Pisegna, J.R.; Padua, D. Gastrointestinal manifestations of hereditary hemorrhagic telangiectasia (HHT): A systematic review of the literature. *Dig. Dis. Sci.* **2017**, *62*, 2623–2630. [CrossRef]

32. De Gussem, E.M.; Edwards, C.P.; Hosman, A.E.; Westermann, C.J.; Snijder, R.J.; Faughnan, M.E.; Mager, J.J. Life expextancy of parents with hereditary haemorrhagic telangiectasia. *Orphanet J. Rare Dis.* **2016**, *11*, 46. [CrossRef] [PubMed]

33. Vuddanda, V.; Jazayeri, M.A.; Turagam, M.K.; Lavu, M.; Parikh, V.; Atkins, D.; Bommana, S.; Yeruva, M.R.; Di Biase, L.; Cheng, J.; et al. Systemic octreotide therapy in prevention of gastrointestinal bleeds related to arteriovenous malformations and obscure etiology in atrial fibrillation. *Jacc. Clin. Electrophysiol.* **2017**, *3*, 1390–1399. [CrossRef] [PubMed]

34. Brown, C.; Subramanian, V.; Wilcox, C.M.; Peter, S. Somatostatin analogues in the treatment of recurrent bleeding from gastrointestinal vascular malformations: An overview and systematic review of prospective observational studies. *Dig. Dis. Sci.* **2010**, *55*, 2129–2134. [CrossRef] [PubMed]

35. Houghton, K.D.; Umar, B.; Schairer, J. Successful treatment of hereditary hemorrhagic telangiectasia with octreotide. *Acg. Case Rep. J.* **2019**, *6*, e00088. [CrossRef] [PubMed]

36. Kroon, S.; Snijder, R.J.; Mager, J.J.; Post, M.C.; Tenthof van Noorden, J.; van Geenen, E.J.M.; Drenth, J.P.H.; Grooteman, K.V. Octreotide for gastrointestinal bleeding in hereditary hemorrhagic telangiectasia: A prospective case series. *Am. J. Hematol.* **2019**, *28*, 1–3. [CrossRef] [PubMed]

37. Lyer, V.N.; Apala, D.R.; Pannu, B.S.; Kotecha, A.; Brinjikji, W.; Leise, M.D.; Kamath, P.S.; Misra, S.; Begna, K.H.; Cartin-Ceba, R.; et al. Intravenous Bevacizumab for refractory hereditary hemorrhagic telangiectasia related epistaxis and gastrointestinal bleeding. *Mayo Clin. Proc.* **2018**, *93*, 155–166.

38. Ou, G.; Galorport, C.; Enns, R. Bevacizumab and gastrointestinal bleeding in hereditary hemorrhagic telangiectasia. *World J. Gastrointest. Surg.* **2016**, *8*, 792–795. [CrossRef]

39. Buscarini, E.; Botella, L.M.; Geisthoff, U.; Kjeldsen, A.D.; Mager, H.J.; Pagella, F.; Suppressa, P.; Zarrabeitia, R.; Dupuis-Girod, S.; Shovlin, C.L. Safety of thalidomide and bevacizumab in patients with hereditary hemorrhagic telangiectasia. *Orphanet J. Rare Dis.* **2019**, *14*, 28. [CrossRef]

40. Wang, X.Y.; Chen, Y.; Du, Q. Successful treatment of thalidomide for recurrent bleeding due to gastric angiodysplasia in hereditary hemorrhagic telangiectasia. *Eur. Rev. Med. Pharm. Sci.* **2013**, *17*, 1114–1116.

41. Alam, M.A.; Sami, S.; Babu, S. Successful treatment of bleeding gastro-intestinal angiodysplasia in hereditary haemorrhagic telangiectasia with thalidomide. *Case Rep.* **2011**, *2011*. [CrossRef]

42. Albiñana, V.; Sanz-Rodríguez, F.; Recio-Poveda, L.; Bernabéu, C.; Botella, L.M. Immunosuppressor FK506 increases endoglin and activin receptor-like kinase 1 expression and modulates transforming growth factor-β1 signaling in endothelial. *Mol. Pharmacol.* **2011**, *79*, 833–843. [CrossRef] [PubMed]
43. Iriarte, A.; Figueras, A.; Cerdà, P.; Mora, J.M.; Jucglà, A.; Penín, R.; Viñals, F.; Riera-Mestre, A. PI3K (Phosphatidylinositol 3-Kinase) activation and endothelial cell proliferation in patients with hemorrhagic hereditary telangiectasia type 1. *Cells* **2019**, *8*, 971. [CrossRef] [PubMed]
44. Ruiz, S.; Zhao, H.; Chandakkar, P.; Papoin, J.; Choi, H.; Nomura-Kitabayashi, A.; Patel, R.; Gillen, M.; Diao, L.; Chatterjee, P.K.; et al. Correcting Smad1/5/8, mTOR, and VEGFR2 treats pathology in hereditary hemorrhagic telangiectasia models. *J. Clin. Invest.* **2019**, 127425. [CrossRef] [PubMed]

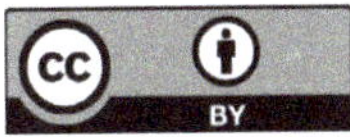

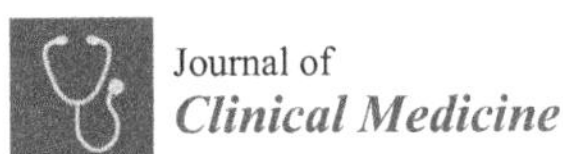

Journal of
Clinical Medicine

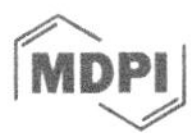

Article

Topical Propranolol Improves Epistaxis Control in Hereditary Hemorrhagic Telangiectasia (HHT): A Randomized Double-Blind Placebo-Controlled Trial

Meir Mei-Zahav [1,2,3,*], Yulia Gendler [1,4], Elchanan Bruckheimer [2,5], Dario Prais [1,2,3], Einat Birk [2,5], Muhamad Watad [2], Neta Goldschmidt [6,†] and Ethan Soudry [2,7,†]

[1]   Pulmonary Institute, Schneider Children's Medical Center of Israel, Petah Tikva 49202, Israel; yulia.gendler@gmail.com (Y.G.); prais@tauex.tau.ac.il (D.P.)
[2]   Sackler Faculty of Medicine, Tel Aviv University, Tel Aviv 69978, Israel; elrealview@gmail.com (E.B.); EBirk@clalit.org.il (E.B.); Watadmohammed@gmail.com (M.W.); ethansoudry@gmail.com (E.S.)
[3]   The National HHT Center, Pulmonary Institute, Schneider CMCI, 14 Kaplan St., Petach Tikva 49202, Israel
[4]   The Department of Nursing, Ariel University, Ariel 40700, Israel
[5]   Cardiology Department, Schneider Children's Medical Center of Israel, Petah Tikva 49202, Israel
[6]   Department of Hematology, Hadassah-Hebrew University Medical Center, Jerusalem 91120, Israel; neta@hadassah.org.il
[7]   Department of Otolaryngology Head and Neck Surgery, Rabin Medical Center, Petah Tikva 49202, Israel
*   Correspondence: mmeizahav@gmail.com
†   Equal senior authorship.

Received: 31 August 2020; Accepted: 26 September 2020; Published: 28 September 2020

Abstract: Epistaxis is a common debilitating manifestation in hereditary hemorrhagic telangiectasia (HHT), due to mucocutaneous telangiectases. The epistaxis can be difficult to control despite available treatments. Dysregulated angiogenesis has been shown to be associated with telangiectases formation. Topical propranolol has demonstrated antiangiogenic properties. We performed a two-phase study, i.e., a double-blind placebo-controlled phase, followed by an open-label phase. The aim of the study was assessment of safety and efficacy of nasal propranolol gel in HHT-related epistaxis. Twenty participants with moderate-severe HHT-related epistaxis were randomized to eight weeks of propranolol gel 1.5%, or placebo 0.5 cc, applied to each nostril twice daily; and continued propranolol for eight weeks in an open-label study. For the propranolol group, the epistaxis severity score (ESS) improved significantly (−2.03 ± 1.7 as compared with −0.35 ± 0.68 for the placebo group, $p = 0.009$); hemoglobin levels improved significantly (10.5 ± 2.6 to 11.4 ± 2.02 g/dL, $p = 0.009$); and intravenous iron and blood transfusion requirement decreased. The change in nasal endoscopy findings was not significant. During the open-label period, the ESS score improved significantly in the former placebo group (−1.99 ± 1.41, $p = 0.005$). The most common adverse event was nasal mucosa burning sensation. No cardiovascular events were reported. Our results suggest that topical propranolol gel is safe and effective in HHT-related epistaxis.

Keywords: hereditary hemorrhagic telangiectasia; epistaxis; propranolol gel; epistaxis severity score; nasal endoscopy; antiangiogenic properties

---

1. Introduction

Hereditary hemorrhagic telangiectasia (HHT) (ORPHA774, HHT 1 OMIM# 187300 and HHT 2 OMIM# 600376) is an autosomal dominant vascular disorder that leads to abnormally dilated blood vessels and arteriovenous malformations. Telangiectases tend to rupture and result in recurrent gastrointestinal bleeding and spontaneous epistaxis, the latter being the most common clinical presentation of patients with HHT [1]. Severely affected individuals may have gushing bleeds several times a day, with consequent iron deficiency anemia and transfusion dependency [1]. Severe epistaxis is associated with significant impairment in daily life activity and decreased quality of life (QOL) [2–4], and is often resistant to standard measures [5].

Although the precise mechanism of arteriovenous malformations and telangiectases formation in HHT is unknown, dysregulation of angiogenesis has been shown to result in an unbalanced generation of abnormal blood vessels [6]. Several antiangiogenic therapeutic agents have been proposed. Bevacizumab, the most frequently used, has demonstrated limited success as a topical treatment of epistaxis [7,8], and significant side effects with systemic use [9].

The non-selective beta-blocker propranolol is commonly used as a topical and systemic treatment for infantile hemangioma [10], with proven anti-angiogenic effects [11]. We previously reported the efficacy of topical propranolol in an open-label study with six participants [12]. That report led us to conduct the current trial to evaluate the safety and efficacy of topical propranolol gel in the treatment of moderate to severe HHT-related epistaxis.

2. Experimental Section

This study was comprised of a double-blind placebo-controlled phase, with continuation to an open-label phase (Figure 1). Patients with HHT having refractory moderate to severe epistaxis were recruited from the Israeli National HHT Center at Schneider Children's Medical Center of Israel and Beilinson Medical Center. Study inclusion and exclusion criteria are summarized in Table 1. Patients with concomitant significant gastrointestinal bleeding were referred for systemic treatment and were not included in the study.

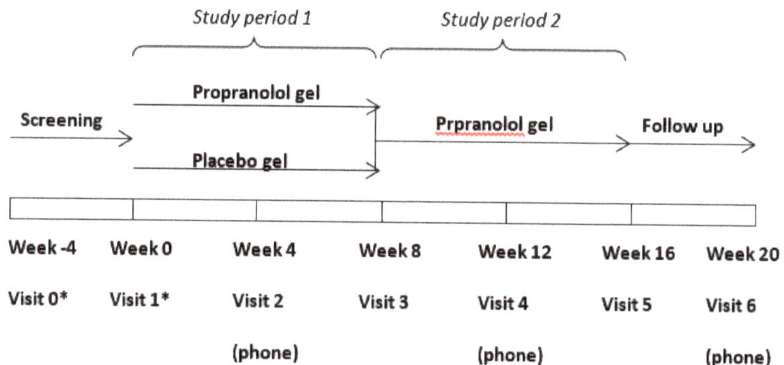

*Visit 0 and visit 1 were allowed at the same day.

Figure 1. Study design.

Table 1. Inclusion and exclusion criteria.

Inclusion criteria:
- Adults, 18 years and older
- Confirmed clinical [13] or genetic diagnosis of HHT
- Epistaxis severity score (ESS, range of scores: 0–10, 10 indicates greatest severity) [14]) ≥4
- Refractory to standard measures that control bleeding

Exclusion criteria:
- Congestive heart failure, baseline bradycardia (heart rate (HR) < 50/min), heart block, asthma or known sensitivity to propranolol)
- Treatment with beta-blockers for other reasons
- Change in epistaxis care in the month prior to enrolment
- Use of any antiangiogenic medication in the month prior to enrolment
- Use of antiplatelet or anticoagulant medications

The study was approved by the local ethics committee (RMC-0191-15) and by the Israel Ministry of Health (MOH, Clinical Trial Registration 20173382, www.health.gov.il/clinicaltrials). All the participants signed an inform consent.

Propranolol gel was prepared with propranolol HCl 1.5% in an isotonic solution and preserved hydroxyethyl cellulose 2% gel. The placebo gel was prepared with preserved hydroxyethyl cellulose 2% gel only. Patients were instructed to apply 0.5 cc propranolol or a placebo gel via a supplied 1 mL syringe, to the nasal mucosa of each nostril, twice daily.

Following screening, the patients were randomly assigned, at a 1:1 ratio, to be treated with propranolol gel or a placebo gel for a period of 8 weeks (the double-blind phase). Randomization was performed by the pharmacy, and the treatment team was blinded to the process. Following the double-blind phase, all the patients were offered to continue an open-label phase for an additional 8 weeks.

The study participants were examined at screening and randomization, and at the end of each treatment phase (the 8th and 16th weeks). Each visit included a recent medical history and physical examination; monitoring of side-effects; measurements of heart rate (HR), blood pressure (BP), blood hemoglobin (HB), and iron and ferritin levels; a rhinology examination; assessment of epistaxis severity according to the epistaxis severity score (ESS); and quality of life (QOL) according to the 12-Item Short Form Health Survey (SF-12) questionnaire. An electrocardiogram was performed at screening and repeated at the primary investigator's discretion.

Nasal endoscopy was performed at screening, and at the 8th and 16th weeks, by a highly trained rhinologist (ES), who was blinded to treatment allocation.

Patients' nasal cavities were decongested with lidocaine 1.5% and phenylephrine 1% spray prior to endoscopic examination with a zero-degree 4 mm endoscope connected to a high definition camera and monitor (Storz). Endoscopies were recorded and representative photographs of the nasal cavities were captured in a de-identified manner. Thus, all patient images were subsequently graded in an anonymized fashion at the conclusion of the study. Nasal involvement with disease at recruitment was graded as follows: mild-few punctate telangiectases, moderate-multiple telangiectases/large arteriovenous malformations involving the anterior nasal septum, and severe-diffuse involvement of the nasal mucosa with telangiectases. During follow up, endoscopies were defined as improved versus no change or worsened.

A telephone interview was performed at each mid-treatment period (4th and 12th week) and 4 weeks after the open-label phase (20th week) to assess efficacy and safety.

Participants were instructed at recruitment to fill out a daily epistaxis diary indicating the severity, frequency, and duration of the epistaxis episodes. Severity was recorded as mild-drops of blood (1), moderate- mild bleed and clots (2), or severe gushing or major clots (3).

Bleeding frequency was recorded as the number of episodes per day. The total minutes of epistaxis per day was recorded as the daily epistaxis duration. Participants were asked to mark in the diary when the medication was applied. Compliance was measured using the diary and by counting the empty syringes returned at every visit. Participants were instructed to measure their BP and HR weekly by their local health provider and to document these results in their diary. Participants were also asked to document any local or systemic symptoms and report them to the investigators.

Indications to terminate the study were any of the following criteria: a systolic BP drop to less than 80 mmHg or a drop of ≥20% from baseline systolic BP, a drop of HR to less than 50/min, any signs of heart block on the electrocardiogram, grade > 2 (CTCAE [15]) local or systemic side effects such as local irritation or an allergic reaction to the medication, and patient's or physician's request.

The primary outcome was the difference in ESS drop between both groups. ESS was first calculated at randomization and was related to the prior 8 weeks, and then at the end of the double-blind period. The change in ESS from randomization to the end of the first 8-week period was compared between the propranolol and control groups. The secondary outcome measures were changes in blood hemoglobin (Hb) levels and intravenous iron, packed cell transfusion (PC) requirements, a change in the intensity of telangiectases in the nasal mucosa as documented by one otolaryngology surgeon (ES), and the change in QOL. In the open-label period the secondary outcome was ESS change from the beginning and the end of the open-label phase.

Statistical Analysis

The sample size was calculated from a pilot study [12], in which ESS improved by 2.85 ± 1.75 following the use of propranolol gel. We anticipated a similar improvement in the current study. We assumed an improvement in ESS of 0.5 in the placebo group. Power analysis calculation (α of 0.05 and 1-β of 0.8) required 9 patients in each arm. Assuming that two participants would drop out of the study per group, 11 participants were planned to be recruited in each group (for a total of 22 participants in the study).

Data were analyzed using SPSS, version 25. Armonk (NY, USA) (SPSS Inc., Chicago, IL, USA). Demographic factors and clinical outcomes were summarized with percentage breakdown. For comparing outcomes between the treatment groups, an independent samples *t*-test was used, with a normal distribution assumed. Otherwise, Mann–Whitney or Wilcoxon rank-sum tests were used. Changes in ESS and clinical parameters between two visits were analyzed using a paired *t*-test. To analyze the improvement in nasal rhinology scoring between the two groups (improved/not improved), the McNemar test was used. Normality assessment was performed using a Shapiro–Wilk test. Normal distribution was assumed when $p > 0.05$.

3. Results

3.1. Study Participants

Twenty-three patients were recruited between April 2018 and March 2019, of whom, 18 (78%) were female. The mean age at study entry was 54.6 ± 10.8 years (range 35–74 years).

Ten participants were randomized to the propranolol group, and 13 to the placebo group. Three participants from the placebo group withdrew from the study, two because of low compliance and one after the development of acute otitis media. None of the participants in the propranolol group withdrew.

Twenty participants completed the double-blind phase, 10 participants in each study group. Their baseline characteristics are presented in Table 2. Differences in the baseline ESS, and in demographic and clinical parameters between the groups were not statistically significant.

Table 2. Baseline characteristics.

	Placebo (*n* = 10)	Propranolol (*n* = 10)	*p*
Age—years (mean ± SD)	51 ± 9	57 ± 11	0.262
Gender (F,M)	9:1	6:4	0.152
Gene mutation (number of participants)	ACVRL1-8 Endoglin-1 ND-1	ACVRL1-5 Endoglin-3 ND-2	0.223
ESS	5.68 ± 1.8	6.50 ± 1.84	0.323
QOL	34.75 ± 10.9	35.1 ± 6.7	0.932
Hemoglobin (g/dL)	10.7 ± 2.52	10.57 ± 2.6	0.918
IV iron */IV PC *	16/3	9/7	0.739/0.481
Ferritin	65.4 ± 86.19	89.65 ± 212.04	0.715
Rhinology grading (number of patients)			0.601
Grade I	4	3	
Grade II	5	5	
Grade III	1	2	
Systolic BP mmHg (mean ± SD)	110.2 ± 9.6	119.3 ± 12.3	0.09
Diastolic BP mmHg (mean ± SD)	63.3 ± 9.2	69.0 ± 9.2	0.20
HR per minute (mean ± SD)	76.0 ± 12.9	73.9 ± 111.7	0.71

* Total number of units of IV iron (Ferinject 500 mg)/IV packed cells (PC) in the 2 months prior to screening. ESS, epistaxis severity score; ACVRL1, activin receptor-like 1; ND, not done; QOL, quality of life; IV, intravenous; PC, packed cells; BP, blood pressure; HR, heart rate.

Compliance was high for both groups (propranolol 90.2 ± 10.3% vs. placebo 94.2 ± 8.1%, *p* = 0.371).

3.2. Primary Outcome

During the first phase of the study, the ESS showed a significant improvement in the propranolol group (from a mean of 6.50 ± 1.84 to 4.47 ± 1.75, *p* = 0.004) and no change in the placebo group (5.68 ± 1.8 to 5.33 ± 2.1, *p* = 0.133, Table 3). The change in ESS was −2.03 ± 1.7 in the propranolol group as compared with −0.35 ± 0.68 in the placebo group, *p* = 0.009 (Figure 2, Table 4).

Table 3. Outcome measures during the double-blind phase of the study. (Placebo group and propranolol group are analyzed separately).

Outcome Measure	Placebo (*n* = 10)			Propranolol (*n* = 10)		
	Baseline	End of DB Phase	*p*	Baseline	End of DB Phase	*p*
Primary outcome						
ESS	5.68 ± 1.8	5.33 ± 2.1	0.133	6.50 ± 1.84	4.47 ± 1.75	0.004
Secondary outcomes						
Hb g/dL	10.7 ± 2.5	10.7 ± 2.3	0.91	10.5 ± 2.6	11.4 ± 2.02	<0.001
Total PC units required *	3	5	0.346	7	3	<0.001
Total IV iron ** doses required *	16	14	0.233	9	4	0.15
QOL	34.75 ± 10.9	40.6 ± 9.11	0.03	35.1 ± 6.7	41 ± 7.39	0.048

ESS, epistaxis severity score; DB, double-blind; Hb, hemoglobin; PC, packed cells; IV, intravenous; QOL, quality of life. * In the 2 prior months and ** dose, Ferinject 500 mg.

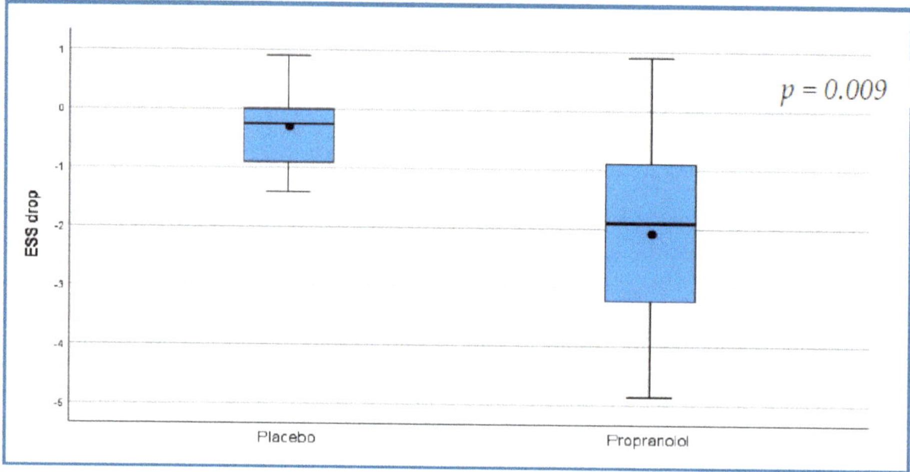

Figure 2. Demonstrating a statistically significant decrease in epistaxis severity score in the propranolol group in the randomized, double-blind phase of the trial.

Table 4. Comparison of the change in outcome measures during the double-blind period among the placebo and propranolol groups.

Outcome Measure	Placebo	Propranolol	p
Primary outcome			
Change in ESS	-0.35 ± 0.68	-2.03 ± 1.7	0.009
Secondary outcomes			
Change in Hb level (g/dL)	0.68 ± 0.01	1.96 ± 0.85	0.216
Change in number of PC required	-0.20 ± 0.63	-0.40 ± 0.69	0.029
Change in number of IV iron doses required *	-0.20 ± 0.63	-0.50 ± 0.97	0.304
QOL	6.11 ± 5.85	6.06 ± 5.90	0.986

ESS, epistaxis severity score; Hb, hemoglobin; PC, packed cells; IV, intravenous; QOL, quality of life. * Dose, Ferinject 500 mg.

Box and whisker plots of the decreases in ESS in the placebo and propranolol groups during the double-blind phase of the study. The black horizontal lines represent the median values of decrease and the range. The dots represent the mean and the boxes represent the interquartile range of decrease (25% to 75%). ESS change of 0.71 was suggested to be the MID (minimal important difference) [16].

3.3. Secondary Outcomes

Significant improvement in Hb level was observed in the propranolol group but not in the placebo group (Table 3). PC transfusion requirement decreased significantly in the propranolol group. Changes were not observed in these parameters in the placebo group. The change in intravenous iron units required was not statistically significant in both groups. QOL improved significantly in both groups.

We also compared the change in the secondary outcomes during the study period between the placebo and the propranolol groups (Table 4). The propranolol group had a significant decrease in PC requirement as compared with the placebo group. There was no significant change in the other secondary outcome measures.

3.4. Nasal Endoscopy

Four patients in the placebo group improved (40%), of whom three were grade I at study entry. Improvement was observed in seven patients (70%) in the propranolol group, of whom five were grade II/III at study entry. One patient in the propranolol group worsened. The difference in improvement between the groups at the end of the placebo-controlled phase was not significant ($p = 0.18$). Among patients with higher grading (II and III) of nasal involvement, improvement was observed in 71.4% of the propranolol group as compared with 16.7% of the placebo group ($p = 0.078$).

3.5. Side Effects

Hypotension or bradycardia were not observed among participants in the placebo and propranolol groups. Mean BP measures were similar between the groups (systolic BP 108.5 ± 8.1 mmHg vs. 111.3 ± 5.95 mmHg, $p = 0.402$ and diastolic BP 60.2 ± 7.6 mmHg vs. 67.5 ± 12.6 mmHg, $p = 0.137$), as was the mean heart rate (73.6 ± 9.7 beats per minute vs. 74.4 ± 13.45, $p = 0.876$).

The most important side effect observed was a burning sensation in the nasal mucosa and the pharynx (Table 5). Five patients in the propranolol group and two in the placebo group had mild and transient burning sensations that resolved during treatment. Four patients in the propranolol and none in the placebo group complained of a substantial burning sensation. Overall, 9 patients in the propranolol group and 2 in the placebo group had some burning sensation ($p = 0.005$). All the patients had a thorough otolaryngologic examination and no visible mucosal injuries were observed. Rhinorrhea was observed in three patients in the propranolol group and in none in the placebo group ($p = 0.06$). Nasal dryness was observed in one participant in the placebo group.

Table 5. Side effects of the double-blind period.

	Placebo (10)	Propranolol (10)	p
Any burning sensation	2	9	0.005
Sustained burning sensation	0	4	0.086
Rhinorrhea	0	3	0.06
Nasal dryness	1	0	1
Otitis media	0	1	1

One patient in the propranolol group had acute otitis media. One patient in the placebo group withdrew the study because of otitis media which led to her hospitalization. The patients both recovered. No other side effects were observed.

3.6. Results of the Open-Label Phase of the Study

Fifteen participants completed the open-label phase, seven in the propranolol group and eight in the placebo group. Two patients in the placebo group withdrew from the study at this phase, as they were awaiting a Young's procedure prior to the study and decided to proceed with this process. Three patients in the propranolol group withdrew from the open-label label phase because of a burning sensation; two of them also had rhinorrhea.

During the open-label phase, the former placebo group, now receiving propranolol gel, showed significant improvement in the ESS score, with a mean drop of 1.99 ± 1.41 from 4.86 ± 1.85 to 2.87 ± 1.6 ($p = 0.005$). During this phase, the propranolol group maintained the decrease in ESS (open-label period 4.6 ± 2.05 to 4.18 ± 0.99, $p = 0.51$) and completed a mean drop of 2.76 ± 1.52 in the 16 weeks of treatment ($p = 0.001$). In addition, the entire cohort showed significant improvement in epistaxis control, frequency and severity, and in daily duration of epistaxis (Table 6).

Table 6. Diary outcome measures in the open label phase, diary comparison.

Outcome Measure (mean ± SD) $n = 15$	Double Blind Period	Open-Label Period	p
Epistaxis frequency, bleeds/day	1.71 ± 1.34	1.24 ± 1.24	<0.001
Epistaxis severity	1.42 ± 0.64	1.03 ± 0.55	<0.001
Epistaxis duration, minutes/day	10.68 ± 9.01	6.13 ± 4.67	<0.001

There was no significant improvement in hemoglobin levels (11.42 ± 2.06 to 11.86 ± 1.79, $p = 0.317$) and QOL (41.38 ± 7.38 to 42.92 ± 8.12, $p = 0.17$).

Compliance for the entire cohort during the open-label phase was a mean 78.74 ± 25.2%. Six patients (40%) reported a burning sensation. One participant reported nasal dryness. There was no sign of mucosal damage in any of the participants on rhinology examination, and all chose to continue treatment. No significant change in BP or HR, nor any other side effects, were observed between the beginning and the end of the open label period (systolic BP 110.4 ± 5.9 to 114.6 ± 13.8 mmHg, $p = 0.27$; diastolic BP 63.5 ± 8.4 mmHg to 64.4 ± 9.1 mmHg, $p = 0.54$; HR 72.6 ± 11.8 to 71.6 ± 13 per minute, $p = 0.55$, all respectively).

4. Discussion

In a randomized double-blind placebo-controlled study, we demonstrated a significant improvement in epistaxis control in persons with HHT treated with topical propranolol gel for moderate-severe epistaxis. A considerable proportion of persons with HHT have mutations in the endoglin (ENG) and ACVLR1 genes, which encode components of the transforming growth factor (TGF)-β receptor [1]. Recently, a Knudsonian two-hit mechanism was suggested for telangiectases formation [17]. Nonetheless, increased blood and tissue levels of VEGF have been found in persons with HHT [18], suggesting a role for this protein in the abnormal angiogenesis process [6]. The non-selective beta blocker propranolol is used routinely to treat infantile hemangiomas [10,11,19]. The possible mechanisms of action for propranolol include both vasoconstrictive and antiangiogenic effects. The latter are related to VEGF expression, which is controlled by adrenergic stimulation. Propranolol's antiadrenergic properties directly reduce VEGF-stimulated angiogenesis [11]. In addition, propranolol causes apoptosis of endothelial cells and reduces VEGF tissue expression [11]. Infantile hemangioma resembles HHT in several aspects, including dysregulated angiogenesis and high levels of tissue VEGF [20,21]. These similarities suggest a role for propranolol in the treatment of HHT. Furthermore, propranolol has been demonstrated to decrease in vitro migration and angiogenesis of HHT endothelial cells [22].

Oral and topical propranolol for epistaxis in HHT has been reported in several uncontrolled studies. In a retrospective study, followed by a prospective case series, 21 persons with HHT were treated with oral propranolol, with daily doses of 80–160 mg. In the retrospective arm, a significant decrease in ESS was observed, with improvement in both epistaxis duration and frequency. In the prospective arm, 11 patients were treated with propranolol for three months, which led to a significant decrease in epistaxis duration and in the number of episodes per month. Side effects caused one patient to discontinue propranolol due to hypotension. Other side effects included asthenia, nightmares, and erectile dysfunction [23]. Our group published a case series of six HHT patients treated with nasal propranolol gel. All the patients reported improvement, with a mean decrease of ESS from 6.43 ± 2.11 to 3.47 ± 1.75 during 12 weeks of treatment ($p = 0.007$). Mean hemoglobin levels increased from 8.42 ± 3.06 g/dL to 10.98 ± 1.78 g/dL ($p = 0.01$), and the number of blood transfusions over a 24-week period decreased ($p = 0.01$). One patient reported a burning sensation during the first week of treatment, which resolved during the second week. No other local or systemic effects were observed [12]. A recent observational report demonstrated the efficacy of combined treatment of sclerotherapy and propranolol on epistaxis control in persons with HHT [24]. Anecdotal use of topical timolol has also been reported [25,26].

The targeting of VEGF for treatment of epistaxis in HHT has been attempted with the antibody bevacizumab [27–29]. Systemic administration of bevacizumab was found to control nosebleeds and other HHT symptoms [27,28,30,31]. However, systemic bevacizumab caused undesired side effects such as fever, headache, rash, and chills, and notably, epistaxis occurred [32]. Local nasal mucosal injections or spray of bevacizumab have been shown to have a beneficial effect in several case studies and uncontrolled studies, but failed to show an advantage in randomized trials [29]. Recent systematic reviews summarizing the published studies suggest that intranasal bevacizumab treatment does not have a significant effect on epistaxis in persons with HHT [7,8]. Other therapeutic options based on the role of PI3K and mTOR role in telangiectases formation have been recently suggested [33,34]. Severe epistaxis may cause gushing bleeds several times a day, resulting in iron deficiency anemia and transfusion dependency [1]. Response is sometimes inadequate to standard measures of nasal packing, laser coagulation, and arterial embolization. Surgical procedures including septal dermoplasty and Young's nasal closure may be effective; however, these are partly irreversible and can result in significant morbidity [27].

This randomized placebo-controlled study corroborates previous non-randomized uncontrolled findings of a significant improvement in the ESS score in persons with HHT treated with propranolol. Propranolol was superior to the placebo for improving epistaxis, measured by a significant drop in the ESS. The improvement in epistaxis control with propranolol gel treatment was also demonstrated by the significant increase in HB levels, and decreases in PC transfusions and IV iron requirements in the treatment group but not in the placebo group. These results are strengthened by the significant improvement in epistaxis control in the participants in the placebo group when they were switched to propranolol treatment in the open-label phase. It should be noted that the propranolol group maintained the decrease in ESS during the open label phase, and overall, demonstrated a significant improvement during the 16 weeks of treatment.

Although a one-month run-in period was an option in the protocol, since patients recruited had moderate to severe epistaxis, they were reluctant to have a run-in period. As there was no run-in period, a diary was not available prior to medication administration to measure changes in epistaxis severity, duration, and frequency in the double-blind phase; however, these outcome measures improved in both groups in the open-label phase.

Nasal endoscopy findings in our study groups were defined during follow up visits as no change, improved, or worsened. The rationale for these definitions was based on our experience that improvement was mostly associated with flattening and paling of the lesions and much less often with a change in grading. Improvement in nasal endoscopy findings was observed in 70% of the propranolol and 40% of the placebo group. The improvement in the placebo arm may have been associated with the rigorous regimen of daily nasal lubrication. Daily intranasal application of propranolol gel was associated with improvement in an additional 30% of patients as compared with the placebo group. Although these results were not statistically significant, a larger cohort may show endoscopic improvement in patients treated with topical propranolol. QOL improved in both groups. The improvement in the placebo group could be related to several factors. First, a major component of the SF-12 questionnaire relates to the emotional state of the patient and its influence on their general health. The close follow up and care, the hope for improvement when joining the open-label phase, as well as the moistening effect of the gel, might have contributed to improvement in the patients' well-being and in QOL. A questionnaire that is more specific to the effects of epistaxis might have shown a statistically significant difference between the groups.

We did not observe any systemic side effects with propranolol treatment. A major side effect was a burning sensation, which affected most of the participants, and led to the withdrawal of three participants from the open-label study. However, the majority of participants reported disappearance or reduction in this sensation with continued treatment. This side effect was less pronounced in the open-label phase. While 40% of the patients reported a burning sensation, all chose to continue treatment, and reported improvement in this side effect. Furthermore, no visible damage was observed in any of the participants in otolaryngologic examination. We believe that propranolol is a mucosal irritant. Since this treatment might be given for longer periods of time, this side effect, as well as other systemic side effects and dose adjustment, should be addressed in future studies.

One patient in the propranolol group and one who withdrew the study from the placebo group developed otitis media. Whether or not methylcellulose gel is the cause is unknown.

Our study is limited due to the relatively small number of patients. Thus, we were unable to reach conclusions regarding some secondary outcomes, as the need for iron infusion. Moreover, important parameters that may affect bleeding such as clinical variants of HHT, type of mutations, as was previously shown by Lesca et al. [35], family relations of the participants, age, and gender were not evaluated. Notably, we had female predominance and, although recent publication did not find a difference in epistaxis frequency between genders [36], a match for gender should be considered in a larger study.

Our novel findings justify and urge a further study with a larger number of patients that could refer to these matters. Further studies should also include a run-in period with an epistaxis diary. The lack of this period in our study precluded assessing the improvement based on these diaries in the placebo-controlled phase.

In summary, our novel findings suggest that topical propranolol gel is safe and effective for epistaxis treatment in patients with HHT-related epistaxis. Larger studies are required to assess the efficacy and safety of systemic and topical propranolol treatment for epistaxis and other HHT related phenomena.

Author Contributions: Conceptualization, M.M.-Z., N.G., E.B. (Elchanan Bruckheimer), and D.P.; methodology, M.M.-Z., N.G., E.B. (Elchanan Bruckheimer), Y.G., E.S., and D.P.; software, Y.G., M.W.; validation, M.M.-Z., N.G., E.B. (Elchanan Bruckheimer), M.W., and E.S.; formal analysis, M.M.-Z., Y.G., N.G., E.S., E.B. (Elchanan Bruckheimer), and E.B. (Einat Birk); writing—original draft preparation, M.M.-Z. and N.G.; writing—review and editing, E.S., E.B. (Elchanan Bruckheimer), D.P., E.B. (Einat Birk), and Y.G.; funding acquisition, M.M.-Z. and N.G. All authors have read and agreed to the published version of the manuscript.

Funding: This research received no external funding.

Acknowledgments: The authors thank the Levi Family for their donation to this study in the memory of their son Oriki.

Conflicts of Interest: The authors declare no conflict of interest. The funders had no role in the design of the study; in the collection, analyses, or interpretation of data; in the writing of the manuscript, or in the decision to publish the results.

References

1. McDonald, J.; Bayrak-Toydemir, P.; Pyeritz, R.E. Hereditary hemorrhagic telangiectasia: An overview of diagnosis, management, and pathogenesis. *Genet. Med. Off. J. Am. Coll. Med. Genet.* **2011**, *13*, 607–616. [CrossRef] [PubMed]
2. Merlo, C.A.; Yin, L.X.; Hoag, J.B.; Mitchell, S.E.; Reh, D.D. The effects of epistaxis on health-related quality of life in patients with hereditary hemorrhagic telangiectasia. *Int. Forum Allergy Rhinol.* **2014**, *4*, 921–925. [CrossRef] [PubMed]
3. Ingrand, I.; Ingrand, P.; Gilbert-Dussardier, B.; Defossez, G.; Jouhet, V.; Migeot, V.; Dufour, X.; Klossek, J.M. Altered quality of life in Rendu-Osler-Weber disease related to recurrent epistaxis. *Rhinology* **2011**, *49*, 155–162. [CrossRef] [PubMed]
4. Loaëc, M.; Morinière, S.; Hitier, M.; Ferrant, O.; Plauchu, H.; Babin, E. Psychosocial quality of life in hereditary haemorrhagic telangiectasia patients. *Rhinology* **2011**, *49*, 164–167. [CrossRef]
5. Sautter, N.B.; Smith, T.L. Treatment of Hereditary Hemorrhagic Telangiectasia-Related Epistaxis. *Otolaryngol. Clin. N. Am.* **2016**, *49*, 639–654. [CrossRef]
6. Ardelean, D.S.; Letarte, M. Anti-angiogenic therapeutic strategies in hereditary hemorrhagic telangiectasia. *Front. Genet.* **2015**, *6*, 35. [CrossRef]
7. Stokes, P.; Rimmer, J. Intranasal bevacizumab in the treatment of HHT -related epistaxis: A systematic review. *Rhinology* **2018**, *56*, 3–10. [CrossRef]

8. Halderman, A.A.; Ryan, M.W.; Marple, B.F.; Sindwani, R.; Reh, D.D.; Poetker, D.M. Bevacizumab for Epistaxis in Hereditary Hemorrhagic Telangiectasia: An Evidence-based Review. *Am. J. Rhinol. Allergy* **2018**, *32*, 258–268. [CrossRef]

9. Rosenberg, T.; Fialla, A.D.; Kjeldsen, J.; Kjeldsen, A.D. Does severe bleeding in HHT patients respond to intravenous bevacizumab? Review of the literature and case series. *Rhinology* **2019**, *57*, 242–251. [CrossRef]

10. Léauté-Labrèze, C.; Dumas de la Roque, E.; Hubiche, T.; Boralevi, F.; Thambo, J.-B.; Taïeb, A. Propranolol for severe hemangiomas of infancy. *N. Engl. J. Med.* **2008**, *358*, 2649–2651. [CrossRef]

11. Storch, C.H.; Hoeger, P.H. Propranolol for infantile haemangiomas: Insights into the molecular mechanisms of action. *Br. J. Dermatol.* **2010**, *163*, 269–274. [CrossRef] [PubMed]

12. Mei-Zahav, M.; Blau, H.; Bruckheimer, E.; Zur, E.; Goldschmidt, N. Topical propranolol improves epistaxis in patients with hereditary hemorrhagic telangiectasia—A preliminary report. *J. Otolaryngol. Head Neck Surg. J. Oto-Rhino-Laryngol. Chir. Cervico-Faciale* **2017**, *46*, 58. [CrossRef] [PubMed]

13. Shovlin, C.L.; Guttmacher, A.E.; Buscarini, E.; Faughnan, M.E.; Hyland, R.H.; Westermann, C.J.; Kjeldsen, A.D.; Plauchu, H. Diagnostic criteria for hereditary hemorrhagic telangiectasia (Rendu-Osler-Weber syndrome). *Am. J. Med. Genet.* **2000**, *91*, 66–67. [CrossRef]

14. Hoag, J.B.; Terry, P.; Mitchell, S.; Reh, D.; Merlo, C.A. An epistaxis severity score for hereditary hemorrhagic telangiectasia. *Laryngoscope* **2010**, *120*, 838–843. [CrossRef]

15. Common Terminology Criteria for Adverse Events (CTCAE)|Protocol Development|CTEP. Available online: https://ctep.cancer.gov/protocolDevelopment/electronic_applications/ctc.htm (accessed on 28 August 2020).

16. Yin, L.X.; Reh, D.D.; Hoag, J.B.; Mitchell, S.E.; Mathai, S.C.; Robinson, G.M.; Merlo, C.A. The minimal important difference of the epistaxis severity score in hereditary hemorrhagic telangiectasia. *Laryngoscope* **2015**, *126*, 1029–1032. [CrossRef]

17. Snellings, D.A.; Gallione, C.J.; Clark, D.S.; Vozoris, N.T.; Faughnan, M.E.; Marchuk, D.A. Somatic Mutations in Vascular Malformations of Hereditary Hemorrhagic Telangiectasia Result in Bi-allelic Loss of ENG or ACVRL1. *Am. J. Hum. Genet.* **2019**, *105*, 894–906. [CrossRef]

18. Sadick, H.; Naim, R.; Gössler, U.; Hörmann, K.; Riedel, F. Angiogenesis in hereditary hemorrhagic telangiectasia: VEGF165 plasma concentration in correlation to the VEGF expression and microvessel density. *Int. J. Mol. Med.* **2005**, *15*, 15–19. [CrossRef]

19. Xu, G.; Lv, R.; Zhao, Z.; Huo, R. Topical propranolol for treatment of superficial infantile hemangiomas. *J. Am. Acad. Dermatol.* **2012**, *67*, 1210–1213. [CrossRef]

20. Przewratil, P.; Sitkiewicz, A.; Andrzejewska, E. Local serum levels of vascular endothelial growth factor in infantile hemangioma: Intriguing mechanism of endothelial growth. *Cytokine* **2010**, *49*, 141–147. [CrossRef]

21. Zhang, L.; Lin, X.; Wang, W.; Zhuang, X.; Dong, J.; Qi, Z.; Hu, Q. Circulating level of vascular endothelial growth factor in differentiating hemangioma from vascular malformation patients. *Plast. Reconstr. Surg.* **2005**, *116*, 200–204. [CrossRef]

22. Albiñana, V.; Recio-Poveda, L.; Zarrabeitia, R.; Bernabéu, C.; Botella, L.M. Propranolol as antiangiogenic candidate for the therapy of hereditary haemorrhagic telangiectasia. *Thromb. Haemost.* **2012**, *108*, 41–53. [CrossRef] [PubMed]

23. Contis, A.; Gensous, N.; Viallard, J.F.; Goizet, C.; Léauté-Labrèze, C.; Duffau, P. Efficacy and safety of propranolol for epistaxis in hereditary haemorrhagic telangiectasia: Retrospective, then prospective study, in a total of 21 patients. *Clin. Otolaryngol. Off. J. ENT-UK Off. J. Neth. Soc. Oto-Rhino-Laryngol. Cervico-Facial Surg.* **2017**, *42*, 911–917. [CrossRef] [PubMed]

24. Esteban-Casado, S.; Martín de Rosales Cabrera, A.M.; Usarralde Pérez, A.; Martínez Simón, J.J.; Zhan Zhou, E.; Marcos Salazar, M.S.; Pérez Encinas, M.; Botella Cubells, L. Sclerotherapy and Topical Nasal Propranolol: An Effective and Safe Therapy for HHT-Epistaxis. *Laryngoscope* **2019**, *129*, 2216–2223. [CrossRef] [PubMed]

25. Epperla, N.; Brilliant, M.H.; Vidaillet, H. Topical timolol for treatment of epistaxis in hereditary haemorrhagic telangiectasia associated with bradycardia: A look at CYP2D6 metabolising variants. *BMJ Case Rep.* **2014**, *2014*. [CrossRef]

26. Olitsky, S.E. Topical timolol for the treatment of epistaxis in hereditary hemorrhagic telangiectasia. *Am. J. Otolaryngol.* **2012**, *33*, 375–376. [CrossRef]

27. Garg, N.; Khunger, M.; Gupta, A.; Kumar, N. Optimal management of hereditary hemorrhagic telangiectasia. *J. Blood Med.* **2014**, *5*, 191–206. [CrossRef]

28. Dupuis-Girod, S.; Ginon, I.; Saurin, J.-C.; Marion, D.; Guillot, E.; Decullier, E.; Roux, A.; Carette, M.-F.; Gilbert-Dussardier, B.; Hatron, P.-Y.; et al. Bevacizumab in patients with hereditary hemorrhagic telangiectasia and severe hepatic vascular malformations and high cardiac output. *JAMA* **2012**, *307*, 948–955. [CrossRef]
29. Riss, D.; Burian, M.; Wolf, A.; Kranebitter, V.; Kaider, A.; Arnoldner, C. Intranasal submucosal bevacizumab for epistaxis in hereditary hemorrhagic telangiectasia: A double-blind, randomized, placebo-controlled trial. *Head Neck* **2015**, *37*, 783–787. [CrossRef]
30. Iyer, V.N.; Apala, D.R.; Pannu, B.S.; Kotecha, A.; Brinjikji, W.; Leise, M.D.; Kamath, P.S.; Misra, S.; Begna, K.H.; Cartin-Ceba, R.; et al. Intravenous Bevacizumab for Refractory Hereditary Hemorrhagic Telangiectasia-Related Epistaxis and Gastrointestinal Bleeding. *Mayo Clin. Proc.* **2018**, *93*, 155–166. [CrossRef]
31. Al-Samkari, H.; Kasthuri, R.S.; Parambil, J.G.; Albitar, H.A.; Almodallal, Y.A.; Vázquez, C.; Serra, M.M.; Dupuis-Girod, S.; Wilsen, C.B.; McWilliams, J.P.; et al. An international, multicenter study of intravenous bevacizumab for bleeding in hereditary hemorrhagic telangiectasia: The InHIBIT-Bleed study. *Haematologica* **2020**. [CrossRef]
32. Kabbinavar, F.; Hurwitz, H.I.; Fehrenbacher, L.; Meropol, N.J.; Novotny, W.F.; Lieberman, G.; Griffing, S.; Bergsland, E. Phase II, randomized trial comparing bevacizumab plus fluorouracil (FU)/leucovorin (LV) with FU/LV alone in patients with metastatic colorectal cancer. *J. Clin. Oncol. Off. J. Am. Soc. Clin. Oncol.* **2003**, *21*, 60–65. [CrossRef] [PubMed]
33. Iriarte, A.; Figueras, A.; Cerdà, P.; Mora, J.M.; Jucglà, A.; Penín, R.; Viñals, F.; Riera-Mestre, A. PI3K (Phosphatidylinositol 3-Kinase) Activation and Endothelial Cell Proliferation in Patients with Hemorrhagic Hereditary Telangiectasia Type 1. *Cells* **2019**, *8*, 971. [CrossRef]
34. Ruiz, S.; Zhao, H.; Chandakkar, P.; Papoin, J.; Choi, H.; Nomura-Kitabayashi, A.; Patel, R.; Gillen, M.; Diao, L.; Chatterjee, P.K.; et al. Correcting Smad1/5/8, mTOR, and VEGFR2 treats pathology in hereditary hemorrhagic telangiectasia models. *J. Clin. Investig.* **2020**, *130*, 942–957. [CrossRef] [PubMed]
35. Lesca, G.; Olivieri, C.; Burnichon, N.; Pagella, F.; Carette, M.-F.; Gilbert-Dussardier, B.; Goizet, C.; Roume, J.; Rabilloud, M.; Saurin, J.-C.; et al. Genotype-phenotype correlations in hereditary hemorrhagic telangiectasia: Data from the French-Italian HHT network. *Genet. Med. Off. J. Am. Coll. Med. Genet.* **2007**, *9*, 14–22. [CrossRef]
36. Mora-Luján, J.M.; Iriarte, A.; Alba, E.; Sánchez-Corral, M.A.; Cerdà, P.; Cruellas, F.; Ordi, Q.; Corbella, X.; Ribas, J.; Castellote, J.; et al. Gender differences in hereditary hemorrhagic telangiectasia severity. *Orphanet J. Rare Dis.* **2020**, *15*, 63. [CrossRef] [PubMed]

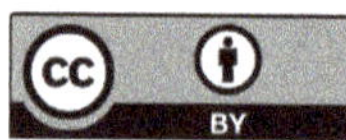

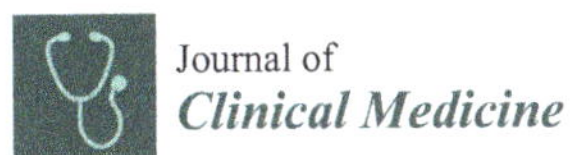 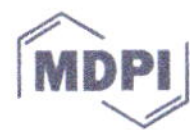

Journal of **Clinical Medicine**

Article

Antithrombotic Therapy in Hereditary Hemorrhagic Telangiectasia: Real-World Data from the Gemelli Hospital HHT Registry

Eleonora Gaetani [1,2,*], Fabiana Agostini [1,2], Igor Giarretta [1,2], Angelo Porfidia [1,3], Luigi Di Martino [1,2], Antonio Gasbarrini [1,2], Roberto Pola [1,4] and on behalf of the Multidisciplinary Gemelli Hospital Group for HHT [1,†]

[1] Multidisciplinary Gemelli Hospital Group for HHT, Fondazione Policlinico Universitario A. Gemelli IRCCS Università Cattolica del Sacro Cuore, 00168 Rome, Italy; fabiana.agostini@libero.it (F.A.); igor.giarretta@unicatt.it (I.G.); angelo.porfidia@policlinicogemelli.it (A.P.); luigidimartino7@gmail.com (L.D.M.); antonio.gasbarrini@unicatt.it (A.G.); roberto.pola@unicatt.it (R.P.)

[2] Department of Translational Medicine and Surgery, Fondazione Policlinico Universitario A. Gemelli IRCCS Università Cattolica del Sacro Cuore, 00168 Rome, Italy

[3] Division of Internal Medicine, Fondazione Policlinico Universitario A. Gemelli IRCCS Università Cattolica del Sacro Cuore, 00168 Rome, Italy

[4] Department of Cardiovascular Sciences, Fondazione Policlinico Universitario A. Gemelli IRCCS Università Cattolica del Sacro Cuore, 00168 Rome, Italy

[*] Correspondence: eleonora.gaetani@unicatt.it; Tel.: +39-06-30157075

[†] Multidisciplinary Gemelli Hospital Group for HHT: Giulio C. Passali, Maria E. Riccioni, Annalisa Tortora, Veronica Ojetti, Daniela Feliciani, Leonardo Stella, Clara De Simone, Luigi Corina, Alfredo Puca, Carmelo L. Sturiale, Laura Riccardi, Aldobrando Broccolini, Carmine Di StasiAndrea Contegiacomo, Annemilia Del Ciello, Pietro M. Ferraro, Emanuela Lucci-Cordisco, Giuseppe Zampino, Valentina Giorgio, Giuseppe Marrone, Gabriele Spoletini, Gabriella Locorotondo, Gaetano Lanza, Erica De Candia, Elisabetta Peppucci, Marianna Mazza, Giuseppe Marano, Maria T. Lombardi, Maria G. Brizzi, Silvia D'Ippolito, Mariaconsiglia Santantonio, Nico Attempati, Guido Costamagna.

Received: 2 May 2020; Accepted: 27 May 2020; Published: 2 June 2020

Abstract: Although Hereditary Hemorrhagic Telangiectasia (HHT) is characterized by an overwhelming bleeding propensity, patients with this disease may also present medical conditions that require antithrombotic therapy (AT). However, precise information on indications, dosage, duration, effectiveness, and safety of AT in HHT patients is lacking. We performed a retrospective analysis of the HHT Registry of our University Hospital and found 26 patients who received AT for a total of 30 courses (19 courses of anticoagulant therapy and 11 courses of antiplatelet therapy). Indications to treatments included: atrial fibrillation, venous thrombosis and pulmonary embolism, heart valve replacement, retinal artery occlusion, secondary prevention after either stroke or myocardial infarction, and thromboprophylaxis for surgery. The total time of exposure to antiplatelet therapy was 385 months and to anticoagulant therapy 169 months. AT was generally well tolerated, with no fatal bleedings and no significant changes in hemoglobin levels. However, we found three major bleedings, with an incidence rate of 6.5 per 100 patients per year. When only patients treated with anticoagulants were considered, the incidence rate of major bleedings increased to 21.6 per 100 patients per year. Our study indicates that major bleeding may occur in HHT patients receiving AT, with a substantially increased rate in those treated with anticoagulants. Further studies are needed to fully estimate the tolerability of antithrombotic drugs in HHT.

Keywords: Hereditary Hemorrhagic Telangiectasia; antithrombotic therapy; anticoagulants; antiplatelets; bleeding; safety

---

1. Introduction

Hereditary Hemorrhagic Telangiectasia (HHT) is a rare autosomal dominant disease characterized by recurrent spontaneous epistaxis, visceral arteriovenous malformations (AVMs), and mucocutaneous telangiectases [1–3]. Five genetic types of HHT are recognized, with three being linked to particular genes. More than 80% of all cases of HHT are due to mutations in either *ENG* or *ACVRL1*, which cause HHT1 and HHT2, respectively [1–3]. About 2% of HHT are instead due to *SMAD4* mutations, which cause colonic polyposis in addition to HHT [1–3].

Although the hallmark of HHT is an overwhelming bleeding propensity, it is well known that patients with this disease are not devoid of medical conditions that require antithrombotic therapy (AT). For instance, they may have coronary artery disease (CAD), venous thromboembolism (VTE), or atrial fibrillation (AF) [4–8]. Additionally, they may require thromboprophylactic anticoagulation when they are hospitalized for an acute medical illness or when they undergo surgical procedures [9,10]. However, precise information on the indications, dosage, duration, and effectiveness of AT in HHT patients is lacking. Additionally, it is not clear whether subjects with HHT are able to tolerate AT, neither is it known if bleedings associated with AT are more common in some HHT phenotypes than other. Finally, no studies have been carried out to evaluate whether there are differences in AT tolerability between subjects with HHT1 or HHT2. The consequence is that clinicians are often afraid to prescribe AT to HHT patients, especially if they are not familiar with the disease. It may also happen that patients are reluctant to take these drugs, since they have been advised to avoid the use of medications that may worsen their risk of bleeding.

One of the most recent studies that evaluated the safety of AT in subjects with HHT was carried out by the European Reference Network for Rare Multisystemic Vascular Diseases (VASCERN), which retrospectively analyzed 28 HHT subjects treated with direct oral anticoagulants (DOACs) for either AF or VTE [11]. The result was that epistaxis worsened in 24 cases and in 11 cases patients had to discontinue treatment. Another recent study analyzed the RIETE Registry—which specifically consists of subjects affected by VTE—and found 23 patients with HHT (in a time frame of approximately 10 years), who presented 2 major bleedings and 6 non major bleedings during anticoagulant treatment [12]. More recently, we published the interim results of a prospective study conducted on 12 HHT subjects treated with either antiplatelet or anticoagulant therapy for various clinical indications for a mean period of approximately 6 months, who did not present any bleeding different from epistaxis while on treatment [13]. In addition, there was not epistaxis worsening and there were not significant changes in hemoglobin levels after initiation of AT [13].

Here, we carried out a retrospective analysis of the "Gemelli Hospital HHT Registry", which contains demographic and clinical information of more than 200 subjects managed at the HHT Center of our University Hospital, with the goal to provide real-world data on indications, dosage, duration, effectiveness, and safety of AT in subjects with HHT.

2. Materials and Methods

We searched the Gemelli Hospital HHT Registry, which contains all the demographic and clinical information of the patients followed at the HHT Center of the 'Fondazione Policlinico Universitario A. Gemelli IRCCS', Rome, Italy. The creation of the Registry was approved by the Ethics Committee of the above-mentioned hospital (protocol number 2999). The time frame of the search was from 1 June 2016 (opening day of the HHT Center) to 31 December 2018.

First, we looked for subjects with a 'definite' diagnosis of HHT, i.e., those with genetic confirmation of the disease and/or those displaying at least 3 of the following 4 Curaçao criteria, as established in the literature [14]: (1) recurrent and spontaneous nosebleeds (epistaxis); (2) multiple telangiectases on the skin of the hands, lips, or face, or inside of the nose or mouth; (3) AVMs or telangiectases in one or more internal organs, including the lungs, brain, liver, intestine, stomach, and spinal cord; (4) a family history of HHT (i.e., first-degree relative, such as brother, sister, parent, or child, who meet these same criteria for definite HHT or has been genetically diagnosed).

Next, we identified subjects who were treated, or had been treated in the past, with AT. We registered the indications to prescription and the type and dosage of the prescribed drug. Duration of treatment and patient compliance to treatment were also registered. Since there were cases of patients that were treated with AT more than once and/or with different drugs for different indications, each course of AT was separately analyzed. We also assessed AT effectiveness and safety, evaluating whether thrombotic/ischemic events or hemorrhagic events occurred while patients were taking AT. To identify all the events, in addition to searching the Registry, we also asked patients to come to our HHT Center to undergo a detailed medical interview and fill out a questionnaire, upon signature of an informed consent. Hemorrhagic events were classified according to the criteria of the International Society on Thrombosis and Haemostasis (ISTH) [15,16]: major bleedings were defined as fatal bleedings, or symptomatic bleedings in critical areas or organs (such as intracranial, intraspinal, intraocular, retroperitoneal, intraarticular or pericardial, or intramuscular with compartment syndrome), or bleedings causing a fall in hemoglobin level of 2 g/dL or more, or leading to transfusion of two or more units of whole blood or red cells; clinically relevant non-major (CRNM) bleedings were defined as acute or subacute clinically overt bleedings that did not satisfy the criteria for major bleedings but led to hospital admission for bleeding, or physician-guided medical or surgical treatment for bleeding, or a change in AT due to bleeding; minor bleedings, with the exception of epistaxis, were defined as acute clinically overt bleedings that did not meet the criteria for either major or CRNM bleedings. We also assessed possible changes in hemoglobin levels after initiation of AT (determined by comparing hemoglobin levels measured within the three months that preceded the initiation of AT with the hemoglobin levels measured after at least 1 month of AT).

The study was approved by the Ethics Committee of the 'Fondazione Policlinico Universitario A. Gemelli IRCSS' (Rome, Italy) (protocol number 49901/18, ID 2329, approval date 20 December 2018).

Statistical Analysis

The SPSS 20.0 and GraphPad Prism 7.0 software were used to perform statistical analysis. Descriptive statistics were used to outline patients' characteristics. Results are expressed as mean ± SD or *n* (%). Incidence rate was calculated as number of bleeding events per 100 patients per year. For parametric variables, we compared means using paired samples Student's t test. P values less than 0.05 were considered statistically significant.

3. Results

3.1. Characteristics of the Study Population

The search of the Registry led to the identification of 29 subjects with a definite diagnosis of HHT who had received AT. Of these, three were deceased at the time of study, for reasons unrelated to AT. In particular, one patient died from severe liver cirrhosis, one from progressive heart failure, and one suffered sudden cardiac death. In the first patient, the indication to AT was AF. He was treated with anticoagulants for a short period of time and then therapy was stopped due to worsening of liver failure. The second patient had AF, but he underwent left atrial appendage closure and therefore was initially treated with anticoagulants and later with aspirin. He tolerated both treatments well. In the third patient, the indication to AT was surgical VTE prophylaxis, for which he was treated with prophylactic doses of enoxaparin for 1 month, without complications.

The 26 remaining patients accepted to participate and were included in the study. The demographical and clinical characteristics of the study population are presented in Table 1. There were 14 males and 12 females with a mean age of 59.3 ± 17.0 years. Nine patients had HHT1 due to *ENG* mutations, while 15 patients had HHT2 due to mutations of *ACVRL1*, consistent with the proportion of the two types of HHT previously found in Italy [17]. A genetic confirmation of the diagnosis was not available in 2 patients, but both fulfilled the Curaçao criteria for a 'definite' diagnosis of HHT. All patients (100.0%) had epistaxis. Twenty-three patients (88.5%) had mucocutaneous telangiectases. There were 10 patients with pulmonary AVMs (pAVMs) (on a total of 22 who had been screened by CT scan of the chest), 5 patients with hepatic AVMs (on a total of 24 who had been screened by either abdominal ultrasound, CT scan, and/or MRI), and 2 patients with cerebral AVMs (on a total of 20 who had been screened by either CT scan and/or MRI of the brain and spinal cord). Ten patients (38.5%) had a history of GI bleeding due to the presence of GI AVMs (on a total of 15 who had been screened by endoscopic procedures).

Table 1. Characteristics of the study population.

Mean age (years ± SD)	59.3 ± 17.0
Gender (male/female ratio)	14/12
HHT1/HHT2/Clinical diagnosis (*n*)	9/15/2
Epistaxis (*n*/total)	26/26
Mucocutaneous telangiectases (*n*/total)	23/26
Family history of HHT (*n*/total)	24/26
Pulmonary AVMs (*n*/screened)	10/22
Hepatic AVMs (*n*/screened)	5/24
Cerebral AVMs (*n*/screened)	2/20
Gastrointestinal AVMs (*n*/screened)	10/15
Previous gastrointestinal bleeding (*n*/total)	10/26

AT: antithrombotic therapy; HHT: Hereditary Hemorrhagic Telangiectasia; AVMs: arteriovenous malformations; SD: standard deviation.

3.2. Antithrombotic Therapy (AT): Indications, Type, Dosage, Duration, and Reasons for Therapy Discontinuation

The 26 HHT patients included in this study received a total of 30 AT courses. As shown in Table 2, there were 19 courses of anticoagulant therapies and 11 courses of antiplatelet therapies. The drugs used were the following: enoxaparin (6 courses), fondaparinux (4 courses), vitamin K antagonists (VKA) (4 courses), direct oral anticoagulants (DOACs) (5 courses), acetylsalicylic acid (ASA) (9 courses), clopidogrel (1 course), and indobufen (1 course).

The indications for treatment are also presented in Table 2. We found that anticoagulant drugs were prescribed to our patients for the following reasons: AF ($n = 6$), heart valve bioprosthesis ($n = 2$), pulmonary embolism (PE) ($n = 1$), cerebral vein thrombosis (CVT) ($n = 1$), superficial vein thrombosis (SVT) ($n = 3$), retinal artery occlusion (RAO) in a patient with Horton's diseases ($n = 1$), secondary prevention after stroke in a patient with pAVMs ($n = 1$), surgical VTE prophylaxis ($n = 4$). The reasons for prescribing antiplatelet medications were: secondary prevention after stroke in patients with pAVMs ($n = 3$), secondary prevention after stroke or transient ischemic attack (TIA) ($n = 3$), secondary prevention after a myocardial infarction (MI) ($n = 2$), prevention of cardiovascular (CV) events in Horton's disease ($n = 1$), primary CV prevention ($n = 2$).

Information regarding dosage and duration of any single AT course is presented in Table 3, along with data regarding the genetic type of HHT and the reasons for possible cessation of therapy. The total time of exposure to AT courses was 554 months. The total time of exposure to antiplatelet courses was 385 months. The total time of exposure to anticoagulant courses was 169 months. In three cases, AT was discontinued by the patient, without medical advice.

Table 2. Type and number of AT courses and reasons for prescription.

Anticoagulant drug	Number of therapeutic courses ($n = 19$)
enoxaparin	6
fondaparinux	4
VKA	4
DOAC	5
Antiplatelet drug	**Number of therapeutic courses ($n = 11$)**
ASA (number of courses)	9
clopidogrel (number of courses)	1
indobufen (number of courses)	1
Reasons why anticoagulant therapy was prescribed	
AF	6
Heart valve bioprosthesis	2
PE	1
CVT	1
SVT	3
RAO in a patient with Horton's disease	1
Secondary prevention after stroke/TIA in a patient with pAVMs	1
Surgical VTE prophylaxis	4
Reasons why antiplatelet therapy was prescribed	
Secondary prevention after stroke in patients with pAVMs	3
Secondary prevention after stroke/TIA	3
Secondary prevention after MI	2
Horton's disease	1
Primary CV prevention	2

AT: antithrombotic therapy; VKA: vitamin K antagonist; DOAC: direct oral anticoagulant; ASA: acetylsalicylic acid; AF: atrial fibrillation; PE: pulmonary embolism; CVT: cerebral vein thrombosis; SVT: superficial vein thrombosis; VTE: venous thromboembolism; TIA: transient ischemic attack; pAVMs: pulmonary arteriovenous malformations; RAO: retinal artery occlusion; MI: myocardial infarction; CV: cardiovascular.

Table 3. Dosage, duration of treatment, compliance to AT, and reasons for therapy discontinuation.

Drug	Genetic Mutation	Indication for Treatment	Dosage Prescribed	Treatment Duration	Ongoing Treatment at the Time of Study	Reason for Therapy Cessation	Therapy Cessation Decided by Doctor or Patient
warfarin	*ACVRL1* (HHT2)	AF	variable, based on INR	6 months	No	hematuria	doctor
rivaroxaban	*ACVRL1* (HHT2)	AF	15 mg o.d.	6 months	No	GI bleeding	doctor
rivaroxaban	*ACVRL1* (HHT2)	AF	15 mg o.d.	27 months	No	GI bleeding	doctor
rivaroxaban	*ACVRL1* (HHT2)	AF	15 mg o.d.	13 months	Yes	—	—
dabigatran	*ACVRL1* (HHT2)	AF	110 mg b.i.d.	21 months	Yes	—	—
apixaban	*ACVRL1* (HHT2)	AF	2.5 mg b.i.d.	20 months	Yes	—	—
acenocoumarol	*ENG* (HHT1)	stroke in pAVM	variable, based on INR	46 months	Yes	—	—
enoxaparin	*ENG* (HHT1)	SVT	4000 U b.i.d.	1 month	No	completion of treatment	doctor
enoxaparin	*ACVRL1* (HHT2)	SVT	4000 U b.i.d.	1 month	No	completion of treatment	doctor
fondaparinux	*ACVRL1* (HHT2)	SVT	2.5 mg o.d.	1 month	No	completion of treatment	doctor
warfarin	*ENG* (HHT1)	heart valve bioprosthesis	variable, based on INR	3 months	No	completion of treatment	doctor
fondaparinux	Clinical diagnosis	heart valve bioprosthesis	2.5 mg o.d.	3 months	No	completion of treatment	doctor
warfarin	*ACVRL1* (HHT2)	PE	variable, based on INR	1 month	No	shift to DOAC	doctor
enoxaparin	*ENG* (HHT1)	RAO in Horton's disease	6000 U b.i.d	5 months	No	completion of treatment	doctor
fondaparinux	*ENG* (HHT1)	CVT	5 mg o.d.	6 months	No	completion of treatment	doctor
enoxaparin	*ACVRL1* (HHT2)	surgical VTE prophylaxis	4000 U o.d.	1 month	No	completion of treatment	doctor
enoxaparin	*ACVRL1* (HHT2)	surgical VTE prophylaxis	4000 U o.d.	3 months	No	completion of treatment	doctor
enoxaparin	*ACVRL1* (HHT2)	surgical VTE prophylaxis	4000 U o.d.	4 months	No	completion of treatment	doctor
enoxaparin	*ACVRL1* (HHT2)	surgical VTE prophylaxis	4000 U o.d.	1 month	No	completion of treatment	doctor
ASA	*ENG* (HHT1)	stroke in pAVM	100 mg o.d.	43 months	No	worsening of epistaxis	patient
ASA	*ENG* (HHT1)	stroke in pAVM	100 mg o.d.	72 months	No	pAVM embolization	doctor
ASA	*ENG* (HHT1)	stroke in pAVM	100 mg o.d.	14 months	Yes	—	—
ASA	Clinical diagnosis	Stroke	100 mg o.d.	30 months	No	worsening of epistaxis	patient
ASA	*ACVRL1* (HHT2)	Stroke	100 mg o.d.	5 months	Yes	—	—
indobufen	*ENG* (HHT1)	TIA	200 mg o.d.	21 months	Yes	—	—
ASA	*ACVRL1* (HHT2)	secondary prevention after MI	100 mg o.d.	94 months	Yes	—	—
ASA	*ACVRL1* (HHT2)	secondary prevention after MI	100 mg o.d.	50 months	Yes	—	—
ASA	*ACVRL1* (HHT2)	primary CV prevention	100 mg o.d.	24 months	No	worsening of epistaxis	patient
ASA	*ACVRL1* (HHT2)	primary CV prevention	100 mg o.d.	18 months	No	medical decision	doctor
clopidogrel	*ENG* (HHT1)	Horton's disease	75 mg o.d.	14 months	Yes	—	—

AT: antithrombotic therapy; AF: atrial fibrillation; INR: international normalized ratio; o.d.: once daily; GI: gastrointestinal; b.i.d.: bis in die; pAVM: pulmonary arteriovenous malformation; SVT: superficial vein thrombosis; PE: pulmonary embolism; DOAC: direct oral anticoagulant; RAO: retinal artery occlusion; CVT: cerebral vein thrombosis; VTE: venous thromboembolism; ASA: acetylsalicylic acid; TIA: transient ischemic attack; MI: myocardial infarction; CV: cardiovascular.

3.3. AT: Effectiveness and Safety

The effectiveness of anticoagulant therapy was high. In particular, patients receiving anticoagulant therapy for AF did not experience embolic stroke or systemic embolism during treatment. Patients treated with anticoagulants for PE, SVT, or CVT did not display thrombotic recurrences during treatment. There were no thrombotic complications during the two courses of anticoagulant therapy prescribed for heart valve bioprosthesis. The patient with pAVM who was treated with acenocoumarol after stroke did not experience new ischemic events during treatment. The patient with Horton's disease that had RAO and was treated with enoxaparin lost vision on the affected eye, but therapy was started many days after onset of symptoms. Finally, patients receiving thromboprophylaxis for surgery did not have thrombotic events while on treatment.

The effectiveness of antiplatelet therapy was also high. In particular, patients with and without pAVMs who started therapy with ASA after stroke or MI did not experience new ischemic events during treatment. The same happened to the patient treated with indobufen after TIA. Finally, the two patients receiving ASA for primary CV prevention and the patient with Horton's disease receiving clopidogrel did not experience ischemic events while on treatment.

Safety data are reported in Table 4. In total, there were three major bleedings. Of these, two were GI bleedings that occurred in the same patient during two different treatment courses with the DOAC rivaroxaban. This patient had already experienced GI bleeding before starting anticoagulation and bleeding while on rivaroxaban occurred after 6 months of treatment in one occasion and after 27 months of the treatment in another occasion. The other case of major bleeding consisted of severe hematuria in a patient treated with warfarin for AF. In the whole population, the incidence rate of major bleeding was 6.5 per 100 patients per year. In the population of patients taking anticoagulants, the incidence rate of major bleeding was 21.6 per 100 patients per year. There were no CRNM bleedings and no minor bleedings different from epistaxis. Likewise, there were no differences in the mean hemoglobin levels measured in the three months that preceded AT and those measured during AT (11.1 ± 2.5 vs. 10.8 ± 2.2 respectively, 95% CI −0.90–0.31, $p = 0.3256$) (Table 4 and Figure 1).

Table 4. Bleeding complications during AT.

Minor bleedings different from epistaxis (*n*/total of AT courses)	0/30
CRNM bleedings (*n*/total of AT courses)	0/30
Major bleedings (*n*/total of AT courses) - in subjects taking anticoagulants (*n*/total of anticoagulant courses) - in subjects taking antiplatelets (*n*/total of antiplatelet courses)	3/30 3/19 0/11
Hb levels (g/dL) during AT versus prior to AT (mean ± SD)	10.8 ± 2.2 vs. 11.1 ± 2.5 (95% CI −0.90–0.31) $p = 0.3256$

AT: antithrombotic therapy; CRNM: clinically relevant non-major; Hb: hemoglobin; SD: standard deviation.

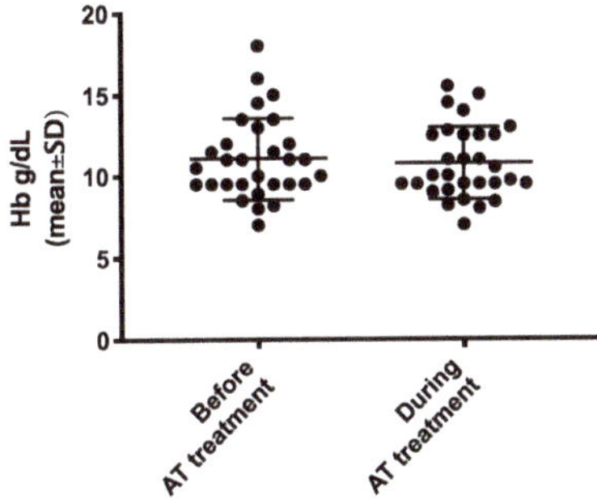

Figure 1. Distribution of hemoglobin (Hb) levels before and during AT.

4. Discussion

This study presents data on the way AT is managed in the real-world in patients with HHT. One interesting point of discussion is the variety of medical conditions requiring AT that we found in subjects with HHT. While some of these conditions, such as secondary CV prevention, and surgical thromboprophylaxis, are relatively common for most physicians, other, such as AF, PE, CVT, RVO, Horton's disease, and stroke in subjects with pAVMs, may be more challenging and require specialized expertise to be properly managed. For instance, in the case of AF, we found that four different anticoagulants were used, which reflects the complexity of the therapeutic choices that can be made in these patients. When the chosen anticoagulant was a DOAC, we found that a low dose was always prescribed: rivaroxaban 15 mg o.d., dabigatran 110 mg b.i.d., and apixaban 2.5 mg b.i.d. It is important to note that precise rules exist for the prescription of low doses of DOACs in patients with AF, based on age, body weight, and kidney function [18,19]. We retrospectively assessed whether the prescription of reduced doses in our patients was respectful of these rules and found that in three cases (two therapeutic courses with rivaroxaban and one therapeutic course with apixaban) prescriptions were off-label. It is known that the prescription of inappropriately low doses of DOACs may increase the risk of stroke and systemic embolism and therefore it should be avoided [20]. It is possible to speculate that the physicians that prescribed these DOACs were more concerned with the hemorrhagic, rather than the thrombotic, risk of their patients and this led to the inappropriate use of low-dose anticoagulant medications. However, it should be noted that, in the population that we analyzed, the effectiveness of these therapies were high and no thrombotic events were registered. Of course, this may be due to the limited number of patients and therefore it is not enough to justify the use of off-labeled doses of DOACs in HHT patients.

Attention should also be paid to the way secondary prevention was managed in patients with pAVMs that had an ischemic stroke. In three cases, it was prescribed an antiplatelet medication, while in another patient it was prescribed the anticoagulant acenocoumarol. This is odd, since the most recent recommendations on the medical treatment of stroke in subjects with pAVMs (produced by the British Thoracic Society) state that, as in the general population, ischemic strokes in patients with pAVM should be treated with antiplatelet agents, while anticoagulants should be used if other indications, such as AF or VTE, coexist [21].

Regarding safety, our study shows that 90% of AT courses was completed without the occurrence of significant hemorrhagic events and that only 10% of them was complicated by episodes of major bleeding. Importantly, there were no episodes of fatal bleeding. Additionally, hemoglobin levels, which are an objective outcome, did not change between before and after starting AT. However, when the incidence of major bleeding was calculated, based on time of exposure to AT, it resulted to be as high as 6.5/100 patients/year. Importantly, the incidence of major bleeding raised to 21.6/100 patients/year when only patients taking anticoagulants were considered. On the other hand, there were no episodes of major bleeding among HHT subjects treated with antiplatelet medications, although the total exposure time to antiplatelet therapy (385 months) was approximately twice the total exposure time to anticoagulant therapy (169 months).

As already mentioned in the Introduction section, two other studies have recently evaluated whether HHT subjects tolerate AT [11,12]. These studies and ours have many similarities. First, they include a similar number of HHT patients: 28 in the study by Shovlin et al. [11], 23 in the study by Riera-Mestre et al. [12], and 26 in our study. Additionally, all these studies have a retrospective design: Shovlin et al. utilized the databases of VASCERN-participating centers [11], Riera-Mestre et al. analyzed the RIETE Registry [12], and we studied the database of the HHT Center of our University Hospital. However, there are also important differences between our study and the other two. For instance, in the study of Riera-Mestre et al., the authors were not able to retrospectively assess Curaçao criteria and/or collect genetic data for all patients [12]. In contrast, in our study, all patients had a 'definite' diagnosis of HHT and a genetic confirmation of the disease was present in 24 out of 26 patients. Another difference is that Shovlin et al. and Riera-Mestre et al. only studied subjects treated with anticoagulants (and only with DOACs in the case of Shovlin et al.) [11,12], while we included individuals treated with antiplatelet medications. Additionally, the indications to treatment were different between these three studies. In Shovlin's study, all patients were affected by either AF or VTE [11], while Riera-Mestre et al. only evaluated subjects with VTE [12]. In contrast, the patients investigated in our study had more heterogeneous indications to AT, which included stroke, MI, thromboprophylaxis, and other diseases. Regarding the results of these studies, Shovlin et al. found that epistaxis worsened in 24 cases and in 11 cases patients had to discontinue treatment, on a total of 28 patients [11]. However, all their subjects were treated exclusively with DOACs. In addition, they did not provide precise information on the medical regimen followed by patients and did not carry out a distinction between bleedings, in terms of severity [11]. On the other hand, Riera-Mestre et al. found two major bleedings and six non major bleedings during anticoagulant treatment, on a total of 23 patients [12]. Precise information on the medical regimen followed by patients was not provided in this case either. Numerically speaking, our results (three major bleedings on a total of 26 patients who received a total of 30 AT courses) appear similar to those reported by Riera-Mestre et al. However, as mentioned above, our population is different, because it did not only include subjects with VTE who were treated with anticoagulants. Therefore, no direct comparisons can be made.

Other important reports available in the literature on this topic are those published by Edwards et al. in 2012 and Devlin et al. in 2013 [22,23]. A main difference between these two studies and ours is that we were able to distinguish between major, CRNM, and minor bleedings, thus providing data not only on the number of hemorrhagic complications, but also on their severity and clinical impact, while this was not done in the study by Devlin et al. [23]. Additionally, the subjects studied by Devlin et al. did not always have a 'definite' diagnosis of HHT [23] and those investigated by Edwards et al. had lower rates of epistaxis, GI bleeding, anemia, and visceral AVMs compared to our patients [22].

Our study has some limitations. It has a small sample size and a retrospective nature. It is possible that some HHT subjects did not receive a prescription of AT despite the presence of a clinical indication, and this might be a selection bias of our study. Additionally, the difference that we saw in the safety of antiplatelet drugs compared to anticoagulant therapies might depend on the small sample size, which also did not allow us to make distinctions between different types of antiplatelet and anticoagulant medications. It is also possible that HHT subjects requiring anticoagulation are different from those requiring antiplatelet therapy and that the increased rate of bleeding that we observed in subjects treated with DOACs depends on the intrinsic characteristics of the patients rather than on the drugs used. Finally, the small sample size did not allow us to investigate whether HHT1 and HHT2 patients have different tolerability to AT, which is a very intriguing issue that deserves further investigation.

In conclusion, our study presents real-world data on HHT subjects treated with AT, providing novel information on the way antiplatelet and anticoagulant medications are used in this unique population, which has an intrinsically high hemorrhagic risk. Our results indicate that major bleeding may occur in HHT patients receiving AT, especially those treated with anticoagulants. Further studies are needed to better define the optimal use of these medications and fully assess the safety profile of various types of AT agents in HHT patients.

Author Contributions: Conceptualization, E.G., A.G., and R.P.; Methodology, E.G. and R.P.; Software, I.G. and A.P.; Validation, E.G. and R.P.; Formal Analysis, F.A., A.P. and I.G.; Investigation, F.A. and L.D.M.; Resources, F.A. and L.D.M.; Data Curation, F.A., A.P. and I.G.; Writing—Original Draft Preparation, E.G. and R.P.; Writing—Review & Editing, E.G., A.G., and R.P.; Visualization, E.G., R.P., A.P. and I.G.; Supervision, E.G. and R.P.; Project Administration, E.G., A.G., and R.P. All authors have read and agreed to the published version of the manuscript.

Funding: This research received no external funding.

Conflicts of Interest: The authors declare no conflict of interest.

References

1. Shovlin, C.L.; Buscarini, E.; Kjeldsen, A.D.; Mager, H.J.; Sabba, C.; Droege, F.; Geisthoff, U.; Ugolini, S.; Dupuis-Girod, S. European reference network for rare vascular diseases (VASCERN) outcome measures for hereditary haemorrhagic telangiectasia (HHT). *Orphanet J. Rare Dis.* **2018**, *13*, 136. [CrossRef] [PubMed]
2. McDonald, J.; Bayrak-Toydemir, P.; Pyeritz, E.R. Hereditary hemorrhagic telangiectasia: An overview of diagnosis, management, and pathogenesis. *Genet. Med.* **2011**, *13*, 607–616. [CrossRef] [PubMed]
3. Sharathkumar, A.A.; Shapiro, A. Hereditary haemorrhagic telangiectasia. *Haemophilia* **2008**, *14*, 1269–1280. [CrossRef] [PubMed]
4. Sulaiman, N.L.; Govani, F.S.; Jackson, J.E.; Begbie, M.E.; Shovlin, C.L. Elevated factor VIII in hereditary haemorrhagic telangiectasia (HHT): Association with venous thromboembolism. *Thromb. Haemost.* **2007**, *98*, 1031–1039. [CrossRef]
5. Livesey, J.A.; Manning, R.A.; Meek, J.H.; Jackson, J.E.; Kulinskaya, E.; Laffan, M.A.; Shovlin, C.L. Low serum iron levels are associated with elevated plasma levels of coagulation factor VIII and pulmonary emboli/deep venous thromboses in replicate cohorts of patients with hereditary haemorrhagic telangiectasia. *Thorax* **2011**, *67*, 328–333. [CrossRef] [PubMed]
6. Buscarini, E.; Leandro, G.; Conte, D.; Danesino, C.; Daina, E.; Manfredi, G.; Lupinacci, G.; Brambilla, G.; Menozzi, F.; de Grazia, F.; et al. Natural history and outcome of hepatic vascular malformations in a large cohort of patients with hereditary hemorrhagic teleangiectasia. *Dig. Dis. Sci.* **2011**, *56*, 2166–2178. [CrossRef]
7. Ginon, I.; Decullier, E.; Finet, G.; Cordier, J.-F.; Marion, D.; Saurin, J.-C.; Dupuis-Girod, S. Hereditary hemorrhagic telangiectasia, liver vascular malformations and cardiac consequences. *Eur. J. Intern. Med.* **2013**, *24*, e35–e39. [CrossRef]
8. Shovlin, C.L.; Awan, I.; Cahilog, Z.; Abdulla, F.N.; Guttmacher, A.E. Reported cardiac phenotypes in hereditary hemorrhagic telangiectasia emphasize burdens from arrhythmias, anemia and its treatments, but suggest reduced rates of myocardial infarction. *Int J. Cardiol.* **2016**, *215*, 179–185. [CrossRef]
9. Schünemann, H.J.; Cushman, M.; Burnett, A.E.; Kahn, S.R.; Beyer-Westendorf, J.; Spencer, F.A.; Rezende, S.M.; Zakai, N.A.; Bauer, K.A.; Dentali, F.; et al. American society of hematology 2018 guidelines for management of venous thromboembolism: Prophylaxis for hospitalized and nonhospitalized medical patients. *Blood Adv.* **2018**, *2*, 3198–3225. [CrossRef]
10. Anderson, D.R.; Morgano, G.P.; Bennett, C.; Dentali, F.; Francis, C.W.; Garcia, D.A.; Kahn, S.R.; Rahman, M.; Rajasekhar, A.; Rogers, F.B.; et al. American society of hematology 2019 guidelines for management of venous thromboembolism: Prevention of venous thromboembolism in surgical hospitalized patients. *Blood Adv.* **2019**, *3*, 3898–3944. [CrossRef]
11. Shovlin, C.L.; Millar, C.M.; Droege, F.; Kjeldsen, A.; Manfredi, G.; Suppressa, P.; Ugolini, S.; Coote, N.; Fialla, A.D.; Geisthoff, U.; et al. Safety of direct oral anticoagulants in patients with hereditary hemorrhagic telangiectasia. *Orphanet J. Rare Dis.* **2019**, *14*, 210–218. [CrossRef] [PubMed]
12. Riera-Mestre, A.; Mora-Luján, J.M.; Trujillo-Santos, J.; Toro, J.D.; Nieto, J.A.; Pedrajas, J.M.; López-Reyes, R.; Soler, S.; Ballaz, A.; Cerdà, P.; et al. Natural history of patients with venous thromboembolism and hereditary hemorrhagic telangiectasia. Findings from the RIETE registry. *Orphanet J. Rare Dis.* **2019**, *14*, 196. [CrossRef] [PubMed]
13. Gaetani, E.; Agostini, F.; Porfidia, A.; Giarretta, I.; Feliciani, D.; Martino, L.D.; Tortora, A.; Gasbarrini, A.; Pola, R.; Passali, G.; et al. Safety of antithrombotic therapy in subjects with hereditary hemorrhagic telangiectasia: Prospective data from a multidisciplinary working group. *Orphanet J. Rare Dis.* **2019**, *14*, 1–5. [CrossRef] [PubMed]
14. Shovlin, C.L.; Guttmacher, A.E.; Buscarini, E.; Faughnan, M.E.; Hyland, R.H.; Westermann, C.J.J.; Kjeldsen, A.D.; Plauchu, H. Diagnostic criteria for hereditary hemorrhagic telangiectasia (Rendu-Osler-Weber syndrome). *Am. J. Med. Genet.* **2000**, *91*, 66–67. [CrossRef]
15. Schulman, S.; Kearon, C. Definition of major bleeding in clinical investigations of antihemostatic medicinal products in non-surgical patients. *J. Thromb. Haemost.* **2005**, *3*, 692–694. [CrossRef]
16. Kaatz, S.; Ahmad, D.; Spyropoulos, A.C.; Schulman, S.; Anticoagulation, F.T.S.O.C.O. Definition of clinically relevant non-major bleeding in studies of anticoagulants in atrial fibrillation and venous thromboembolic disease in non-surgical patients: Communication from the SSC of the ISTH. *J. Thromb. Haemost.* **2015**, *13*, 2119–2126. [CrossRef]

17. Lesca, G.; Olivieri, C.; Burnichon, N.; Pagella, F.; Carette, M.-F.; Gilbert-Dussardier, B.; Goizet, C.; Roume, J.; Rabilloud, M.; Saurin, J.-C.; et al. Genotype-phenotype correlations in hereditary hemorrhagic telangiectasia: Data from the French-Italian HHT network. *Genet. Med.* **2007**, *9*, 14–22. [CrossRef]
18. Kirchhof, P.; Benussi, S.; Kotecha, D.; Ahlsson, A.; Atar, D.; Casadei, B.; Castella, M.; Diener, H.-C.; Heidbuchel, H.; Hendriks, J.; et al. 2016 ESC guidelines for the management of atrial fibrillation developed in collaboration with EACTS. *Eur. J. Cardiothorac. Surg.* **2016**, *50*, e1–e88. [CrossRef]
19. Steffel, J.; Verhamme, P.; Potpara, T.S.; Albaladejo, P.; Antz, M.; Desteghe, L.; Haeusler, K.G.; Oldgren, J.; Reinecke, H.; Roldán-Schilling, V.; et al. The 2018 European heart rhythm association practical guide on the use of non-vitamin K antagonist oral anticoagulants in patients with atrial fibrillation. *Eur. Hear. J.* **2018**, *39*, 1330–1393. [CrossRef]
20. Yao, X.; Shah, N.D.; Sangaralingham, L.R.; Gersh, B.J.; Noseworthy, P.A. Non–Vitamin K antagonist oral anticoagulant dosing in patients with atrial fibrillation and renal dysfunction. *J. Am. Coll. Cardiol.* **2017**, *69*, 2779–2790. [CrossRef]
21. Shovlin, C.L.; Condliffe, R.; Donaldson, J.W.; Kiely, D.G.; Wort, S.J. British thoracic society clinical statement on pulmonary arteriovenous malformations. *Thorax* **2017**, *72*, 1154–1163. [CrossRef] [PubMed]
22. Edwards, C.P.; Shehata, N.; Faughnan, M.E. Hereditary hemorrhagic telangiectasia patients can tolerate anticoagulation. *Ann. Hematol.* **2012**, *91*, 1959–1968. [CrossRef] [PubMed]
23. Devlin, H.L.; Hosman, A.E.; Shovlin, C.L. Antiplatelet and anticoagulant agents in hereditary hemorrhagic telangiectasia. *New Engl. J. Med.* **2013**, *368*, 876–878. [CrossRef] [PubMed]

MDPI
St. Alban-Anlage 66
4052 Basel
Switzerland
Tel. +41 61 683 77 34
Fax +41 61 302 89 18
www.mdpi.com

Journal of Clinical Medicine Editorial Office
E-mail: jcm@mdpi.com
www.mdpi.com/journal/jcm